CORONARY INTERVENTIONS

Edited by **Neville Kukreja**

Coronary Interventions
Edited by Neville Kukreja

Published by InTech

Janeza Trdine 9, 51000 Rijeka, Croatia

Publishing Process Manager Martina Blecic

Technical Editor Teodora Smiljanic

Cover Designer InTech Design Team

Additional hard copies can be obtained from orders@intechopen.com

Coronary Interventions, Edited by Neville Kukreja
p. cm.
ISBN 978-953-51-0498-8

Meet the editor

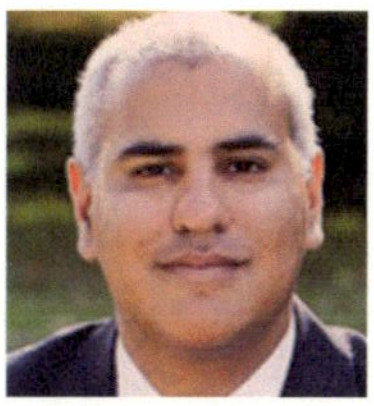

Dr Neville Kukreja is a Consultant Interventional Cardiologist at the East & North Hertfordshire NHS Trust and the Royal Brompton & Harefield NHS Foundation Trust. He did his undergraduate studies in Cambridge and London before completing his basic medical and cardiology training in London. He underwent training in Interventional Cardiology at St Mary's Hospital and the Royal Brompton Hospital in London and also at the internationally renowned Thoraxcenter in Rotterdam. He is currently on the General Medical Council's specialist register with accreditation in both Cardiology and General Internal Medicine. He is a member of the British Cardiovascular Society, British Cardiovascular Intervention Society, European Society of Cardiology and European Association of Percutaneous Coronary Intervention. He has co-authored more than 40 original research articles, 10 review articles and 6 book chapters. He has also been a co-author of more than 45 scientific abstracts which have been presented at major national and international cardiology scientific meetings. He is a peer- reviewer for a number of high-impact journals. He has been an invited speaker and faculty member at major international cardiology meetings, including the American College of Cardiology (ACC), European Society of Cardiology (ESC) and American Heart Association (AHA). His clinical interests include general medicine, general cardiology with particular expertise in all aspects of Percutaneous Coronary Intervention. His main research interests are the evaluation of new and existing drug-eluting stents and invasive coronary imaging (intravascular ultrasound and optical coherence tomography). He currently contributes towards the general and interventional cardiology service at the East & North Hertfordshire NHS Trust, including the provision of daytime primary percutaneous coronary intervention for local patients suffering a heart attack. He also participates in the on call rota at the Harefield Heart Attack Centre, one of the busiest PPCI units in the country providing 24hr emergency treatment for heart attack patients from Northwest London, Hertfordshire, Bedfordshire and Berkshire.

Contents

1

Transradial Approach for Coronary Interventions: The New Gold Standard for Vascular Access?

Antoine Guédès
CHU Mont-Godinne, University of Louvain
Belgium

1. Introduction

The perfect cardiac catheterization technique, including good diagnostic and therapeutic qualities, without risk and with no recovery time for the patient, does not exist. Obtaining initial access to the arterial circulation is the first and most frequent catheterization difficulty encountered by the interventional cardiologist during the procedure. Often, it is also the only difficult part of the exam for the patient because it may cause a vagal reaction or painful spasm. These procedural problems inevitably increase catheterization time and are sometimes the underlying causes of more significant complications. Arterial access is a crucial step of percutaneous cardiac procedures and therefore requires special attention.

Today, percutaneous coronary intervention (PCI) are usually performed via the femoral or radial arteries (a brachial approach may occasionally be required as third choice vascular access). Since the first demonstration of transradial approach feasibility in 1989, by Lucien Campeau, many studies have confirmed this initial experience and especially its safety and performances compared to transfemoral route. Nevertheless, a recent study reports that less than 2% of percutaneous coronary interventions were performed by a transradial approach in the United States between 2004 and 2007(1). The persistent discrepancy between current practice in vascular access site choice and known advantages of a radial access needs to be clarified, enlightened by recent data.

2. Short overview of complications related to arterial access site choice for PCI

Over the last three decades, advances in percutaneous coronary interventions techniques and contemporary pharmacotherapy have made these procedures safer and more reliable in a wide range of patients, often older and sicker than before.

2.1 Bleeding after percutaneous coronary interventions

In routine clinical practice, bleeding complications are a frequent non-cardiac outcome of therapy for acute coronary syndromes even in the case of an adequate arterial puncture technique. Aggressive antithrombotic regimens used in this setting even if highly powerful in reducing ischemic events, also expose patients to a higher rate of bleeding (related or not to the vascular access site).

More than two thirds of all bleeding complications involve the arterial access site and range from a local non significant hematoma to life-threatening bleeding (Fig. 1). The most common origins of bleedings not related to arterial access are gastrointestinal followed by cardiac tamponade and intracranial haemorrhage (2,3).

Retroperitoneal haemorrhage is more difficult to classify because of its double potential aetiology (often linked to manipulations related to a femoral approach but rarely occurring spontaneously in the case of anticoagulation and/or antiplatelet therapy). Retroperitoneal bleeding leading to a major bleed is reported to occur in approximately 0.1% to 0.3% of patient treated by a femoral access but is maybe an underestimate (2,4).

Risk factors for such complications are now well identified and could be divided in four categories (see Table 1).

Clinical Factors	- Advanced age - Female gender - Low body weight/obesity - Prior bleeding - Severe hypertension - Heart failure - Peripheral vascular disease - Acute coronary syndrome
Biochemical Factors	- Renal insufficiency - Anemia - Diabetes
Procedural Variations	- Femoral Access (versus Radial Access) - Increased sheath /Catheter size - Prolonged sheath time after procedure - Intra aortic Balloon Pump - Concomitant venous sheath - Need for repeat intervention
Treatment Combinations	- Antiplatelet therapy (dosage, efficacy, timing, duration) - Overdose of anticoagulants (+/- GP IIb/IIIa inhibitors) - Crossover / combinations of anticoagulants -Thrombolytic agents

Table 1. Factors associated with a higher bleeding risk (5-10)

Large randomized trials and registries with "real world" populations of patients have clearly identified clinical characteristics conferring a higher risk of bleeding: advanced age, female gender, obesity, low body weight, chronic renal disease, peripheral vascular disease and a previous history of bleeding. Procedural predictors for an increased bleeding risk include faulty puncture technique, sheath size, prolonged sheath time, use of glycoprotein (GP) IIb/IIIa inhibitors, vascular closure devices, intensity/duration of anticoagulation with heparin, but also vascular access strategy using femoral rather than radial artery(3,9,11-17).

The main difficulty encountered when comparing trials which study the true incidence of haemorrhagic events linked to vascular access options remains the lack of a precise definition for this complication (18-20) or at least of a consensus taking into account main parameters in order to establish a bleeding severity score (clear identification of bleeding site, haematocrit / haemoglobin drop, hemodynamic consequences, treatments required...).

Even if some authors (21) report a significant reduction in the incidence of major femoral bleeding complications over time (from 8.4 % in 1995 to 3.5 % in 2005), the single effective way to reduce majors bleeding related to a coronary angiography or intervention procedure, according to recent data, is to use radial access (2,11,22-24). In experts hands, this strategy allows a 50 to 75 % reduction in major bleeding events (24) with the greatest absolute benefit for obese patients and in the setting of acute myocardial infarction (primary or rescue coronary angioplasty). Therefore, radial access should be promoted as the preferential access site for percutaneous coronary interventions. Nevertheless the keys to preventing bleeding complications are well known: good knowledge and recognition of predisposing factors, meticulous examination of the access site before the puncture follow by a careful sheath placement in the artery without forceful manoeuvre and discontinuation of heparin at the end of the procedure.

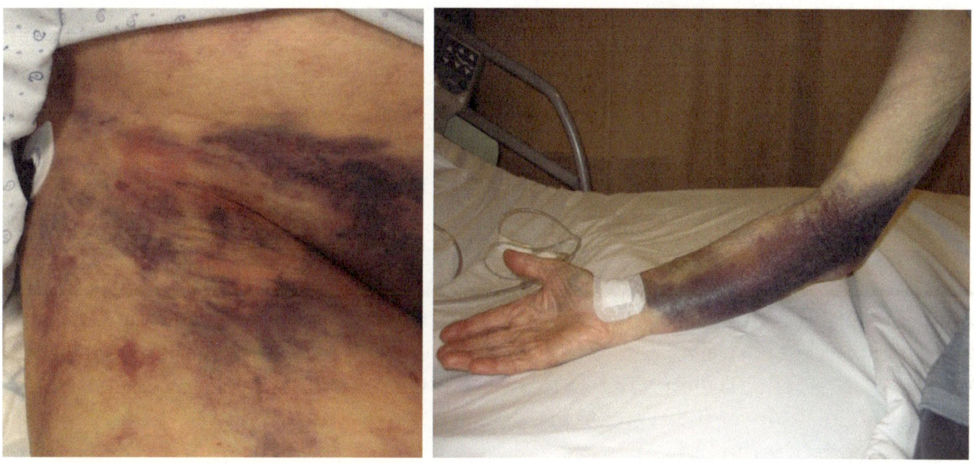

Fig. 1. Large right groin and forearm hematomas.

2.2 Other frequent complications related to arterial access site

Other significant access site related complications encountered after a catheterization procedure are pseudoaneurysm, arterio-venous fistula, femoral laceration, femoral thrombosis with or without distal embolization, and any need for a surgical exploration or repair. Less frequently groin infection (puncture site abscess), neural damage and venous thrombosis are observed.

2.2.1 Pseudonaneurysm

A pseudoaneurysm is defined as an encapsulated hematoma or cavity (contained by surrounding tissues) communicating with the lumen of an artery because of a localized disruption of the media (Fig. 2). It mainly occurs after an inadequate artery compression following sheath withdrawal. Predisposing factors for this iatrogenic arterial trauma are impaired hemostasis and factors known to be associated with difficult and prolonged procedures (peripheral vascular disease, large sheath use, aggressive anticoagulation and/or fibrinolytic therapy, prolonged sheath and anticoagulation times) and in case of a femoral approach the concomitant use of an intra aortic balloon pump and an early ambulation after catheterization. The reported incidence for femoral access seems to be around 1% (maybe higher), and is lower in the case of radial access (≤ 0.2 %) (2,25-28).

An adequate recognition of this complication, which may occur more than one year after the catheterization procedure, is mandatory because of the risk of rupture estimated at approximately 4 % for large pseudoaneurysms (> 3cm) (29-31).

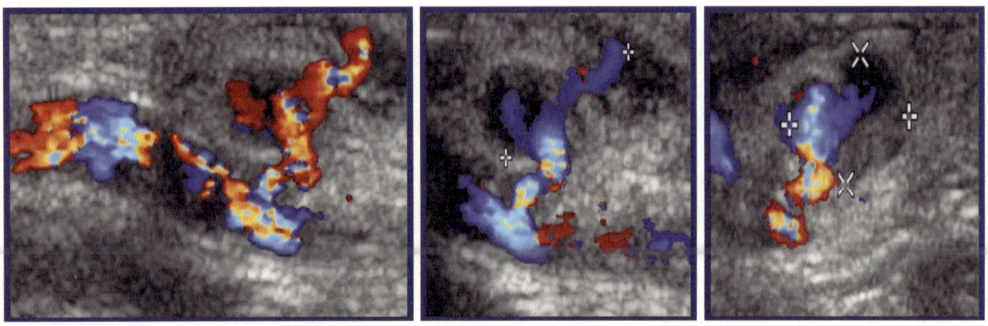

Fig. 2. Pseudoaneurysm of the radial artery (2D color-Doppler flow imaging)

2.2.2 Arteriovenous fistula

An arteriovenous fistula results from an overlying vein puncture during femoral artery catheterization, creating a communication between the two vessels after sheath removal. A high velocity and continuous jet originating from the artery and going into the vein lumen, is often easily demonstrated by color flow Doppler examination if clinical manifestations exist at the access site. The reported incidence is low in recent trials studying patients after a coronary angiography or intervention by femoral approach (0.1-2.2%) and extremely rare for radial approach (< 0.1%) (2,4,26).

By femoral approach, the occurrence of arteriovenous fistula and pseudonaneurysm is reported to be significantly higher if the puncture site is located distal to the division of the deep and superficial femoral arteries (25).

2.2.3 Arterial wall dissection

Arterial wall dissection is probably frequently unrecognized especially in cases of local dissection although its true incidence is hard to establish. Regarding published and already historical data for recognized dissection, the incidence of this arterial wall injury varies from 0.01% to 0.5% (32,33). However, when considering the fact that, as demonstrated by angiographic studies, 25% of patients admitted for a catheterization procedure had common femoral artery atherosclerotic plaques determining at least a 20 % stenosis, it is easy to understand that all intravascular foreign body as a needle or catheter may easily deflect off some of these plaques.

2.2.4 Arterial thrombosis

Due to the increasing number of percutaneous cardiac procedures performed annually and to the worldwide operator preference for this vascular access, most arterial thromboses occur in the common femoral artery. Nevertheless the incidence of this serious adverse event remains very low after coronary intervention (<0.5%) probably because of the widespread use of high dose multi-drug antithrombotic therapy for percutaneous interventions (2,4).

The common femoral artery being the unique blood supply to the leg, an urgent diagnostic of this complication followed by immediate heparinization and mechanical or surgical thrombectomy are usually required. On the contrary, radial artery thrombosis is a relatively frequent asymptomatic condition (incidence: 3-6 %). It is a benign issue, with nearly no clinical sequelae observed after occlusion of this vessel, because of the double blood supply to the hand insured by the palmar arch. Many of these radial occlusions (40-60%) are spontaneously recanalized after one month (11,34). This specific point will be discussed later in the chapter.

2.3 Impact of vascular closure devices on vascular access site complications

Today, closure devices are widely used to obtain a rapid hemostasis after percutaneous transfemoral approach but their safety remains largely controversial. Marginal evidences concerning the effectiveness of these devices are derived from pooled analyses of a heterogeneous group of small randomized trials, many of poor methodological quality (26,35).

All of the approved arterial closure devices have proven their efficacy in obtaining immediate hemostasis after sheath removal, in allowing early ambulation, and in improving patient comfort (36). However, there is no report showing a clear reduction of access site complications related to their use (compared to efficacy of manual compression) especially after diagnostic angiography. In the setting of percutaneous coronary interventions, meta-analysis of randomized trials only showed a trend towards less access site related complications with some of these devices but also an increased risk with others (26,35). Additionally, four separate prospective studies have found that bleeding complications were more frequent with transfemoral access and closure device than with transradial access (up to 3.7% versus less than 0.7%, respectively) (37-40).

There are still matters of concern about the use of these devices. For example they may increase the risk of hematoma and pseudoaneurysm formation (26,35,36,41-43). Moreover, early device failure rates and their impact on vascular access site complications are not always clearly reported in these trials but may decrease after the initial learning curve. Recently, data with the last generation of vascular closure devices suggest that their use may decrease vascular complications but these points had to be confirmed once again by large randomized trials because it maybe simply reflects a better patient selection and operator experience with these devices over time (4,42,44).

When an arteriotomy closure device is used, some specific complications may occur in addition to those previously described for manual compression. A higher rate of access site infections (0.3% versus 0.05 % with manual compression) and more episodes of acute or late limb ischemia (0.4% versus 0.1% for manual compression) are reported. The need for surgery, in case of device failure, is not commonly reported with details in the great majority of previous published trials. Nevertheless, surgery for partial embolization, to remove trapped components of these devices or after vessel laceration is uncommon(4,35).

Given the remaining uncertainty about their true impact on vascular complications and the difficulty to assess costs induced by specific vascular access complications, the widespread adoption of these devices following endovascular interventions is still controversial and needs to be clarified in the future (4,45).

2.4 Conclusions

All vascular access techniques, even if perfectly handled by the interventional cardiologist are linked with a minimal but inevitable rate of complications arising because materials enter atherosclerotic vessels. To avoid more serious clinical consequences for the patients, it is particularly important to give meticulous attention to the access site not only before the puncture but also in the hours following the procedure and to recognize predisposing factors for such complications.

3. Anatomical considerations and technical aspects of a transradial approach

3.1 Favorable anatomical characteristics of the radial artery

Differences observed in terms of vascular complications after radial and femoral percutaneous interventions are mainly based on favorable anatomical characteristics of the radial artery (compared to those describe for the common femoral artery) (Table 2 and Fig. 3).

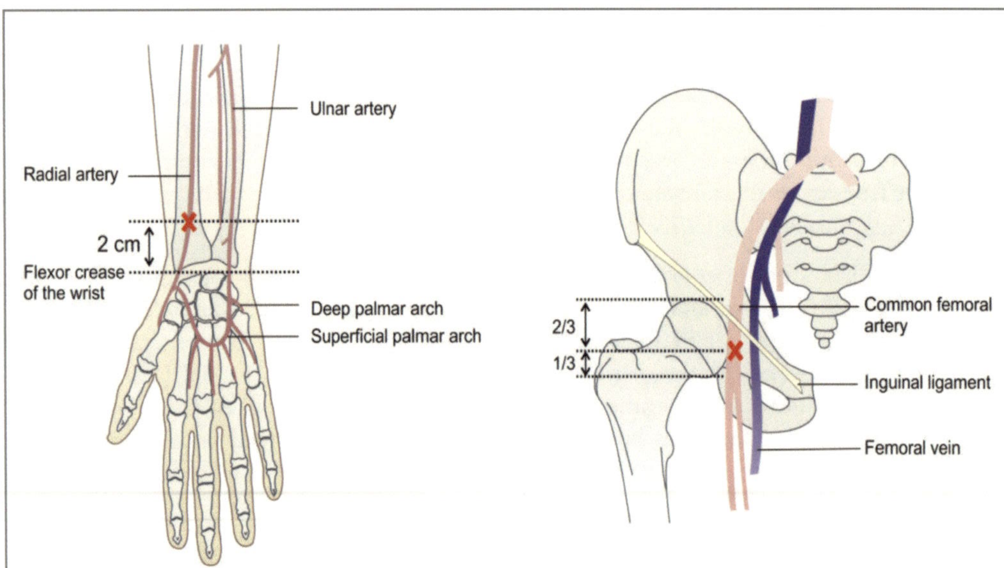

Fig. 3. Landmarks for vascular access (48,50,51)

Common Femoral Artery (CFA)	Radial Artery (RA)
CFA is relatively deep. • The ideal site of puncture may be hard to identify especially in obese patients. • The inguinal crease is an unreliable landmark in more than two thirds of patients. • The strongest femoral pulse correctly identified the mid-CFA in 90 % of cases	Distal RA had a superficial course, • This artery is easy to palpate even in obese patients • At the level of the puncture site, the artery lies just under skin and fascias
Puncture site is over the hip joint • The most reliable landmark is probably the junction between the middle and the lower third of the femoral head (radiographic landmark)	Puncture site is not over a joint • The most reliable landmark is ideally 2-3 cm proximal to the flexor crease of the wrist (clinical landmark)
Compression of the CFA may be hard • No hard and fixed structures behind the artery	RA can easily be compressed with minimal pressure • At the puncture site, radial bone is just beneath the artery
CFA lies just near a major vein (Femoral Vein) and nerve (Femoral Nerve)	RA is separated from median nerve and major veins
CFA is the unique blood supply to the leg	Double blood supply to the hand insured by the palmar arch

Table 2. Comparison of access site characteristics (46-48)

Its superficial course makes this artery easily accessible to puncture and, after the procedure, more amenable to compression (because of bone support beneath), even in obese patients. The puncture site is not over a joint, so compression devices are always stable and effective to ensure good hemostasis after sheath removal. Also wrist movements are not impaired after a transradial percutaneous intervention, which facilitates rapid recovery and makes an outpatient strategy feasible. Moreover, the radial artery is separated from median nerve and major veins of the forearm making post-catheter injuries of these structures rare. Lastly, the double blood supply to the hand makes hand ischemia an almost impossible complication if the presence of functional collaterals between the radial and the ulnar arteries, as judged by the Modified Allen's Test (49) or alternative tests, has been assessed.

3.2 Learning curve and prerequisite conditions for a safe technique conversion

The same catheterization laboratory set up and patient preparation as for femoral procedures can be used for the radial approach and only minor adaptations to improve patient and operator comfort, especially for the puncture, are required. A good arm support system is the only inescapable element needed and a pulse oximeter (finger plethysmography) may be required to perform alternative tests in case of an abnormal modified Allen's test (50,51).

Transradial access is known to be technically more demanding and time consuming, especially during the early learning curve (52).

The small caliber (2-3.5 mm in diameter) and the alpha–adrenergic innervations of the artery make the puncture task the key point of a successful transradial procedure.

When the accurate site of puncture has been correctly identified, the most critical step of the radial catheterization procedure begins. Different puncture techniques exist but the most commonly used today by experienced radial operators is the over-the-needle technique (50,51).

As described in many papers dedicated to transradial approach (53) puncture remains, for beginners, the cornerstone of the learning curve and it takes time to develop all the skills required, even for experienced interventionalists. Obtaining arterial access by a single or a limited number of puncture attempts is probably the best way to avoid difficulties linked to a refractory spasm following a difficult puncture.

This is the reason why, it is strongly recommended to take extra time to prepare and realize the puncture and to keep in mind that gentle and cautious manipulations will always pay off later. Failure of the puncture task (inability to puncture or to wire the artery) accounts for more than 50 % of transradial approach failures. Even if it takes approximately 200-300 cases to overcome initial difficulties, several studies confirms the reality of a long learning curve (53). During the beginner's phase of radial access experience, good patient selection with a readily palpable radial pulse is necessary to help perfect all the skills needed for this elegant technique. Weak radial pulses, small radial arteries, old patients, patients with known peripheral vascular disease or post CABG surgery should be avoided at this time. All these elements, required to identify patients with the most difficult access, are given by the bedside clinical evaluation of the patient, even if puncture is frequently less difficult than anticipated.

During the procedure, inability to cross forearm, arm or intra thoracic vasculature difficulties accounts for 10 % of transradial approach failures, inability to reach a coronary or graft ostia due to difficulties in rotating and manipulating the catheters for 10% and the remaining failures are related to the inability to reach a contra-lateral mammary graft.

An access site crossover, related to failure of initial strategy, is required in 6-7% of transradial procedures compared to less than 2% in case of femoral approach (including PCI procedures). For high volume radial operators or centers, lower crossover rates are reported (4-6%) (2,11,24,53). Once again, these data confirm the importance of experience and expertise when interventionalists are dealing with this approach.

In these conditions, with growing experience and state of the art materials, and if there is a systematic use of the contra-lateral radial artery in case of puncture failure on the initial side (the same technique is applied for femoral access) a very high success rate can be expected by this technique, approximately 98 % or more, with no significant differences among subgroups of patients (53).

After a while, when experience and confidence in the technique has grown, more adequate catheter choice and skills in their manipulations will ensure similar clinical results as in the femoral approach (2,11).

Indeed, PCI success rate is similar for the two approaches. The RIVAL study, the largest randomized trial comparing radial and femoral access for acute coronary syndromes, demonstrates the equivalence of the two techniques in terms of complications at the level of the coronary tree (2). The number of guiding catheters required for the procedure, the rate of abrupt coronary closure, no reflow, dissection with reduced flow, perforation, catheter thrombus and stent thrombosis were similar in the two arms of the study. These observations had already emerged from the meta-analysis performed by Agostoni in 2004 (11), which did not show statistically significant differences in terms of procedural failure for studies performed after 1999. Similarly, no differences were shown in PCI procedural time and contrast volumes used for the procedures.

3.3 Difficult cases by transradial approach and limits of the technique

Transradial approach is considered to be a difficult approach, first because of the puncture task but also for the frequent occurrence of spasm, difficult catheter selection or inability to overcome difficult radial or vascular anatomy, especially during the learning curve.

Spasm is usually related to prolonged or excessive catheter manipulation but may already occur during puncture or after sheath insertion. By using adequate doses of spasmolytic drugs (intra-arterial verapamil) at the beginning and during the procedure and small catheter size (5 French), refractory spasm becomes rare (1,1% versus 4,8% with 6 French catheters) (54). Interestingly, spasm more frequently occurs where difficulties are encountered in advancing the wire or the catheter and not only at the level of the radial artery (it can also be seen at the level of the upper limb or of the brachio-cephalic trunk). For experienced radial operators, spasm is not reported as a pertinent cause of radial approach failure during percutaneous coronary interventions (11,53). However, when resistance occurs, it is strongly recommended to perform an angiogram to adequately define the anatomy, spasm level or rarely stenosis or occlusion levels. Several studies have shown that intra-arterial verapamil and nitroglycerine are the most effective medications to prevent or to relieve spasms. Moreover, selective angiograms of the left and right coronary arteries (as well as left ventriculography) are possible with only one catheter by transradial approach (Optitorque TIG™ catheter, Terumo corp.). Thus, there should not be a need for three different catheter exchanges, which also helps in reducing the occurrence of spasm. In the same way, sheath-induced spasms are minimized and far less frequent when hydrophilic-coated materials are used. Hydrophilic coating also helps to reduce patient discomfort and facilitates sheath withdrawal (55). Finally, a higher incidence of radial artery thrombosis is documented in patients with periprocedural spasm (56).

Beginners frequently evoke loops, tortuosities and anatomic variants as one other major hurdle to overcome during learning curve. These unpredictable abnormalities are quite rare in current practice but the most challenging ones may require an alternative vascular access site. Tips and tricks, state of the art materials (especially hydrophilic wire and 0.014" PTCA guidewires) are helpful in overcoming these difficulties in a large majority of these cases. Solutions that work are often those associated with gentle wire and catheter manipulations in order to prevent vascular injury and perforation.

Another frequently advanced argument against transradial intervention is inadequate guiding support. Randomized trials performed after 2000 do not advocate this point when procedural success is compared to those reported for transfemoral PCI studies, especially when dedicated radial materials are used (2,11,37,57). Most radial arteries have a lumen large enough to accommodate 6 French catheters and some large radial arteries are able to eventually accept 7 French catheters or larger, but these sizes are not often required.

Large lumen 6 French guiding catheters with dedicated radial shapes give good back up support and allow to perform a wide range of the most complex intracoronary procedures (ostial or bifurcation lesions, left main stenosis, chronic total occlusions, thrombectomy, rotational atherectomy, saphenous vein graft lesions, acute coronary syndromes and ST-elevation myocardial infarction) (2,58-63) but standard curves designed for femoral approach also work well in most cases.

Nevertheless, in routine clinical practice, 5 French guiding catheters make direct stenting easily feasible in the great majority of procedures. In a randomized comparison study, Dahm had even shown a trend in favor of the superiority of 5 French guiding catheters over 6 French guiding catheters in terms of procedural (95.4 versus 92.9 %, p =0,097) and clinical success (93.1 versus 90.5 %, p=0,097) (54).On the other hand, today, with larger sheathless guiding catheter technology, coronary techniques only accessible by a femoral way are far less numerous than before (64,65). For example, sheathless 7.5 French guiding catheters open the way for the most complex PCI techniques, in nearly all patients, by transradial approach but had smaller outer diameters than 6 French radial introducer sheaths.

As with the femoral approach, the ideal sizing and shape of guiding catheters is still, and will stay a matter for debate.

The side to choose for the first radial approach in a given patient also remains a controversial issue with no clear answer. In most centers, transradial coronary interventions are performed through the right radial artery, because this side offers a more comfortable working position for the operator, but on a technical point of view there is some evidence that catheter manipulation could be easier by a left-sided approach, because of similar sensations compared to a femoral way and perhaps offering more back-up support for guiding catheters. In the TALENT study, a randomized comparison of right versus left radial approach for diagnostic procedures, the left approach was associated with lower fluoroscopy time and radiation dose, reflecting an easier procedure, particularly in older patients (> 70 years) and for operators in training (66). The absence of a radial artery pulse or a negative Modified Allen's Test on one side, as well as the need to selectively cannulate a mammary bypass graft also frequently influence the choice. Today, long catheters allow to easily reach the infradiaphragmatic arterial system (renal, mesenteric, iliac, femoral or lower limb arteries but also for example a gastro-epiploic bypass graft). If these catheters are not available, a left radial approach saves ten centimeters of catheter length (by this route, catheters do not cross the arch of aorta).Similarly, the cerebrovascular pathology (carotid and vertebral arteries) can be imaged and eventually treated by transradial approach.

In routine clinical practice, the control of bypass grafts is also a frequent request. Angiography of the left internal mammary artery is easy to perform by the left radial approach (as for a right internal mammary artery by the right radial approach). In case of a bilateral mammary artery bypass graft, a right radial approach should be preferred but left internal mammary artery opacification by the right radial remains challenging even for skilled operators (53,67). A successful selective opacification of the contra-lateral mammary artery can be expected in 50% of these particular cases if performed by an experienced operator using dedicated catheters (53).In our institution, we mainly use for this purpose the Outlook™ 4 French diagnostic catheter (Terumo corp.).To reach saphenous vein grafts, either left or right radial approaches can be chosen, with a similar success rate using standard catheter curves (63). Sometimes, a bilateral radial approach, during the same procedure, is necessary to obtain adequate images of the grafts.

Finally, there are only a few relative contraindications to a transradial approach: patients with a negative Allen test in both hands, patients with end-stage renal disease (just before the creation of an arteriovenous fistula for haemodialysis) and patients with known severe obstructive atherosclerotic disease at the level of the innominate, subclavian or upper limb arteries. Finally, some patients may have had previous coronary artery bypass surgery using a radial artery as a conduit which precludes radial access by this side.

3.4 Conclusions

One challenge encountered with radial access is the steep learning curve, but this hurdle can be more easily overcome by following an educational program dedicated to this approach and addressed to interventionalists and fellows in training. The widespread diffusion of the technique in teaching centers as well as the growing interest of major cardiovascular societies and device industry for this approach will also progressively ensure its greater penetration in the interventional cardiologists' community.

4. Specific complications of transradial approach

Despite a proven safety profile leading to a drastic reduction of vascular access site bleeding, the transradial approach is not totally free of complications. Catheterizers must be aware of some rare complications, which are often minor and localized if recognized without any delay.

4.1 Post procedural radial artery thrombosis: The main pitfall of transradial approach?

Although radial artery thrombosis is still a matter of concern after a transradial approach, this complication is usually benign because of the double blood supply to the hand insured by the two forearm arteries inter-connected at the level of the palmar arch. Moreover, hand-threatening ischemia, with necrosis or clinical sequelae, has not been reported after a transradial procedure to this day.

As shown by studies that have planned post catheterization Doppler ultrasound examinations, the incidence of radial artery thrombosis ranges, in general, from 3% to 6% but one study reports a rate of 9.5% (34,56,68-71). A loss of radial pulse is reported in up to 9% of patients in other studies.

The occlusion rate increases with the size of catheters used for the procedure (54,72) and is more precisely related to the ratio between the inner radial artery diameter and the sheath outer diameter (73) . The incidence of occlusion is 4% if the ratio is higher than 1 and rises dramatically to 13% in patients with a ratio of less than 1.

Other factors have been found to affect occlusion rate. Repeat cannulation (74) and older age are known to be predisposing factors but heparinization is effective in reducing its occurrence as well as the use of hydrophilic materials. For transradial procedure, adequate anticoagulation is extremely important and should be immediately started in all patients after sheath insertion; at least 5000 units of intra-arterial heparin are recommended. In patients receiving only 1000 units for a diagnostic coronary angiography, the incidence of radial occlusion climbs up to 30% (34). Intra-arterial or intravenous heparin administration provide comparable efficacy in preventing radial artery occlusion (75).

Nearly 50% of the patients in whom the radial artery is shown occluded at hospital discharge may expect a spontaneous recanalization of the vessel in the first month after procedure. Therefore, the true definitive incidence of radial artery thrombosis is probably between 2 and 3% (34).

Short procedure duration and immediate sheath removal at the end of the procedure, whatever the dose of heparin or the use of GP IIbIIa inhibitors, also contribute in maintaining radial permeability. In the same way, it seems to be relevant to avoid prolonged post-procedure compression times, especially if a mechanical device applying high pressures is used. Moreover, with some of these compression devices, a fine pressure adjustment, in order to always maintain blood flow in the radial artery during the compression, is feasible and may contribute to radial artery protection (76). In the PROPHET trial, guided compression that allowed antegrade flow, using the Barbeau's test to document radial artery patency at time of hemostasis, was shown to be highly effective in preventing radial artery occlusion (incidence decreased by 75% at 30 days after radial access) when compared to usual care (1.8% versus 7%, $p<0.05$) (77).

Nevertheless, even if radial occlusion is a fairly infrequent outcome of transradial approach, the radial artery patency should be checked in all patients after the procedure. Bernat et al. have shown recently that an early and short (1-hour) ipsilateral ulnar artery compression using TR band™ (Terumo corp.) could be an effective and safe non-pharmacologic method for the treatment of acute radial artery occlusion (78).

4.2 Post-procedural non-occlusive radial artery injury

As demonstrated by several studies, permanent radial artery damage without occlusion may sometimes follow transradial procedure.

In a first study, ultrasound examinations of the radial artery showed no significant difference in the mean radial artery internal diameter between pre and early post-procedure measurements (at 1 day). Conversely, after a mean follow up of 4.5 months, internal diameter significantly decreased from 2.63 ± 0.35 to 2.51 ± 0.29 mm ($p = 0.01$). Moreover the mean radial artery diameter was smaller and the radial occlusion rate higher (2.6% versus 0%; $p = 0.01$) in patients undergoing repeat transradial approach as compared to a first-time procedure (79).

Further intravascular ultrasound (IVUS) studies have explained that this progressive narrowing is secondary to an intima-media thickening (hyperplasia), especially in the distal radial artery, presumably induced by trauma from sheath or catheter insertion (80,81). Sanmartin et al. reported that soon after a transradial catheterization the vasoreactivity is impaired, but generally recovers as early as 1 month after the procedure (82). Edmunson et al. have also demonstrated that the vessel vasoreactivity was maintained despite the fact that post procedural non occlusive radial artery injury was a quiet common observation after transradial interventions (80). Therefore, the main underlying process of this permanent arterial wall injury is certainly catheter-based.

4.3 Forearm hematoma

Radial artery perforation, if not early recognized and managed, can lead to severe forearm hematoma and compartment syndrome. Prompt detection of the complication and precise localization of the bleeding source are of prime importance to adequately manage the problem with a pressure bandage dressing or a blood pressure sphygmomanometer inflated just over systolic pressure and placed over the bleeding area (83,84). In the great majority of cases this maneuver permits an easy, rapid and effective hemostasis. Afterwards, a careful observation of the forearm is required especially if the procedure is completed with the same initial access.

The most common etiology of hematoma is radial or small side branch perforation by the guidewire during sheath insertion or loops crossing especially in patients receiving multiple antiplatelet therapies (85).

Inadequate catheter manipulations or forceful maneuvers during guidewire or catheter advancement can also cause small radial side branch avulsions or dissections leading to hematomas. Hydrophilic guidewires easily entering these small arteries should always be advanced carefully because of their high perforation risk profiles.

Delayed recognition of a quiet but prolonged bleeding may lead to a large hematoma formation and sometimes to a compartment syndrome by pressure induced occlusion of the two major forearm arteries (ulnar and radial) (83,86).This severe complication must be treated by urgent fasciotomy and hematoma drainage to prevent ischemic injuries (Fig. 4). Fortunately, this very infrequent complication more often occurs during the learning curve of the technique and can be partially avoided by adequate nursing staff education and training.

4.4 Miscellaneous complications

Radial artery eversion or rupture during sheath removal or when catheters are drawing back, are due to a severe and refractory spasm of the radial artery blocking material retrieval (87). This complication should never occur by using hydrophilic-coated sheaths/catheters and with gentle manipulations.

Extremely rare cases of axillary, infraclavicular or even mediastinal hematomas due to perforation of a small arterial branch have also been reported (88).Late rebleeding occurring several hours or days after the procedure, as well as pseudo-aneurysms and arterio-venous fistula are quiet rare after transradial approach (see below paragraph 2.2).

Causalgia (uncommon) is secondary to nerve injury during arterial puncture or sometimes secondary to aggressive haemostatic compression (50). Residual pain is often transient but may be permanent. Similarly, but with a more severe clinical pattern, instances of chronic regional pain syndrome are described at the whole arm level (89).

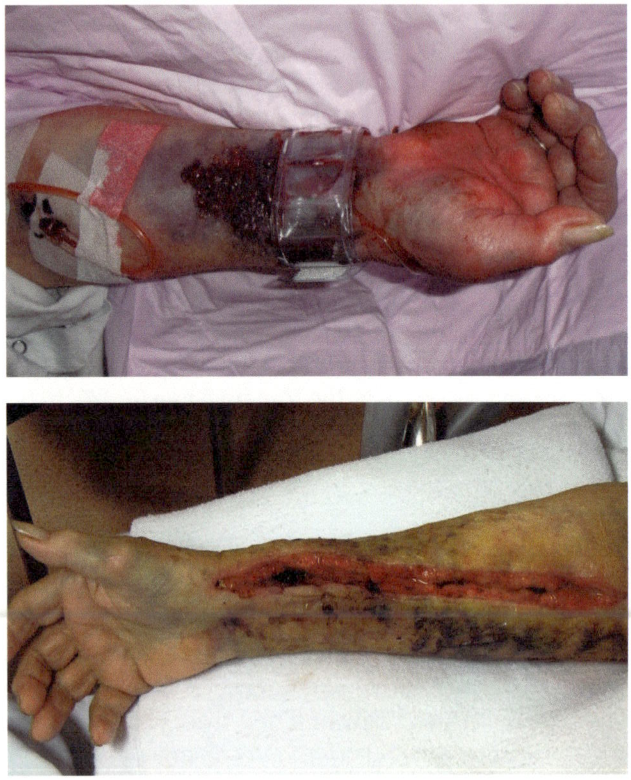

Fig. 4. Rare case of compartment syndrome (The same patient before and after urgent fasciotomy)

4.5 Conclusions

Long term consequences of radial artery occlusion or injury have to be further investigated, not only in patients requiring repeated percutaneous coronary interventions but also for patients in whom a radial conduit may be used for a surgical myocardial revascularization or the creation of an arterio-venous fistula.

To defend the use of radial access for coronary interventions, the conclusions of some recent major trials do not advocate the superiority of the radial artery over venous conduits for CABG surgery in terms of usefulness as well as for short or long-term patency (90). Nevertheless a retrospective study has shown a reduced early graft patency (77% versus 98%, $p=0.017$) in patients who had experienced a previous radial procedure before radial artery harvesting but without early clinical impact (91).

5. Clinical results and outcomes with transradial approach

5.1 Drastic reduction of periprocedural bleeding complications with transradial approach potentially drives reduction in mortality

Initially based on limited observational studies, followed by small single center or limited multicenter randomized studies, data concerning the safety of transradial approach and the lack of severe access site bleeding when compared to transfemoral approach are now supported by large registries (22), several meta-analyses (11,24) and more recently by a large, randomized and multicenter trial (2). According to these data, when compared with the transfemoral approach, a 27% (2) to 80% (11) reduction of entry-site bleeding complications may be expected with transradial approach.

As a result of these observations and of the progressive widespread endorsement of guidelines related to antithrombotic therapies for coronary procedures, attention has progressively turned to periprocedural bleeding complications and how to reduce the risk. If post-PCI bleeding events not related to the arterial access site are more difficult to anticipate, current literature, as Rao et al. have written, provides more and more data suggesting that the choice of the radial rather than the femoral access is associated with comparatively larger reductions in bleeding risk than those ever achieved with any anticoagulant strategy (92).

In parallel, according to several important studies, major bleeding events occurring after percutaneous coronary interventions have been shown to be independently associated with a marked increased risk of death and recurrent ischemic events in patients with an acute coronary syndrome or undergoing an elective revascularization (13,15,17,21,24,93). More precisely, bleeding in the 30 days after a percutaneous coronary intervention is strongly associated with mortality as late as 1 year after the procedure. This bleeding in the first 30 days after the procedure is comparatively as strong as the 30-day occurrence of other events such as post-procedural myocardial infarction and the need for an urgent revascularization. Not only major but also minor bleedings have been shown to be associated with late mortality (15). Before these observations, the composite endpoint of efficacy and safety used to assess PCI procedures was, traditionally, the combined incidence of death, myocardial infarction and urgent repeat revascularization of the target vessel at 30-days. To take into account post PCI bleeding impact on mortality, the "quadruple endpoint" that includes 30-days incidence of death, myocardial infarction, urgent revascularization and major bleeding has been recently introduced and should be promoted for the assessment of outcome after PCI.

Finally, as expected, a link between the reduction of bleeding complications with transradial interventions and a potential mortality reduction had recently emerged from data analysis. In the MORTAL study, Chase et al. found, by data linkage of three databases collecting clinical and procedural outcomes of 38,872 PCI patients of the British Columbia Cardiac Registry, that patients treated by transradial approach had a significantly lower rate of post-procedural blood transfusions (1.4% versus 2.8% for femoral, $p<0.01$) and a significant reduction in 30-day and 1-year mortality, odds ratio = 0.71 [95% CI 0.61 to 0.82] and 0.83 [95% CI 0.71 to 0.98], respectively (all $p<0.001$). In this study, the absolute increase in risk of death at 1 year associated with receiving a transfusion was 6.78% and the number needed to treat was 14.74 (prevention of 15 transfusions required to "avoid" one death). Therefore, transradial approach could potentially save one life for one thousand percutaneous coronary interventions performed by this way rather than by transfemoral approach (22). A large international registry provided similar results and demonstrated that transradial approach was independently associated with a lower risk of death or myocardial infarction after PCI (odds ratio = 0.52 [95% CI 0.31 to 0.89]) (94). Subsequently, the PRESTO ACS vascular substudy, including patients with non-ST-elevation acute coronary syndromes, also showed significant reduction in bleedings with the radial approach (0.7% versus 2.4% for femoral, p=0.05) and for the combined endpoint of 1-year mortality or re-infarction (4.9% versus 8.3%, p=0.05)(95). In patients suffering ST-segment elevation myocardial infarction (STEMI), the meta-analysis conducted by Vorobcsuk demonstrated a significant mortality reduction with transradial PCI (2.04% versus 3.06% for femoral, odds ratio= 0.54 [95% CI 0.33-0.86], p=0.01) (96). In the meta-analysis conducted by Jolly et al., despite the confirmation of a dramatic reduction of major access site bleedings with the transradial approach (0.05% versus 2.3% for femoral, odds ratio= 0.27 [95% CI 0.16, 0.45], $p < 0.001$), no significant association between this approach and a reduced 1-year mortality was found (24). In the same way, in the RIVAL study including patients with acute coronary syndromes, radial access did not reduce the primary outcome of death, myocardial infarction, stroke or non-CABG-related major bleeding compared with femoral approach even if radial access significantly reduced vascular access complications and insured similar procedural success rates (but patients presented with cardiogenic shock, known severe peripheral vascular disease precluding a femoral approach or previous coronary bypass surgery using the two internal mammary artery were ineligible for this trial). Nevertheless when the results of the RIVAL study ,restricted to centers with the highest radial tertile in this study, are included in an updated meta-analysis of all randomized trials conducted by known radial experts, the composite of death, myocardial infarction, or stroke was lower in the radial group than in the femoral group (2.3% versus 3.5%, p=0.005) (2). These observations suggest that the effectiveness of radial access might be linked to operator's or center's expertise in transradial PCI.

5.2 Does transradial approach influence the occurrence of silent cerebral injuries or post-procedural strokes?

Stroke is also a subject that people are worried about with the radial approach but previous studies have never demonstrated higher rates of TIAs or strokes with this technique even if used in higher risk subgroups of patients, such as the octogenarians (2,24,27).

Lund et al. and more recently Jurga et al. raised concern about the possibility that transradial access may induce subclinical solid cerebral microemboli at a higher extent than the transfemoral approach (97,98). As assessed by magnetic resonance imaging, 15% of patients suffered embolization toward the brain when the catheter passed from the right arm to the aorta in those examined with transradial access compared with none in the transfemoral group (p=0.567)(98). Transcranial Doppler showed that significantly more microemboli passed the right middle cerebral artery with right radial access than with the femoral (for radial median number of microemboli was 10 (1-120) and 6 (1-19) for femoral) (97).

Nevertheless, these two small studies have to be interpreted with caution for many reasons. The limited number of patients, the not so well reported operators experience for transradial approach but also the restricted use of the right radial artery may have negatively influenced the results. The clinical implications of these observations and the risk of cognitive impairment have not been explored further.

5.3 What about operator and patient radiation exposure during a transradial approach?

Interventional cardiology is known to be one of the professions with the greatest exposure to radiation. This is currently a growing problem for the cardiologist's health. Therefore, data regarding transradial technique are of great interest.

When interventional cardiologists, or fellows during their training, are dealing with a new technique they are often confronted with a higher level of radiation. When skills improve, catheter manipulations are more efficient and procedures are shortened which finally helps minimize radiation exposure.

For the transradial approach the problem is the same but, being technically more demanding, this technique is associated with a longer learning curve. However, in current literature, radial access is consistently associated, when compared to femoral, with longer procedural and fluoroscopic times which slightly but significantly increase occupational radiation exposure for operators but also irradiation for patients (1,2,11,24,99). In the RIVAL study, median fluoroscopy time was higher in the radial group than in the femoral group (9.8 min versus 8.0 min, $p<0.0001$) and these results were similar to those reported by Agostoni et al. (8.9 min versus 7.8 min, $p< 0.001$) or Rao et al. (13.5 versus 11.3 min, $p<0.01$).Jolly et al. have reported a mean difference of 0.4 minutes of fluoroscopy between the two techniques ([95% CI 0.3-0.5], $p<0.001$). The main limitation of previous observations is the significant variability among operators' performances. Some other confounding factors have to be discussed.

First of all, fluoroscopy time does not always correlate well with radiation dose received by operators (100). Secondly, many centers used classic catheter curves (Judkins, Amplatz, etc) for either diagnosis or intervention but the use of a dedicated radial catheter (Optitorque TIG™ catheter, Terumo corp.) may have influenced total fluoroscopic time. Indeed, radial operators have to take advantage of the possibility to complete a full coronary and left ventricular study with only one catheter to reduce radiation exposure (which is a significant difference compared to the femoral technique). Third, the exact puncture site is not always clearly reported in these trials. As mentioned before, a recent randomized trial, designed to evaluate safety and efficacy of left radial approach compared with right radial approach for coronary diagnostic and interventional procedures, showed that the left side was associated with slight but significantly lower fluoroscopy time and radiation dose adsorbed by patients. The left radial access advantages were particularly seen in older patients and for operators in training (66). These results are encouraging and future trials may further explore the potential advantages of a systematic left radial approach with the use of dedicated radial catheters to reduce the amount of fluoroscopy and finally the gap with femoral approach in terms of radiation exposure.

In addition, impact of operator ability in catheters or X-Ray tube manipulations (beam collimation, adequate tube angulations and operator position), as well as the use of radiation protection devices (low leaded flaps, upper mobile leaded glass, lead shields, lead aprons) are not often evaluated. The procedural setting (coronary angiography versus angioplasty, ad-hoc versus staged or urgent coronary interventions) may also influence measurements. Moreover many of these studies have been performed in centers (or by operators) with limited experience in transradial approach and results have not been corrected for probable improvements with greater expertise.

Finally, even if differences in terms of radiation dose beneath the lead apron are minimal between these approaches, their clinical impact in the long term is not known and operators should always apply all efforts to reduce the radiation dose in their daily practice.

5.4 Conclusions

Concerning many points, the debate is not closed and future randomized trials, if correctly powered to demonstrated differences in primary outcomes between the two vascular approaches and designed to avoid confounding factors, will be useful to confirm these findings. However, all the previous authors agree with the fact that clinicians may choose radial access for percutaneous coronary interventions because of its similar performances and above all, its reduced vascular complications.

6. Transradial approach: The perspectives

6.1 Outpatient strategy is feasible with transradial approach

Ad-hoc percutaneous coronary interventions, performed immediately after diagnostic angiography, have been shown to have equivalent short and long term safety when compared to elective interventions (101-105). In current clinical practice, ad-hoc PCI represents the majority of elective coronary interventions in most countries. PCI programs with same day discharge are therefore conceivable.

In accordance with the known benefits of transradial interventions, including less bleeding complications, better quality of care and earlier ambulation after the procedure, it was natural to test the feasibility and safety of an ambulatory discharge strategy in selected patients undergoing transradial coronary procedures. Numerous international studies are now available and even if not always randomized, they have validated this strategy after uncomplicated transradial percutaneous coronary interventions (106-112). No more access site complications are observed and the majority of events occurring 24 hours after discharge would not have been avoided by traditional next-day discharge. Bertrand et al. have also shown in a selected high risk population of patients (two thirds of patients presented with unstable angina and approximately 20% presented with high-risk acute coronary syndrome prior to the procedure) that same-day home discharge after uncomplicated transradial coronary stenting and administration of a bolus of abciximab is not clinically inferior to the standard overnight hospitalization with a bolus of abciximab followed by a 12-hour infusion. The primary composite end point of this study was the 30-day incidence of any of the following events: death, myocardial infarction, urgent revascularization, major bleeding, repeat hospitalization, access site complications, and severe thrombocytopenia. The incidence of the primary end point was 20.4% in the same-day discharge group and 18.2% in the overnight hospitalization group (P=0.017 for non-inferiority).No death occurred and the rate of major bleeding in both groups was extremely low at 0.8% and 0.2%, respectively (106).

Interestingly, similar feasibility and safety data are far less numerous to date for femoral approach, even if the same strategy may likewise be amenable by this access. Previous trials have demonstrated a higher incidence of local vascular complications either with or without the use of a vascular closure device and despite an optimal post-PCI recumbency depending on the vascular access management strategy chosen by the operator. Moreover, patients undergoing a transfemoral access, even if receiving closure devices, more frequently need to be reassured regarding early ambulation compared to those with a transradial approach and an unrestricted post-catheterization ambulation (109).

6.2 Reductions of hospitalizations stays and costs

Several dedicated costs analyses have shown a significant reduction in hospital costs with transradial access compared to other arterial access sites .The economic benefits of the transradial approach are mainly derived from its known advantages: a reduced incidence of vascular access site complications and immediate ambulation after the procedure (45).

A lower rate of access site complications also means decreased length of stay and costs compared with those observed in case of an adverse event (1,113,114). A vascular complication inevitably drives additional charges related to its careful medical evaluation using different diagnostic vascular imaging techniques and because of treatments required. Red blood cell or platelet transfusions (preceded by numerous laboratory tests), thrombin injections or operating room charges for surgical repair rapidly increase hospitalization costs. These adverse outcomes inevitably prolong hospitalization but indirect costs linked with an increased nursing and staff workload must also be considered even if they are more difficult to appreciate. Several authors have evaluated the negative economic impact of vascular access complications and the incremental costs ranged from $ 4000 for minor complications up to $ 14 000 for major events (114-116). Cooper et al. have showed, in a single center randomized study, that transradial access for diagnostic cardiac catheterization led to significant reductions in hospital costs when compared to femoral access ($ 2010 versus $2299 respectively, $p< 0.001$). Lower bed costs, mainly, taking into account nursing workload, but also pharmacy explain the median cost reduction of 289 $ per procedure (117). In the same way, Roussanov et al. have shown that a femoral access with or without the use of a closure device also failed to reduce total hospitalization costs as compare to radial access even in case of similar recovery times (radial =369.5 $ ± 74.6, femoral= 446.9 $ ± 60.2 and femoral with closure device 553.4 $ ± 81.0; $p < 0.001$) (118).

Immediate ambulation, in addition to showing radial approach safety, provides additional cost reductions through different mechanisms. First, transradial approach provides shorter length of stay .A systematic review and meta-analysis of randomized trials showed that radial access reduced hospital stay by a mean of 0.4 days [95% CI 0.2-0.5], $p=0.0001$) which also means an expedited room turn-over (24).Secondly, as reported by Amoroso et al, nursing workload can be significantly reduced inside (86 min versus 174 min for femoral access) as well as outside the catheterization laboratory (386 min versus 720 min for femoral access) when the radial way is systematically used for a catheterization procedure (119).An increased catheterization laboratory throughput can also be expected with radial access because less time is spent for sheath removal. Third, it has been shown that same day home discharge after an uncomplicated transradial percutaneous intervention results in a 50% relative reduction in post-PCI medical costs. In the EASY trial, at 30-day follow-up, the mean cumulative medical cost per outpatient was $1,117 ± $1,554 versus $2,258 ± $1,328 for overnight-stay patients (Canadian dollars). The mean difference of $1,141[95% CI: $962 to $1,320] was mainly due to the extra night for overnight hospital stay (120). Finally, with shorter length of stay and fewer vascular access site complications, a more rapid return to professional activities is insured for working patients.

Dedicated radial equipments (such as micropuncture kits and catheters) are still a little bit more expensive than those used for femoral access. However, the RIVAL study reported the use of a lower mean number of diagnostic catheters per procedure with transradial access and similarly the same number of guiding catheters per PCI for the two techniques (2). Economic implications of these observations are not yet quantified, especially during the early adoption of the radial technique, which is often associated with increased catheter usage because of frequent inadequate choices.

7. Conclusions

Over the last two decades, major improvements have been achieved in pharmacotherapy and device technology making percutaneous coronary interventions safer, despite the increasing complexity of clinical and anatomic conditions treated during these procedures. Numerous trials are now available and show undoubtedly the superiority of the transradial approach with respect to the incidence of vascular access site complications, especially bleeding, and this despite the fact that all transradial procedures are performed immediately after an initial bolus of heparin to prevent radial artery thrombosis. Moreover, transradial percutaneous interventions can be performed with the same success rate as procedures by femoral approach and have shown their capacities to shorten hospitalization duration and offer the possibility for an outpatient strategy. In addition, transradial access has the potential of reducing medical costs and increasing hospital bed utilization without jeopardizing patient safety. The transradial approach also increases peri-procedural patient comfort and is now strongly preferred by patients for subsequent procedures (2,117). All these advantages are maybe a part of the solution to reduce pressure on limited hospital resources facing rising demands. Nevertheless, even if the transradial approach is extremely safe and occlusion of the artery without any clinical consequences, further studies are needed to search for materials minimizing physiological and anatomical changes in the cannulated radial artery. Radial experts underscore the need for other large randomized trials to confirm that radial approach has a favourable impact on the incidence of post procedural ischemic events and cuts mortality as compared to femoral approach. In this case, guidelines relative to percutaneous coronary interventions should be updated and the worldwide practice changed but transradial access is already an essential tool for the interventional cardiologist.

8. Acknowledgments

The author would like to thank Caroline Lepiece, MD, for her expert assistance in the revision of the manuscript and also Vincent Dangoisse, MD, Patrick Chenu, MD, and Erwin Schroeder,MD , my teachers in interventional cardiology.

9. References

[1] Rao SV, Ou FS, Wang TY, et al. Trends in the prevalence and outcomes of radial and femoral approaches to percutaneous coronary intervention: a report from the National Cardiovascular Data Registry. JACC Cardiovasc Interv 2008;1:379-86.

[2] Jolly SS, Yusuf S, Cairns J, et al. Radial versus femoral access for coronary angiography and intervention in patients with acute coronary syndromes (RIVAL): a randomised, parallel group, multicentre trial. Lancet 2011;377:1409-20.

[3] Kinnaird TD, Stabile E, Mintz GS, et al. Incidence, predictors, and prognostic implications of bleeding and blood transfusion following percutaneous coronary interventions. Am J Cardiol 2003;92:930-5.

[4] Resnic FS, Arora N, Matheny M, Reynolds MR. A cost-minimization analysis of the angio-seal vascular closure device following percutaneous coronary intervention. Am J Cardiol 2007;99:766-70.

[5] Geisler T, Gawaz M, Steinhubl SR, Bhatt DL, Storey RF, Flather M. Current strategies in antiplatelet therapy--does identification of risk and adjustment of therapy contribute to more effective, personalized medicine in cardiovascular disease? Pharmacol Ther 2010;127:95-107.

[6] Gunasekaran S, Cherukupalli R. Radial artery perforation and its management during PCI. J Invasive Cardiol 2009;21:E24-6.

[7] Mannucci PM, Franchini M. Mechanism of hemostasis defects and management of bleeding in patients with acute coronary syndromes. Eur J Intern Med 2010;21:254-9.

[8] Ndrepepa G, Keta D, Byrne RA, et al. Impact of body mass index on clinical outcome in patients with acute coronary syndromes treated with percutaneous coronary intervention. Heart Vessels 2010;25:27-34.

[9] Ndrepepa G, Keta D, Schulz S, et al. Characterization of patients with bleeding complications who are at increased risk of death after percutaneous coronary intervention. Heart Vessels 2010;25:294-8.

[10] Wijns W, Kolh P, Danchin N, et al. Guidelines on myocardial revascularization. Eur Heart J 2010;31:2501-55.

[11] Agostoni P, Biondi-Zoccai GG, de Benedictis ML, et al. Radial versus femoral approach for percutaneous coronary diagnostic and interventional procedures; Systematic overview and meta-analysis of randomized trials. J Am Coll Cardiol 2004;44:349-56.

[12] Doyle BJ, Rihal CS, Gastineau DA, Holmes DR, Jr. Bleeding, blood transfusion, and increased mortality after percutaneous coronary intervention: implications for contemporary practice. J Am Coll Cardiol 2009;53:2019-27.

[13] Eikelboom JW, Mehta SR, Anand SS, Xie C, Fox KA, Yusuf S. Adverse impact of bleeding on prognosis in patients with acute coronary syndromes. Circulation 2006;114:774-82.

[14] Moscucci M, Fox KA, Cannon CP, et al. Predictors of major bleeding in acute coronary syndromes: the Global Registry of Acute Coronary Events (GRACE). Eur Heart J 2003;24:1815-23.

[15] Ndrepepa G, Berger PB, Mehilli J, et al. Periprocedural bleeding and 1-year outcome after percutaneous coronary interventions: appropriateness of including bleeding as a component of a quadruple end point. J Am Coll Cardiol 2008;51:690-7.

[16] Osten MD, Ivanov J, Eichhofer J, et al. Impact of renal insufficiency on angiographic, procedural, and in-hospital outcomes following percutaneous coronary intervention. Am J Cardiol 2008;101:780-5.

[17] Rao SV, O'Grady K, Pieper KS, et al. Impact of bleeding severity on clinical outcomes among patients with acute coronary syndromes. Am J Cardiol 2005;96:1200-6.

[18] An international randomized trial comparing four thrombolytic strategies for acute myocardial infarction. The GUSTO investigators. N Engl J Med 1993;329:673-82.
[19] Chesebro JH, Knatterud G, Roberts R, et al. Thrombolysis in Myocardial Infarction (TIMI) Trial, Phase I: A comparison between intravenous tissue plasminogen activator and intravenous streptokinase. Clinical findings through hospital discharge. Circulation 1987;76:142-54.
[20] Stone GW, McLaurin BT, Cox DA, et al. Bivalirudin for patients with acute coronary syndromes. N Engl J Med 2006;355:2203-16.
[21] Doyle BJ, Ting HH, Bell MR, et al. Major femoral bleeding complications after percutaneous coronary intervention: incidence, predictors, and impact on long-term survival among 17,901 patients treated at the Mayo Clinic from 1994 to 2005. JACC Cardiovasc Interv 2008;1:202-9.
[22] Chase AJ, Fretz EB, Warburton WP, et al. Association of the arterial access site at angioplasty with transfusion and mortality: the M.O.R.T.A.L study (Mortality benefit Of Reduced Transfusion after percutaneous coronary intervention via the Arm or Leg). Heart 2008;94:1019-25.
[23] Cox N, Resnic FS, Popma JJ, Simon DI, Eisenhauer AC, Rogers C. Comparison of the risk of vascular complications associated with femoral and radial access coronary catheterization procedures in obese versus nonobese patients. Am J Cardiol 2004;94:1174-7.
[24] Jolly SS, Amlani S, Hamon M, Yusuf S, Mehta SR. Radial versus femoral access for coronary angiography or intervention and the impact on major bleeding and ischemic events: a systematic review and meta-analysis of randomized trials. Am Heart J 2009;157:132-40.
[25] Hirano Y, Ikuta S, Uehara H, et al. Diagnosis of vascular complications at the puncture site after cardiac catheterization. J Cardiol 2004;43:259-65.
[26] Koreny M, Riedmuller E, Nikfardjam M, Siostrzonek P, Mullner M. Arterial puncture closing devices compared with standard manual compression after cardiac catheterization: systematic review and meta-analysis. Jama 2004;291:350-7.
[27] Louvard Y, Benamer H, Garot P, et al. Comparison of transradial and transfemoral approaches for coronary angiography and angioplasty in octogenarians (the OCTOPLUS study). Am J Cardiol 2004;94:1177-80.
[28] Waksman R, King SB, 3rd, Douglas JS, et al. Predictors of groin complications after balloon and new-device coronary intervention. Am J Cardiol 1995;75:886-9.
[29] Corriere MA, Guzman RJ. True and false aneurysms of the femoral artery. Semin Vasc Surg 2005;18:216-23.
[30] Graham AN, Wilson CM, Hood JM, Barros D'Sa AA. Risk of rupture of postangiographic femoral false aneurysm. Br J Surg 1992;79:1022-5.
[31] Kazmers A, Meeker C, Nofz K, et al. Nonoperative therapy for postcatheterization femoral artery pseudoaneurysms. Am Surg 1997;63:199-204.
[32] Sherev DA, Shaw RE, Brent BN. Angiographic predictors of femoral access site complications: implication for planned percutaneous coronary intervention. Catheter Cardiovasc Interv 2005;65:196-202.
[33] Tavris DR, Gallauresi BA, Dey S, Brindis R, Mitchel K. Risk of local adverse events by gender following cardiac catheterization. Pharmacoepidemiol Drug Saf 2007;16:125-31.

[34] Stella PR, Kiemeneij F, Laarman GJ, Odekerken D, Slagboom T, van der Wieken R. Incidence and outcome of radial artery occlusion following transradial artery coronary angioplasty. Cathet Cardiovasc Diagn 1997;40:156-8.

[35] Nikolsky E, Mehran R, Halkin A, et al. Vascular complications associated with arteriotomy closure devices in patients undergoing percutaneous coronary procedures: a meta-analysis. J Am Coll Cardiol 2004;44:1200-9.

[36] Chevalier B, Lancelin B, Koning R, et al. Effect of a closure device on complication rates in high-local-risk patients: results of a randomized multicenter trial. Catheter Cardiovasc Interv 2003;58:285-91.

[37] Mann T, Cowper PA, Peterson ED, et al. Transradial coronary stenting: comparison with femoral access closed with an arterial suture device. Catheter Cardiovasc Interv 2000;49:150-6.

[38] Louvard Y, Ludwig J, Lefevre T, et al. Transradial approach for coronary angioplasty in the setting of acute myocardial infarction: a dual-center registry. Catheter Cardiovasc Interv 2002;55:206-11.

[39] Morice MC, Dumas P, Lefevre T, Loubeyre C, Louvard Y, Piechaud JF. Systematic use of transradial approach or suture of the femoral artery after angioplasty: attempt at achieving zero access site complications. Catheter Cardiovasc Interv 2000;51:417-21.

[40] Sciahbasi A, Fischetti D, Picciolo A, et al. Transradial access compared with femoral puncture closure devices in percutaneous coronary procedures. Int J Cardiol 2009;137:199-205.

[41] Dangas G, Mehran R, Kokolis S, et al. Vascular complications after percutaneous coronary interventions following hemostasis with manual compression versus arteriotomy closure devices. J Am Coll Cardiol 2001;38:638-41.

[42] Dauerman HL, Applegate RJ, Cohen DJ. Vascular closure devices: the second decade. J Am Coll Cardiol 2007;50:1617-26.

[43] Meyerson SL, Feldman T, Desai TR, Leef J, Schwartz LB, McKinsey JF. Angiographic access site complications in the era of arterial closure devices. Vasc Endovascular Surg 2002;36:137-44.

[44] Arora N, Matheny ME, Sepke C, Resnic FS. A propensity analysis of the risk of vascular complications after cardiac catheterization procedures with the use of vascular closure devices. Am Heart J 2007;153:606-11.

[45] Caputo RP. Transradial Arterial Access: Economic Considerations. J Invasive Cardiol. 2009;21:18-20.

[46] Fitts J, Ver Lee P, Hofmaster P, Malenka D. Fluoroscopy-guided femoral artery puncture reduces the risk of PCI-related vascular complications. J Interv Cardiol 2008;21:273-8.

[47] Grier D, Hartnell G. Percutaneous femoral artery puncture: practice and anatomy. Br J Radiol 1990;63:602-4.

[48] Safian RD, Freed M. The manual of interventional cardiology: Physicians' Press, 2001.

[49] Barbeau GR, Arsenault F, Dugas L, Simard S, Lariviere MM. Evaluation of the ulnopalmar arterial arches with pulse oximetry and plethysmography: comparison with the Allen's test in 1010 patients. Am Heart J 2004;147:489-93.

[50] Hamon M, Mc Fadden E. Trans-radial approach for cardiovascular interventions: ESM, 2003.

[51] Patel T. Patel's Atlas of Transradial Intervention: The Basics: Seascript Company, 2007.

[52] Sciahbasi A, Romagnoli E, Trani C, et al. Evaluation of the "learning curve" for left and right radial approach during percutaneous coronary procedures. Am J Cardiol 2011;108:185-8.

[53] Guédès A, Dangoisse V, Gabriel L, et al. Low rate of conversion to transfemoral approach when attempting both radial arteries for coronary angiography and percutaneous coronary intervention: a study of 1,826 consecutive procedures. J Invasive Cardiol 2010;22:391-7.

[54] Dahm JB, Vogelgesang D, Hummel A, Staudt A, Volzke H, Felix SB. A randomized trial of 5 vs. 6 French transradial percutaneous coronary interventions. Catheter Cardiovasc Interv 2002;57:172-6.

[55] Kiemeneij F, Fraser D, Slagboom T, Laarman G, van der Wieken R. Hydrophilic coating aids radial sheath withdrawal and reduces patient discomfort following transradial coronary intervention: a randomized double-blind comparison of coated and uncoated sheaths. Catheter Cardiovasc Interv 2003;59:161-4.

[56] Rathore S, Stables RH, Pauriah M, et al. Impact of length and hydrophilic coating of the introducer sheath on radial artery spasm during transradial coronary intervention: a randomized study. JACC Cardiovasc Interv 2010;3:475-83.

[57] Saito S, Tanaka S, Hiroe Y, et al. Comparative study on transradial approach vs. transfemoral approach in primary stent implantation for patients with acute myocardial infarction: results of the test for myocardial infarction by prospective unicenter randomization for access sites (TEMPURA) trial. Catheter Cardiovasc Interv 2003;59:26-33.

[58] Chodor P, Krupa H, Kurek T, et al. RADIal versus femoral approach for percutaneous coronary interventions in patients with Acute Myocardial Infarction (RADIAMI): A prospective, randomized, single-center clinical trial. Cardiol J 2009;16:332-40.

[59] Egred M. Feasibility and Safety of 7-Fr Radial Approach for Complex PCI. J Interv Cardiol 2011.

[60] Hamon M, Sabatier R, Zhao Q, Niculescu R, Valette B, Grollier G. Mini-invasive strategy in acute coronary syndromes: direct coronary stenting using 5 Fr guiding catheters and transradial approach. Catheter Cardiovasc Interv 2002;55:340-3.

[61] Ochiai M, Isshiki T, Toyoizumi H, et al. Efficacy of transradial primary stenting in patients with acute myocardial infarction. Am J Cardiol 1999;83:966-8, A10.

[62] Rathore S, Hakeem A, Pauriah M, Roberts E, Beaumont A, Morris JL. A comparison of the transradial and the transfemoral approach in chronic total occlusion percutaneous coronary intervention. Catheter Cardiovasc Interv 2009;73:883-7.

[63] Rathore S, Roberts E, Hakeem AR, Pauriah M, Beaumont A, Morris JL. The feasibility of percutaneous transradial coronary intervention for saphenous vein graft lesions and comparison with transfemoral route. J Interv Cardiol 2009;22:336-40.

[64] Mamas MA, Eichhofer J, Hendry C, et al. Use of the Heartrail II catheter as a distal stent delivery device; an extended case series. EuroIntervention 2009;5:265-71.

[65] Mamas MA, Fath-Ordoubadi F, Fraser DG. Atraumatic complex transradial intervention using large bore sheathless guide catheter. Catheter Cardiovasc Interv 2008;72:357-64.

[66] Sciahbasi A, Romagnoli E, Burzotta F, et al. Transradial approach (left vs right) and procedural times during percutaneous coronary procedures: TALENT study. Am Heart J 2011;161:172-9.

[67] Cha KS, Kim MH. Feasibility and safety of concomitant left internal mammary arteriography at the setting of the right transradial coronary angiography. Catheter Cardiovasc Interv 2002;56:188-95.

[68] Benit E, Missault L, Eeman T, et al. Brachial, radial, or femoral approach for elective Palmaz-Schatz stent implantation: a randomized comparison. Cathet Cardiovasc Diagn 1997;41:124-30.

[69] Kiemeneij F, Laarman GJ, Odekerken D, Slagboom T, van der Wieken R. A randomized comparison of percutaneous transluminal coronary angioplasty by the radial, brachial and femoral approaches: the access study. J Am Coll Cardiol 1997;29:1269-75.

[70] Mann JT, 3rd, Cubeddu MG, Schneider JE, Arrowood M. Right Radial Access for PTCA: A Prospective Study Demonstrates Reduced Complications and Hospital Charges. J Invasive Cardiol 1996;8 Suppl D:40D-44D.

[71] Plante S, Cantor WJ, Goldman L, et al. Comparison of bivalirudin versus heparin on radial artery occlusion after transradial catheterization. Catheter Cardiovasc Interv 2010;76:654-8.

[72] Wu SS, Galani RJ, Bahro A, Moore JA, Burket MW, Cooper CJ. 8 french transradial coronary interventions: clinical outcome and late effects on the radial artery and hand function. J Invasive Cardiol 2000;12:605-9.

[73] Saito S, Ikei H, Hosokawa G, Tanaka S. Influence of the ratio between radial artery inner diameter and sheath outer diameter on radial artery flow after transradial coronary intervention. Catheter Cardiovasc Interv 1999;46:173-8.

[74] Sakai H, Ikeda S, Harada T, et al. Limitations of successive transradial approach in the same arm: the Japanese experience. Catheter Cardiovasc Interv 2001;54:204-8.

[75] Pancholy SB. Comparison of the effect of intra-arterial versus intravenous heparin on radial artery occlusion after transradial catheterization. Am J Cardiol 2009;104:1083-5.

[76] Sanmartin M, Gomez M, Rumoroso JR, et al. Interruption of blood flow during compression and radial artery occlusion after transradial catheterization. Catheter Cardiovasc Interv 2007;70:185-9.

[77] Pancholy S, Coppola J, Patel T, Roke-Thomas M. Prevention of radial artery occlusion-patent hemostasis evaluation trial (PROPHET study): a randomized comparison of traditional versus patency documented hemostasis after transradial catheterization. Catheter Cardiovasc Interv 2008;72:335-40.

[78] Bernat I, Bertrand OF, Rokyta R, et al. Efficacy and safety of transient ulnar artery compression to recanalize acute radial artery occlusion after transradial catheterization. Am J Cardiol 2011;107:1698-701.

[79] Yoo BS, Lee SH, Ko JY, et al. Procedural outcomes of repeated transradial coronary procedure. Catheter Cardiovasc Interv 2003;58:301-4.

[80] Edmundson A, Mann T. Nonocclusive radial artery injury resulting from transradial coronary interventions: radial artery IVUS. J Invasive Cardiol 2005;17:528-31.

[81] Wakeyama T, Ogawa H, Iida H, et al. Intima-media thickening of the radial artery after transradial intervention. An intravascular ultrasound study. J Am Coll Cardiol 2003;41:1109-14.

[82] Sanmartin M, Goicolea J, Ocaranza R, Cuevas D, Calvo F. Vasoreactivity of the radial artery after transradial catheterization. J Invasive Cardiol 2004;16:635-8.

[83] Bazemore E, Mann JT, 3rd. Problems and complications of the transradial approach for coronary interventions: a review. J Invasive Cardiol 2005;17:156-9.

[84] Tizon-Marcos H, Barbeau GR. Incidence of compartment syndrome of the arm in a large series of transradial approach for coronary procedures. J Interv Cardiol 2008;21:380-4.

[85] Louvard Y, Lefevre T. Loops and transradial approach in coronary diagnosis and intervention. Catheter Cardiovasc Interv 2000;51:250-2.

[86] Rathore S, Morris JL. The radial approach: is this the route to take? J Interv Cardiol 2008;21:375-9.

[87] Dieter RS, Akef A, Wolff M. Eversion endarterectomy complicating radial artery access for left heart catheterization. Catheter Cardiovasc Interv 2003;58:478-80.

[88] Park KW, Chung JW, Chang SA, Kim KI, Chung WY, Chae IH. Two cases of mediastinal hematoma after cardiac catheterization: A rare but real complication of the transradial approach. Int J Cardiol 2008;130:e89-92.

[89] Papadimos TJ, Hofmann JP. Radial artery thrombosis, palmar arch systolic blood velocities, and chronic regional pain syndrome 1 following transradial cardiac catheterization. Catheter Cardiovasc Interv 2002;57:537-40.

[90] Goldman S, Sethi GK, Holman W, et al. Radial artery grafts vs saphenous vein grafts in coronary artery bypass surgery: a randomized trial. Jama 2011;305:167-74.

[91] Kamiya H, Ushijima T, Kanamori T, et al. Use of the radial artery graft after transradial catheterization: is it suitable as a bypass conduit? Ann Thorac Surg 2003;76:1505-9.

[92] Rao SV, Cohen MG, Kandzari DE, Bertrand OF, Gilchrist IC. The transradial approach to percutaneous coronary intervention: historical perspective, current concepts, and future directions. J Am Coll Cardiol 2010;55:2187-95.

[93] Manoukian SV, Feit F, Mehran R, et al. Impact of major bleeding on 30-day mortality and clinical outcomes in patients with acute coronary syndromes: an analysis from the ACUITY Trial. J Am Coll Cardiol 2007;49:1362-8.

[94] Montalescot G, Ongen Z, Guindy R, et al. Predictors of outcome in patients undergoing PCI. Results of the RIVIERA study. Int J Cardiol 2008;129:379-87.

[95] Sciahbasi A, Pristipino C, Ambrosio G, et al. Arterial access-site-related outcomes of patients undergoing invasive coronary procedures for acute coronary syndromes (from the ComPaRison of Early Invasive and Conservative Treatment in Patients With Non-ST-ElevatiOn Acute Coronary Syndromes [PRESTO-ACS] Vascular Substudy). Am J Cardiol 2009;103:796-800.

[96] Vorobcsuk A, Konyi A, Aradi D, et al. Transradial versus transfemoral percutaneous coronary intervention in acute myocardial infarction Systematic overview and meta-analysis. Am Heart J 2009;158:814-21.

[97] Jurga J, Nyman J, Tornvall P, et al. Cerebral microembolism during coronary angiography: a randomized comparison between femoral and radial arterial access. Stroke 2011;42:1475-7.

[98] Lund C, Nes RB, Ugelstad TP, et al. Cerebral emboli during left heart catheterization may cause acute brain injury. Eur Heart J 2005;26:1269-75.

[99] Brasselet C, Blanpain T, Tassan-Mangina S, et al. Comparison of operator radiation exposure with optimized radiation protection devices during coronary angiograms and ad hoc percutaneous coronary interventions by radial and femoral routes. Eur Heart J 2007.

[100] Sciahbasi A, Romagnoli E, Trani C, et al. Operator radiation exposure during percutaneous coronary procedures through the left or right radial approach: the TALENT dosimetric substudy. Circ Cardiovasc Interv 2011;4:226-31.

[101] Chung WJ, Fang HY, Tsai TH, et al. Transradial approach percutaneous coronary interventions in an out-patient clinic. Int Heart J 2010;51:371-6.

[102] Feldman DN, Minutello RM, Gade CL, Wong SC. Outcomes following immediate (ad hoc) versus staged percutaneous coronary interventions (report from the 2000 to 2001 New York State Angioplasty Registry). Am J Cardiol 2007;99:446-9.

[103] Good CW, Blankenship JC, Scott TD, Skelding KA, Berger PB, Wood GC. Feasibility and safety of ad hoc percutaneous coronary intervention in the modern era. J Invasive Cardiol 2009;21:194-200.

[104] Krone RJ, Shaw RE, Klein LW, Blankenship JC, Weintraub WS. Ad hoc percutaneous coronary interventions in patients with stable coronary artery disease--a study of prevalence, safety, and variation in use from the American College of Cardiology National Cardiovascular Data Registry (ACC-NCDR). Catheter Cardiovasc Interv 2006;68:696-703.

[105] Shubrooks SJ, Jr., Malenka DJ, Piper WD, et al. Safety and efficacy of percutaneous coronary interventions performed immediately after diagnostic catheterization in northern new england and comparison with similar procedures performed later. Am J Cardiol 2000;86:41-5.

[106] Bertrand OF, De Larochelliere R, Rodes-Cabau J, et al. A randomized study comparing same-day home discharge and abciximab bolus only to overnight hospitalization and abciximab bolus and infusion after transradial coronary stent implantation. Circulation 2006;114:2636-43.

[107] Gilchrist IC, Nickolaus MJ, Momplaisir T. Same-day transradial outpatient stenting with a 6-hr course of glycoprotein IIb/IIIa receptor blockade: a feasibility study. Catheter Cardiovasc Interv 2002;56:10-3.

[108] Heyde GS, Koch KT, de Winter RJ, et al. Randomized trial comparing same-day discharge with overnight hospital stay after percutaneous coronary intervention: results of the Elective PCI in Outpatient Study (EPOS). Circulation 2007;115:2299-306.

[109] Jabara R, Gadesam R, Pendyala L, et al. Ambulatory discharge after transradial coronary intervention: Preliminary US single-center experience (Same-day TransRadial Intervention and Discharge Evaluation, the STRIDE Study). Am Heart J 2008;156:1141-6.

[110] Silber S, Albertsson P, Aviles FF, et al. Guidelines for percutaneous coronary interventions. The Task Force for Percutaneous Coronary Interventions of the European Society of Cardiology. Eur Heart J 2005;26:804-47.

[111] Slagboom T, Kiemeneij F, Laarman GJ, van der Wieken R. Outpatient coronary angioplasty: feasible and safe. Catheter Cardiovasc Interv 2005;64:421-7.

[112] Slagboom T, Kiemeneij F, Laarman GJ, van der Wieken R, Odekerken D. Actual outpatient PTCA: results of the OUTCLAS pilot study. Catheter Cardiovasc Interv 2001;53:204-8.

[113] Cohen DJ, Lincoff AM, Lavelle TA, et al. Economic evaluation of bivalirudin with provisional glycoprotein IIB/IIIA inhibition versus heparin with routine

glycoprotein IIB/IIIA inhibition for percutaneous coronary intervention: results from the REPLACE-2 trial. J Am Coll Cardiol 2004;44:1792-800.

[114] Rao SV, Kaul PR, Liao L, et al. Association between bleeding, blood transfusion, and costs among patients with non-ST-segment elevation acute coronary syndromes. Am Heart J 2008;155:369-74.

[115] Kugelmass AD, Cohen DJ, Brown PP, Simon AW, Becker ER, Culler SD. Hospital resources consumed in treating complications associated with percutaneous coronary interventions. Am J Cardiol 2006;97:322-7.

[116] Pinto DS, Stone GW, Shi C, et al. Economic evaluation of bivalirudin with or without glycoprotein IIb/IIIa inhibition versus heparin with routine glycoprotein IIb/IIIa inhibition for early invasive management of acute coronary syndromes. J Am Coll Cardiol 2008;52:1758-68.

[117] Cooper CJ, El-Shiekh RA, Cohen DJ, et al. Effect of transradial access on quality of life and cost of cardiac catheterization: A randomized comparison. Am Heart J 1999;138:430-6.

[118] Roussanov O, Wilson SJ, Henley K, et al. Cost-effectiveness of the radial versus femoral artery approach to diagnostic cardiac catheterization. J Invasive Cardiol 2007;19:349-53.

[119] Amoroso G, Sarti M, Bellucci R, et al. Clinical and procedural predictors of nurse workload during and after invasive coronary procedures: the potential benefit of a systematic radial access. Eur J Cardiovasc Nurs 2005;4:234-41.

[120] Rinfret S, Kennedy WA, Lachaine J, et al. Economic impact of same-day home discharge after uncomplicated transradial percutaneous coronary intervention and bolus-only abciximab regimen. JACC Cardiovasc Interv 2010;3:1011-9.

2

Percutaneous Coronary Intervention and 30-Day Mortality: The CANADA Score

Rohan Poulter and Jaap Hamburger
University of British Columbia
Canada

1. Introduction

Coronary artery disease remains highly prevalent in contemporary society and over 1000000 revascularisation procedures by percutaneous coronary intervention (PCI) are performed annually worldwide. PCI has seen significant improvement in clinical outcomes with the current generation of drug eluting stents. The role of PCI in multivessel coronary disease has been expanded with current trial evidence indicating equipoise between PCI and coronary artery by-pass surgery in selected groups.

Increasingly, coronary artery by-pass surgery (CABG) or PCI is being considered as an equivalent revascularisation strategy within the same patient population. Given the options available to clinicians and patients it is important to have robust tools to accurately compare the risk and benefits of selected strategies when making management decisions. Whilst these tools have been available to the cardiac surgeons for some time (Granton & Cheng, 2008), an equivalent tool for the interventional cardiologist has only recently been published.

The CANADA Score is a risk prediction model for determining 30 day mortality risk in patients undergoing elective, urgent and emergent PCI. Its development and validation will be discussed with reference to the established cardiac surgical risk calculators currently available.

2. Risk prediction models

Risk prediction models are statistical models produced from patient databases using a combination of individual risk predication markers and are used by clinicians and patients for making treatment decisions. Model inaccuracy and ineffectiveness can therefore have negative implications on risk measurement and subsequent patient decisions and outcomes. The accuracy of the model is typically summarised in terms of the model's discrimination and calibration (Janes et al, 2008). The applicability of a risk model to a patient population is determined by validation.

2.1 Discrimination

Discrimination is the ability of the model to correctly classify outcomes (Nathanson & Higgins, 2008). The statistical measures of area under the curve (AUC) or concordance index (C-index) are commonly used to describe how well patients are classified within the model.

Patients typically are assigned a positive classification if the model predicts the probability of an outcome as >0.5. Conversely, a negative classification indicates the model predicts the probability of an outcome is <0.5. A patient is therefore correctly classified when an outcome event occurs in a patient with a positive classification, or when no event occurs in a patient with a negative classification. Sensitivity and specificity are derived from the fraction of correctly classified patients. The receiver operating characteristic (ROC) curve is derived from the plot of specificity against (1 - sensitivity), and the area under the ROC curve (AUC) measures the discriminatory ability of the model. An AUC of 0.5 indicates no discriminatory ability and 1.0 indicates perfect discrimination (Cook, 2008). A good model would have AUC 0.7 - 0.9.

2.2 Calibration

Calibration is determined by comparing the predicted and observed outcomes within subgroups of increasing risk within the dataset and applying the Hosmer-Lemeshow (H-L) statistical test (Hosmer & Lemeshow, 2000) to assess "goodness of fit". The H-L goodness of fit test divides subjects into deciles based on predicted probabilities and calculates a chi-square from observed and expected frequencies. If the H-L statistic has p-value >0.05, it implies there is no significant difference between observed and model-predicted values and therefore the model is well calibrated. Calibration plots can be used to give a graphical representation of model calibration.

2.3 Validation

Strategies to validate statistical models include (Altman & Royston, 2000):

a. Internal - evaluation from a single dataset
   Internal validation refers to the application of a model to the same cohort from which it was derived, often by splitting one dataset into separate training and validation cohorts. This can be problematic as models tend to over fit the data and calibration appears erroneously good (Vickers & Cronin, 2010). Internal validation also does not address real differences that may exist between different cohorts. Methods to improve internal validation include cross validation and bootstrap resampling.
b. Temporal - evaluation of a second dataset after the original cohort
   Temporal validation involves collecting data from the same sources but at a later time point. It is a prospective evaluation of the original model, but it may take considerable time to accrue an adequate number of events in the second dataset.
c. External - evaluation of geographically separate cohorts
   External validation addresses the generalizability of the statistical model by application to a different population from that used to derive the model. It can be performed retrospectively making it attractive for widespread application and can help address issues related to sample selection.

3. Cardiac surgical models

3.1 STS score

The Society of Thoracic Surgeons (STS) National Adult Cardiac Database was established in 1989 and currently contains over 4.5 million records. It represents >90% of adult cardiac surgical procedures performed in the United States. In the interval 1997-1999 there were 503 478 CABG-only procedures identified from 495 participating centres. From this, 30 potential risk factors for mortality were identified on univariate screening (Table 1). The over-all 30 day mortality rate was 3.05%. Using multivariate logistic regression an STS Score model was developed that had good discrimination (c-index 0.78) and modest calibration (H-L $p = 0.0016$) (Table 2) (Shroyer et al, 2003).

3.2 EuroSCORE

A European multi-national database was established in 1995 (Nashef et al, 1999) and information on risk factors and mortality was collected for 19 030 consecutive adult patients undergoing cardiac surgery under cardiopulmonary bypass in 128 surgical centres in eight European states (Roques et al, 2003). Data were collected for 68 preoperative and 29 operative risk factors proven or believed to influence mortality. From this a series of objective risk factors (Table 1) were weighted by regression analysis and developed into an additive score (additive EuroSCORE) to predict mortality. Overall, 14 799 patients were divided into a developmental cohort (n= 13 302) and validation cohort (n= 1479). The 30 day mortality was for the entire cohort was 4.7%. The additive EuroSCORE had good discrimination in both the development (c-index 0.79) and validation (c-index 0.76) cohort, as well as good calibration (H-L p value <0.40 & <0.68 respectively) (Table 2). The additive EuroSCORE was further externally validated in a North American population. Despite demographic differences the model performed well with discriminatory c-index 0.75 and excellent calibration (predicted and observed mortality 4.15%) (Nashef et al, 2002).

A limitation of the additive EuroSCORE was underestimation of risk in very high risk populations (Sergeant et al, 2001). A second model was published using the coefficient of the variables in the logistic regression data rather than additive weights to predict mortality. The logistic EuroSCORE had similar discrimination (c-index 0.785) to the additive model but superior accuracy in high risk populations. The models diverged at a predicted mortality of 8-10% (Michel et al, 2003).

	STS Score	EuroSCORE	CANADA Score
Patient Factors			
Age	X	X	X
Gender	X	X	X
Renal failure	X	X	X [a]
Critical preoperative state	X	X	X
Chronic lung disease	X	X	
PVD / CVD	X	X	
CVA / Neurological dysfunction	X	X	
Previous cardiac surgery	X	X	
Multiple reoperations	X		

	STS Score	EuroSCORE	CANADA Score
Ethnicity	X		
BSA	X		
Diabetes	X		
Hypercholesterolemia	X		
Hypertension	X		
Immunosuppressive Rx	X		
Smoker	X		
Cardiac-Related Factors			
Aortic stenosis	X		X [b]
LV dysfunction (LVEF)	X	X	X
NYHA IV	X	X	X
IABP	X	X	X [c]
LMS	X		X
Triple vessel disease	X		X
Current ACS			X
STEMI recurrent / on-going			X
Prior MI	X	X	
PTCA <6 hrs	X		
Mitral insufficiency	X		
Active endocarditis		X	
Pulmonary hypertension		X	
Operation Related Factors			
Urgent status	X	X	X
Other than isolated CABG		X	
Surgery on thoracic aorta		X	
Post infarct septal rupture		X	

a, Dialysis; b, Contraindications to left ventricular contrast angiography include significant aortic stenosis (valve area <1.0 cm^2); c, Critical pre-procedure state includes the anticipated need for IABP

Table 1. Comparison of Risk Factors Used to Predict 30-Day Mortality in Various Models.

Model	Patients	30 day mortality	C-Index	H-L p-value
STS Score development	503478	3.05%	0.78	.0016
Additive EuroSCORE development	13302	4.7%	0.783	<0.40
Additive EuroSCORE validation	1497	4.7%	0.76	<0.68
Logistic EuroSCORE	14799	4.7%	0.785	N/A
CANADA Score training set (development)	26350	1.5%	0.90	0.84
CANADA Score validation	6549	1.4%	0.91	0.12
NCDR CathPCI Risk Score subset	204111	2.94%	0.86	N/A

Table 2. Comparison of Cohort and Model Performance for Various Risk Calculators.

4. PCI models

Early models examining risk associated with percutaneous coronary interventions were well validated for the predication of in-hospital mortality (Moscucci et al, 2001; Qureshi et al, 2003; Resnic et al, 2001; Shaw et al, 2002; Singh et al, 2002; Wu et al, 2006). However, these models had the potential to miss adverse events due to the nature of contemporary PCI where many patients are discharged within 24 hours of admission. As patients may be suitable for revascularization by either CABG or PCI it was important to develop a tool to facilitate an appropriate comparison of outcomes between these strategies.

4.1 NCDR CathPCI risk score

Contemporary risk scores were developed from the National Cardiovascular Data Registry (NCDR) (Peterson et al, 2010). The NCDR CathPCI Registry catalogues patient characteristics, angiographic and procedural details and in-hospital outcomes. From this, various risk models to predict in-hospital mortality were derived from pre-procedural and procedural data (full model), as well as a simplified model based on pre-procedure data only. To establish 30-day mortality, the NCDR records for patients aged over 65 were linked to claims data from the national Centers for Medicare and Medicaid Services (CMS). Linked data from 204111 patients observed in-hospital mortality as 1.99% and 30 day mortality as 2.94%. The c-index for predicating 30-day mortality using the NCDR in-patient mortality model was 0.86.

5. The CANADA score

The British Columbia Cardiac Registry (BCCR) is a population based database for all invasive cardiac procedures performed in British Columbia, Canada. The registry is used for clinical, administrative and research purposes. The linkage of BCCR data with the death registry of the British Columbia (BC) Vital statistics Agency facilitates outcome research. All procedures were performed at four academic tertiary centres that collectively perform 7500 PCI annually.

All patients who had PCI performed in British Columbia (BC) from 2000 - 2005 who were BC residents were included in the study (Hamburger et al, 2009). PCI was defined as any coronary artery procedure that included balloon angioplasty, stent implantation, atherectomy, brachytherapy and thrombectomy. Second or subsequent PCI were not included for further analysis. All cause mortality data was obtained from the BC Vital Statistics Agency.

The study cohort was divided into two groups. Procedures between January 01, 2000 and December 31, 2004 formed the training set that was used to develop the multivariable predictive model for all-cause 30-day mortality. Procedures from 2005 were used to validate the model.

Variables for predicting 30-day mortality post PCI included patient demographics, co-morbidities and clinical features such as indication for procedure and disease anatomy. Variables that were significantly associated with 30-day mortality in the univariate analysis (Table 3) or that were considered to be clinically important predictors for 30-day mortality were assessed in a stepwise logistic regression analysis. Only significant predictors ($P < 0.05$) in the multiple logistic regression analysis were kept in the final predictive model (Table 4).

A total of 32 899 procedures were performed. These were divided into 26 350 in the training set and 6549 in the validation set. The overall 30-day mortality was 1.5% (n=500), with mortality in the training set 1.5% (n=406) and validation set 1.4% (n=94) respectively. Of note, overall approximately one third of deaths occurred beyond 7 days (161/500, 32.2%) with similar proportions in the training (121/406, 29.8%) and validation sets (40/94, 42.6%) (Figure 1). The discrimination of the CANADA Score was good with the c-index for the training set 0.90 (Figure 2) and 0.91 for the validation set (Figure 3). The calibration was also good (H-L p values 0.84 & 0.12 respectively) (Table 2).

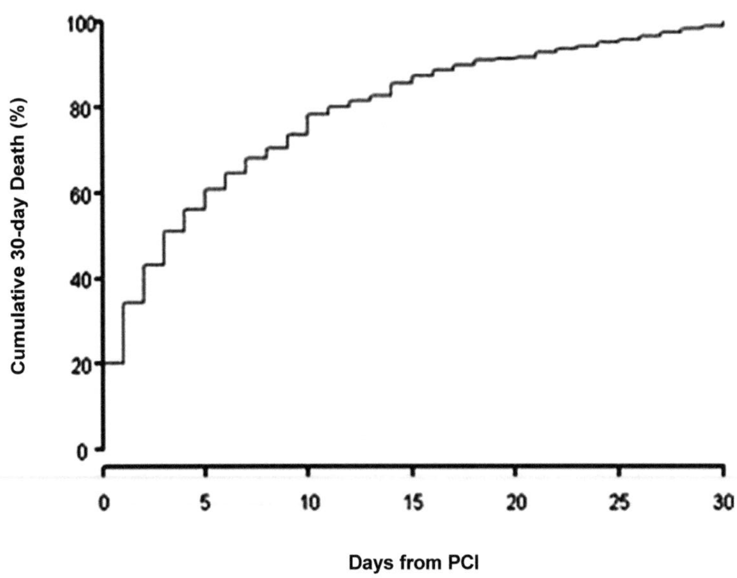

Fig. 1. Cumulative mortality versus time for all deaths in CANADA Score study population.

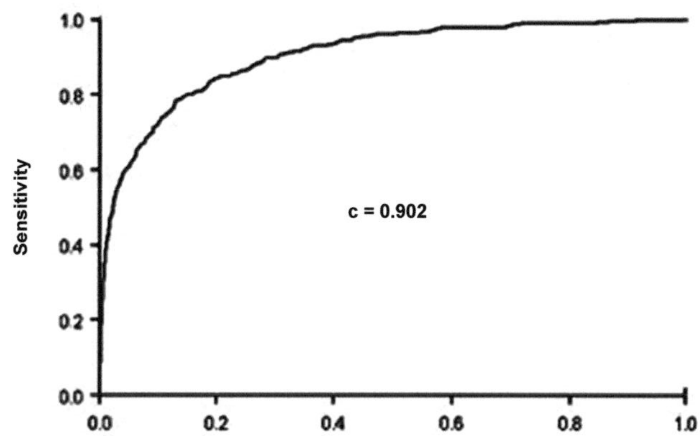

Fig. 2. Receiver operator characteristic (ROC) curve for CANADA Score training set.

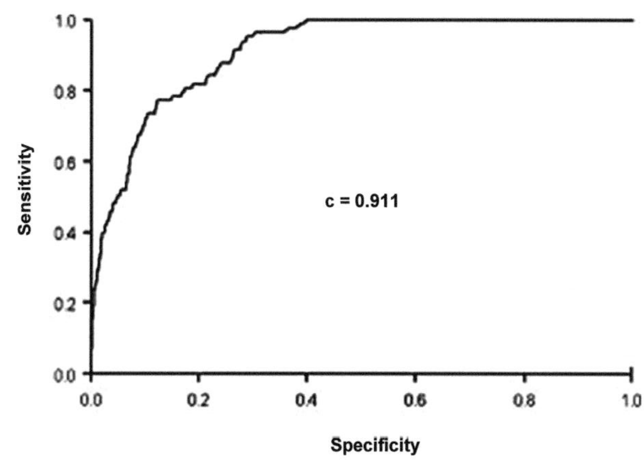

Fig. 3. Receiver operator characteristic (ROC) curve for CANADA Score validation set.

The CANADA Score was further externally validated using data sets from Alberta, Canada, and Massachusetts, United States of America.

The Alberta Provincial Project for outcome Assessment in Coronary Heart Disease (APPROACH) began 15 years ago as a cardiac catheterization and cardiac surgery database. The database includes clinical information on 126,500 patients with diagnostic cardiac catheterization and/or revascularization procedures, and 34000 hospital admissions for ACS (www.approach.org). The Canada Score model was evaluated against 9483 PCI performed from April 2005 - March 2008. The 30-day mortality was 1.8%. The c-index for this cohort was 0.88 (Kurana et al, 2010a).

The Massachusetts Department of Public Health began collecting patient specific outcome data to evaluate all cardiac surgery and coronary intervention programs in 2002. Data were submitted to the Massachusetts Data Analysis Center (Mass-DAC) with data collection for coronary interventions using the ACC-NCDR Instrument beginning in 2003 (www.massdac.org). During the period Jan 2005 - September 2007, 36 341 PCI procedures were performed. The 30-day mortality was 2.05% and c-index for the Canada Score in this cohort was 0.87 (Kurana et al, 2010b).

Category	Number of patients	Number of deaths	30-Day mortality rate (%)	Odds ratio	95% Confidence intervals	*P*
Total number of patients	26,350	406				
Age (continuous)						
Mean ± SD: 64.3 ± 11.5	26,350			1.05	1.04–1.06	<0.001
Gender						
Male	19,283	265	1.37	1.00	Ref.	
Female	7,064	141	2.00	1.46	1.19–1.80	<0.001
Urgency of procedure						
Non-urgent	7,626	219	0.18	1.00	Ref.	
Emergency	2,965	171	7.39	43.36	25.22–74.56	<0.001
Urgent	15,643	14	1.09	6.01	3.48–10.37	<0.001
Extent of coronary artery disease						
Single or two vessel disease	17,420	176	1.01	1.00	Ref.	
Triple-vessel disease	7,830	164	2.09	2.68	2.03–3.54	<0.001
Left main disease	1,100	66	6.00	7.99	5.70–11.22	<0.001
Left ventricular ejection fraction						
<30%	783	48	6.13	18.90	12.63–28.28	<0.001
30%–50%	5,488	82	1.49	4.39	3.08–6.25	<0.001
>50%	14,521	50	0.34	1.00	Ref.	
Clinically Contraindicated	3,989	197	4.94	15.04	11.00–20.55	<0.001
CCS class IV angina						
No	7,395	17	0.23	1.00	Ref.	
Yes	16,364	361	2.21	9.79	6.02–15.94	<0.001
NYHA dyspnoea ≥ 3 or congestive heart failure						
No	25,570	311	1.22	1.00	Ref.	
Yes	776	95	12.24	11.33	8.89–14.43	<0.0001
Indication for procedure						
Stable Angina	8,426	18	0.21	1.00	Ref.	
STEMI Ongoing	2,253	168	7.46	37.64	23.09–61.34	<0.001
STEMI Recurrent	1,216	23	1.89	9.01	4.85–16.74	<0.001
Other ACS	14,440	196	1.36	5.75	3.13–10.55	<0.001

Category	Number of patients	Number of deaths	30-Day mortality rate (%)	Odds ratio	95% Confidence intervals	*P*
Hemodynamically unstable prior to procedure						
No	26,168	349	1.33	1.00	Ref.	
Yes	167	56	33.53	37.33	26.62–52.35	<0.001
Cardiogenic shock						
No	26,149	322	1.23	1.00	Ref.	
Yes	186	83	44.62	64.64	47.44–88.07	<0.001
Anticipated need for IABP						
No	26,065	324	1.24	1.00	Ref.	
Yes	285	82	28.77	32.09	24.28–42.42	<0.001
Critical preprocedural state						
No	25,876	261	1.01	1.00	Ref.	
Yes	474	145	30.59	43.26	34.36–54.47	<0.001
Treated with IIb/IIIa inhibitor preprocedure						
No	25,419	376	1.48	1.00	Ref.	
Yes	931	30	3.22	2.22	1.52–3.24	<0.001
Lytic therapy preprocedure						
No	24,485	358	1.46	1.00	Ref.	
Yes	1,865	48	2.57	1.78	1.31–2.42	<0.001
Ongoing dialysis or serum creatinine >200 μmol/L						
No	25,641	361	1.41	1.00	Ref.	
Yes	604	37	6.13	4.57	3.23–6.47	<0.001
Diabetes mellitus						
No	20,324	283	1.39	1.00	Ref.	
Yes	5,924	115	1.94	1.40	1.13–1.75	0.003
Hypertension						
No	12,022	207	1.72	1.00	Ref.	
Yes	14,226	191	1.34	0.78	0.64–0.95	0.013
Hyperlipidaemia						
No	10,903	266	2.44	1.00	Ref.	
Yes	15,345	132	0.86	0.35	0.28–0.43	<0.001

Category	Number of patients	Number of deaths	30-Day mortality rate (%)	Odds ratio	95% Confidence intervals	*P*
Peripheral vascular disease						
No	24,192	350	1.45	1.00	Ref.	
Yes	2,056	48	2.33	1.63	1.20–2.21	0.002
Cerebrovascular disease						
No	24,433	343	1.40	1.00	Ref.	
Yes	1,815	55	3.03	2.20	1.64–2.93	<0.001
Cigarette smoker						
No	10,137	225	2.22	1.00	Ref.	
Yes	4,542	55	1.21	0.54	0.40–0.73	<0.001
Exsmoker > 3 months	11,569	118	1.02	0.45	0.36–0.57	<0.001
Previous myocardial infarction						
No	18,444	274	1.49	1.00	Ref.	
Yes	7,804	124	1.59	1.07	0.87–1.33	0.531
Previous PCI						
No	19,588	313	1.60	1.00	Ref.	
Yes	6,674	86	1.29	0.80	0.63–1.02	0.075
Previous CABG						
No	23,121	345	1.49	1.00	Ref.	
Yes	3,132	53	1.69	1.14	0.85–1.52	0.3901
History of chronic pulmonary disease requiring treatment						
No	24,235	348	1.44	1.00	Ref.	
Yes	2,013	50	2.48	1.75	1.30–2.36	<0.001
Potentially life-limiting hepatobiliary or gastrointestinal disease						
No	24,923	368	1.48	1.00	Ref.	
Yes	1,325	30	2.26	1.55	1.06–2.25	0.023
Diagnosis of malignancy						
No	24,757	372	1.50	1.00	Ref.	
Yes	1,491	26	1.74	1.16	0.78–1.74	0.460

Table 3. Baseline Variables in CANADA Score Univariate Analysis.

	β Coefficient	Adjusted OR	95% Confidence intervals	
Intercept	−9.89			
Age (per 10 year increase)	0.39	1.48	1.32	1.65
Gender	0.23	1.26	0.98	1.61
Emergency	0.95	2.58	1.87	3.57
Left main disease	1.09	2.98	2.06	4.29
Triple-vessel disease	0.45	1.57	1.22	2.02
LVEF < 30%	1.84	6.27	4.02	9.77
LVEF 30–50%	0.86	2.36	1.63	3.39
LVEF Clinically Contraindicated	1.55	4.71	3.33	6.66
NYHA ≥ 3/CHF	0.82	2.26	1.65	3.10
Critical preprocedural state	1.97	7.20	5.33	9.74
STEMI Ongoing	2.00	7.40	4.07	13.46
STEMI Recurrent	1.43	4.19	2.08	8.43
Other ACS	1.35	3.87	2.30	6.53
Dialysis/Creatinine > 200 μmol/L	0.76	2.13	1.40	3.23

LVEF, Left ventricular ejection fraction; NYHA, New York Heart Association; CHF, Congestive heart failure; STEMI, ST-elevation myocardial infarction; ACS, acute coronary syndrome; Critical preprocedural state, Hemodynamically unstable prior to procedure or Cardiogenic shock or Anticipated need for IABP.

Table 4. Predictors of Mortality in the CANADA Score Multivariable Model.

6. Comparison of risks – Surgical versus percutaneous revascularisation

Increasingly it has become relevant to select the optimal revascularization strategy for patients deemed appropriate for revascularisation by either coronary artery bypass grafting or percutaneous intervention. Published studies of coronary anatomy alone have shown to predict the need for future revascularisation (Serruys et al, 2009; Sianos et al, 2005), but not mortality. The scores derived from an anatomical assessment alone has been shown to have only modest correlation to predicted risk using either surgical (logistic EuroSCORE) or percutaneous (CANADA Score) risk calculators that incorporate clinical and anatomical factors (Hoole & Hamburger, 2011). The same study found comparative risk assessment using either logistic EuroSCORE or CANADA Score has good correlation (R=0.80) and importantly recognised that patients with high predicted risk for surgery may have higher risk for a percutaneous revascularisation strategy (Figure 4). This implies patients declined for surgery should not necessarily default to a PCI treatment strategy. It must be noted that the definition of risk factors in different models may vary and must be considered when applying multiple models to individual patients (Table 5).

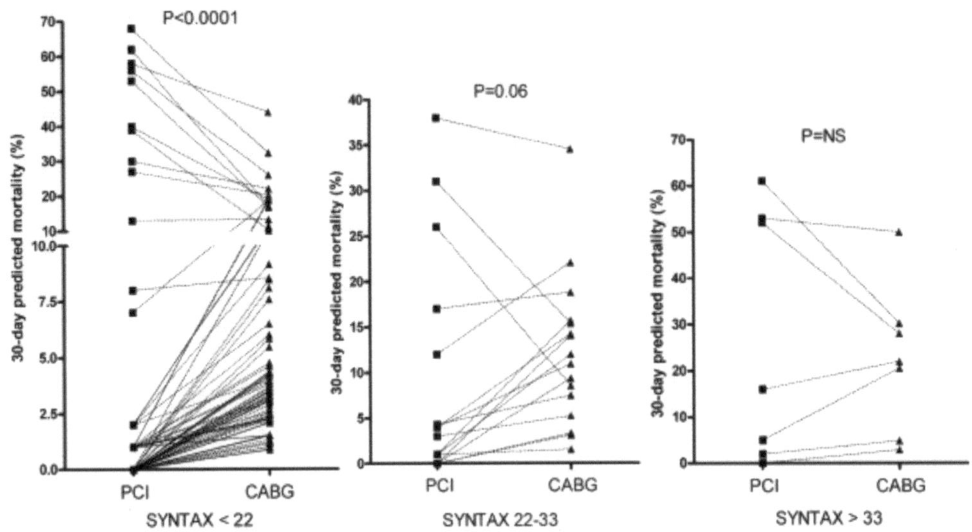

Fig. 4. Comparison of predicted PCI (CANADA Score) and CABG (EuroSCORE) mortality relative to tertiles of subject's anatomical risk (SYNTAX Score).

Risk Factor	EuroSCORE	STS Score	CANADA Score
Age	Per 5 years or part thereof over 60 years	Per 5 years or part thereof over 60 years	Per 10 year increase
Sex	Female	Female	Female
Chronic pulmonary disease	Long-term use of bronchodilators or steroids for lung disease	Patient required pharmacologic therapy for the treatment of chronic pulmonary compromise, or patient has a FEV1 <75% of predicted value	
Extracardiac arteriopathy	Any one or more of the following: claudication, carotid occlusion or >50% stenosis, previous or planned intervention on the abdominal aorta, limb arteries or carotids	Patient has peripheral vascular disease as indicated by claudication either with exertion or rest; amputation for arterial insufficiency; aorto-iliac occlusive disease reconstruction; peripheral vascular bypass surgery, angioplasty or stent; documented AAA, AAA repair, or stent; positive non-invasive testing documented – or –	

Risk Factor	EuroSCORE	STS Score	CANADA Score
		Patient has cerebrovascular disease, documented by any one of the following: Unresponsive coma >24 h; CVA (symptoms >72 h after onset); RIND (recovery within 72 h); TIA (recovery within 24 h); or noninvasive carotid test with >75% occlusion	
Neurological dysfunction disease	Severely affecting ambulation or day to day functioning	A central neurologic deficit persisting more than 24 h	
Previous cardiac surgery	Requiring opening of the pericardium	Prior cardiac surgical operation(s) with or without the use of cardiopulmonary bypass	
Serum creatinine / renal insufficiency	> 200 mmol/l preoperatively	> 200 mmol/l preoperatively	> 200 umol/l or dialysis
Active endocarditis	Patient still under antibiotic treatment for endocarditis at the time of surgery	Patient currently under antibiotic treatment for endocarditis at the time of surgery	
Critical preoperative state	Any one of more of the following: ventricular tachycardia or fibrillation or aborted sudden death, preoperative cardiac massage, preoperative ventilation before arrival in the anaesthetic room, preoperative inotropic support, intra-aortic balloon counterpulsation or preoperative acute renal	Any one or more of the following: sustained ventricular tachycardia or ventricular fibrillation requiring cardioversion and/or IV amiodarone, preoperative inotropic support, preoperative intra-aortic balloon pump, or patient required cardiopulmonary resuscitation within 1 h before the start of the operative procedure	Cardiogenic shock (a systolic blood pressure of <90 mmHg for at least 30 min and/or the need for supportive measures to maintain a systolic blood pressure of >90 mmHg, clinical evidence of end-organ hypoperfusion) or hemodynamic

Risk Factor	EuroSCORE	STS Score	CANADA Score
	failure (anuria or oliguria <10 ml/ h)		instability prior to the procedure (transient hypotension not fulfilling the definition for cardiogenic shock, or caused by sustained arrhythmia) or the anticipated need for an intra-aortic balloon pump.
Unstable angina	Rest angina requiring iv nitrates until arrival in the anaesthetic room	Preoperative use of iv nitrates	STEMI on-going, STEMI recurrent or other ACS
LV dysfunction	Moderate or LVEF 30–50%; Poor or LVEF ,30%	LVEF 30–50%; LVEF <30%	LVEF 30–50%; LVEF <30% or LVEF contraindicated*
Recent myocardial infarction	< 90 days	< 21 days	
Pulmonary hypertension	Systolic PA pressure >60 mmHg	Systolic PA pressure >30 mmHg	
Emergency	Carried out on referral before the beginning of the next working day	Procedure status is emergent or salvage. *Emergent:* The patient's clinical status includes any of the following. a. Ischaemic dysfunction (any of the following): (1) ongoing ischaemia including rest angina despite maximal medical therapy (medical and/or IABP); (2) acute evolving myocardial infarction within 24 h before surgery; or (3) pulmonary oedema requiring intubation. b. Mechanical dysfunction	Procedure has to be done without delay

Risk Factor	EuroSCORE	STS Score	CANADA Score
		(either of the following): (1) shock with circulatory support; or (2) shock without circulatory support. *Salvage: The patient is undergoing CPR en route to the OR or prior to anaesthesia induction*	
Other than isolated CABG	Major cardiac procedure other than or in addition to CABG	Any valve procedure in addition to or separate from CABG	
Surgery on thoracic aorta	For disorder of ascending, arch or descending aorta	Aortic aneurysm/dissection repair	
Post-infarct septal rupture		Ventricular septal defect	
3 vessel disease			Greater than 50% lesion in any three vessels
Left main disease		>= 50% compromise of vessel diameter preoperatively	Greater than 50% lesion
NYHA			≥ 3

*LVEF contraindicated = comorbid conditions preclude left ventricular contrast angiography (significant aortic stenosis (valve area <1.0 cm^2), presence of aortic valve prosthesis, impaired renal function (serum creatinine >200umol/L), a critical preprocedural clinical state, NYHA IV dyspnoea, grossly elevated left ventricular end diastolic pressure (>30 mmHg).

Table 5. Definition of Risk Factors for Various Risk Calculators.

7. Conclusion

Predicting procedural risk enables the correct treatment decisions to be made and allows valid informed consent and accurate patient counselling. This is particularly important as PCI has become accepted as a viable alternative to established surgical intervention. Early assessment of risk with PCI was limited to short term events that ignored important late events and prevented direct comparison with surgical risk predication tools. The CANADA Score was developed to accurately predict 30 day mortality risk and has been externally validated in large North American cohorts demonstrating broad applicability to varied patient groups. The CANADA Score confirms that both anatomical and clinical data are required to provide accurate and discriminatory 30 day mortality risk prediction and it therefore allows comparison with well validated surgical risk prediction models to guide optimal revascularisation strategy. Application of the CANADA Score to patients with high surgical risk demonstrates the potential for equal or greater risk with a percutaneous strategy and challenges the traditional notion that percutaneous revascularization should be a default strategy for these patients. The CANADA Score is available as an on-line calculator (www.canadascore.org) (Figure 5) facilitating easy integration into regular clinical practice.

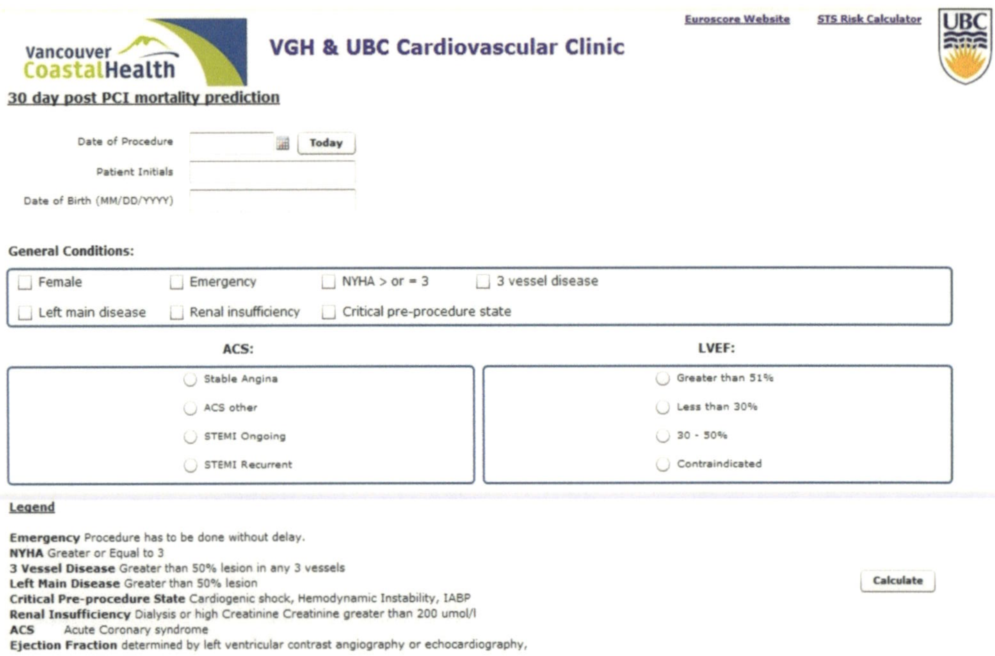

Fig. 5. On-line CANADA Score Calculator. Available at www.canadascore.org

8. References

Altman DG, Royston P. What do we mean by validating a prognostic model? *Stat Med.* 2000;19(4):453-473.

Cook NR. Statistical evaluation of prognostic versus diagnostic models: beyond the ROC curve. *Clin Chem.* 2008;54(1):17-23.

Granton J, Cheng D. Risk stratification models for cardiac surgery. *Semin Cardiothorac Vasc Anesth.* 2008;12(3):167-174.

Hamburger JN, Walsh SJ, Khurana R, Ding L, Gao M, Humphries KH, Carere R, Fung AY, Mildenberger RR, Simkus GJ, Webb JG, Buller CE. Percutaneous coronary intervention and 30-day mortality: the British Columbia PCI risk score. *Catheter Cardiovasc Interv.* 2009;74(3):377-385.

Hoole SP, Hamburger JN. Comparing procedural risks to select the optimal revascularization strategy: certainty in an uncertain anatomical world. *Catheter Cardiovasc Interv.*77(2):313-314.

Hosmer DW, Lemeshow S. *Applied logistic regression.* 2nd ed. New York: Wiley; 2000.

Janes H, Pepe MS, Gu W. Assessing the value of risk predictions by using risk stratification tables. *Ann Intern Med.* 2008;149(10):751-760.

Khurana R NS, Silbaugh T, Humphries KH, Gao M, Ding L, Lovett A, Cohen D, Hamburger JN. INDEPENDENT US VALIDATION OF THE BRITISH COLUMBIA PCI RISK

SCORE. *Journal of the American College of Cardiology.* 2010;55(10, Supplement 1):A134.E1261.

Khurana R NS, Silbuagh T, Humphries K, Gao M, Ding L, Lovett A, Galbraith D, Cohen DJ, Hamburger J. The Canada score: independent US and Canadian validation of the British Columbia PCI risk score. *European Heart Journal.* 2010;31((suppl 1)):19.

Michel P, Roques F, Nashef SA. Logistic or additive EuroSCORE for high-risk patients? *Eur J Cardiothorac Surg.* 2003;23(5):684-687; discussion 687.

Moscucci M, Kline-Rogers E, Share D, O'Donnell M, Maxwell-Eward A, Meengs WL, Kraft P, DeFranco AC, Chambers JL, Patel K, McGinnity JG, Eagle KA. Simple bedside additive tool for prediction of in-hospital mortality after percutaneous coronary interventions. *Circulation.* 2001;104(3):263-268.

Nashef SA, Roques F, Hammill BG, Peterson ED, Michel P, Grover FL, Wyse RK, Ferguson TB. Validation of European System for Cardiac Operative Risk Evaluation (EuroSCORE) in North American cardiac surgery. *Eur J Cardiothorac Surg.* 2002;22(1):101-105.

Nashef SA, Roques F, Michel P, Gauducheau E, Lemeshow S, Salamon R. European system for cardiac operative risk evaluation (EuroSCORE). *Eur J Cardiothorac Surg.* 1999;16(1):9-13.

Nathanson BH, Higgins TL. An introduction to statistical methods used in binary outcome modeling. *Semin Cardiothorac Vasc Anesth.* 2008;12(3):153-166.

Peterson ED, Dai D, DeLong ER, Brennan JM, Singh M, Rao SV, Shaw RE, Roe MT, Ho KK, Klein LW, Krone RJ, Weintraub WS, Brindis RG, Rumsfeld JS, Spertus JA. Contemporary mortality risk prediction for percutaneous coronary intervention: results from 588,398 procedures in the National Cardiovascular Data Registry. *J Am Coll Cardiol.*55(18):1923-1932.

Qureshi MA, Safian RD, Grines CL, Goldstein JA, Westveer DC, Glazier S, Balasubramanian M, O'Neill WW. Simplified scoring system for predicting mortality after percutaneous coronary intervention. *J Am Coll Cardiol.* 2003;42(11):1890-1895.

Resnic FS, Ohno-Machado L, Selwyn A, Simon DI, Popma JJ. Simplified risk score models accurately predict the risk of major in-hospital complications following percutaneous coronary intervention. *Am J Cardiol.* 2001;88(1):5-9.

Roques F, Michel P, Goldstone AR, Nashef SA. The logistic EuroSCORE. *Eur Heart J.* 2003;24(9):881-882.

Sergeant P, de Worm E, Meyns B. Single centre, single domain validation of the EuroSCORE on a consecutive sample of primary and repeat CABG. *Eur J Cardiothorac Surg.* 2001;20(6):1176-1182.

Serruys PW, Morice MC, Kappetein AP, Colombo A, Holmes DR, Mack MJ, Stahle E, Feldman TE, van den Brand M, Bass EJ, Van Dyck N, Leadley K, Dawkins KD, Mohr FW. Percutaneous coronary intervention versus coronary-artery bypass grafting for severe coronary artery disease. *N Engl J Med.* 2009;360(10):961-972.

Shaw RE, Anderson HV, Brindis RG, Krone RJ, Klein LW, McKay CR, Block PC, Shaw LJ, Hewitt K, Weintraub WS. Development of a risk adjustment mortality model using the American College of Cardiology-National Cardiovascular Data Registry (ACC-NCDR) experience: 1998-2000. *J Am Coll Cardiol.* 2002;39(7):1104-1112.

Shroyer AL, Coombs LP, Peterson ED, Eiken MC, DeLong ER, Chen A, Ferguson TB, Jr., Grover FL, Edwards FH. The Society of Thoracic Surgeons: 30-day operative mortality and morbidity risk models. *Ann Thorac Surg.* 2003;75(6):1856-1864; discussion 1864-1855.

Sianos G, Morel MA, Kappetein AP, Morice MC, Colombo A, Dawkins K, van den Brand M, Van Dyck N, Russell ME, Mohr FW, Serruys PW. The SYNTAX Score: an angiographic tool grading the complexity of coronary artery disease. *EuroIntervention.* 2005;1(2):219-227.

Singh M, Lennon RJ, Holmes DR, Jr., Bell MR, Rihal CS. Correlates of procedural complications and a simple integer risk score for percutaneous coronary intervention. *J Am Coll Cardiol.* 2002;40(3):387-393.

Vickers AJ, Cronin AM. Everything you always wanted to know about evaluating prediction models (but were too afraid to ask). *Urology.*76(6):1298-1301.

Wu C, Hannan EL, Walford G, Ambrose JA, Holmes DR, Jr., King SB, 3rd, Clark LT, Katz S, Sharma S, Jones RH. A risk score to predict in-hospital mortality for percutaneous coronary interventions. *J Am Coll Cardiol.* 2006;47(3):654-660.

3

Complications of Coronary Intervention

Seung-Jin Lee
Soonchunhyang University Cheonan Hospital
South Korea

1. Introduction

Drug-eluting stents (DES) substantially reduce restenosis compared with bare metal stents and represent a significant advance in percutaneous coronary interventions (PCIs). Accordingly, DES have been rapidly adopted into practice and are currently used in the vast majority of PCI procedures. As PCIs for more complicated lesions increase, various complications, such as stent thrombosis, fracture, dissection or perforation, are also increase. For example, PCIs for patients who have chronic total occlusion increase and these patients tend to have more risk factors like diabetes mellitus, hypertension, dyslipidemia, and previous myocardial infarction and also have multi-vessel diseases and have decreased left ventricular ejection fraction. If major procedure-related complications were developed in these high risk patients, it may leads to fatal results. So it is important to understand possible complications of PCIs and eliminate potential risk factors before procedures.

1.1 Stent fracture

Drug-eluting stents (DES) have proven very effective in reducing restenosis by suppressing neointimal hyperplasia. However, potentially serious complications such as in-stent restenosis and thrombus still occur. Stent fracture has been identified as a possible contributor to these adverse outcomes. A number of risk factors for the development of stent fracture have been described, although a detailed analysis of the angiographic factors predisposing to stent fracture is lacking.

1.2 Incidence and definition

Stent fracture is defined as the cases where the linear or curvilinear connections of stent struts are interrupted and areas of the stented segment are uncovered by stent struts visible on coronary angiography. The incidence of stent fracture is reported in 0.8-7.7% of cases.[1-8] However, because of limited sensitivity of angiography to detect fracture, its true incidence is still unknown. In a recent report analyzed from autopsy findings, stent fracture was observed in 29% of total patients.[9] So, the real incidence of stent fracture is assumed to be a little higher than what has been clinically reported. Stent fracture from patients treated with Cypher stents is more frequently observed than in cases of Taxus stents. The incidence of stent fracture of Cypher stent was 1.3% in the SIRIUS trial,[9] compared to 0.58% incidence with the Taxus stent is in the Taxus IV/V/VI trials. Stent fracture has previously been recognized in noncoronary vessels, especially in the superficial femoral and popliteal arteries and with bare-metal stents in saphenous vein grafts.[10,11] Because old classifications of stent fracture are originated from in cases of femoropopliteal arteries, Popma *et al.* suggested a more detailed new classification specially designed for coronary arteries (Figure 1, Table 1).[12]

1.3 Predictors and possible mechanisms

Stent fractures in the bare-metal stent era might be overlooked and masked due to the diffuse tissue overgrowth within the stented segment. Because drug-eluting stents can suppress neointimal hyperplasia more effectively thereby stent fracture may now be more obvious in the very localized lesions bordered by segments with no evidence of neointima.[13] As already mentioned, among DESs, Cypher stents showed more frequent stent fractures compared to Taxus stents. The inter-strut angles of the Cypher stent which has a closed-cell design, were significantly smaller than Taxus stent which has an open-cell design.[14] The different stent strut design should be considered as a key mechanism of Cypher stent fracture. To maintain smaller inter-strut angles and a more regular strut distribution, there must be higher shear forces on the struts of Cypher stent. Therefore the closed-cell designed Cypher stent may be more prone to fracture when shear forces are beyond its flexibility. It seems that stent fractures are rare in newer generation stents such as Xience V or Eendeavor stents. Stent fractures most frequently occur in the right coronary artery followed by the left anterior descending artery and finally the left circumflex artery. The predisposition of the right coronary artery for stent fracture is possibly attributed to the vessel anatomy, due to the excessive tortuosity, angulation, or change of angulation after stent implantation. Vessel movement throughout the cardiac cycle creates flexion, stretching, and torsion forces, creating hinge points and can lead to mechanical fatigue and fracture.[2] Procedure related contributing factors are longer and more angulated lesions, lesions that are ostial in location with more proximal tortuosity, calcification, total occlusion, stent overlap, stenting in saphenous vein grafts, and overstretching of the stents with high pressure.[12]

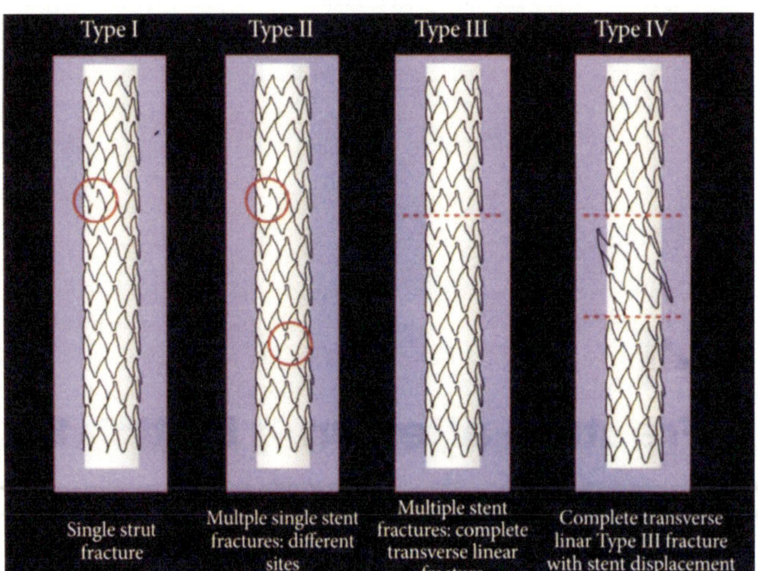

Fig. 1. Definitions used for stent fracture

Classification	Current report	Allie et el	Scheinert et al
Type 0	No strut fracture	-	-
Type I	Single strut fracture or gap between struts greater than 2 times expanded cell diameter	Single strut fracture only	Minor-single strut fracture
Type II	Multiple strut fracture with V-form division of the stent	Multiple single stent fractures occurring at different sites	Moderate-fracture >1 strut
Type III	Complete transverse stent fracture without displacement of fractured fragments more than 1 mm during the cardiac cycle	Multiple single stent fractures resulting in complete transverse linear fracture but without stent displacement	Severe-complete separation of stent segments
Type IV	Complete transverse stent fracture with abundant movement and displacement of fractured fragments of more than 1 mm during the cardiac cycle	Complete transverse linear type III fracture with stent displacement	-

Table 1. Definitions used for stent fracture[12]

1.4 Clinical implications

The complications observed with DES fracture include in-stent restenosis, target lesion revascularization, stent thrombosis, myocardial infarction, stent-related aneurysm, and sudden death. Lee et al. observed binary restenosis in six out of 10 patients (60%) with stent fracture and one patient had stent thrombosis.[5] Local mechanical irritation of the vessel can occur from fractured stent struts, which may result in inflammation and neointimal hyperplasia. Restenosis could also reflect decreased local drug availability secondary to distortion of the stent architecture and polymer coating.[13] Exposure of a free metal strut protruding into the vessel lumen could trigger platelet activation and resultant stent thrombosis. Acute myocardial infarction and sudden death can develop from fracture-related stent thrombosis.

1.5 Diagnosis and treatment

Usually stent fracture can be diagnosed by conventional fluoroscopy or follow-up coronary angiography. If the diagnosis is obscure, Intravascular Ultrasound (IVUS), Multi-Detector Computed Tomography (MDCT), or Optical Coherence Tomography (OCT) can be helpful. Because recently developed stents tend to have thinner struts and less radiopacity, the diagnosis of stent fracture tends to difficult. Unfortunately, there is no consensus of the treatment of stent fracture. It depends on whether or not there is restenosis and its related symptoms.

2. No-reflow phenomenon

The phenomenon of no-reflow is defined as inadequate myocardial perfusion through a given segment of the coronary circulation without angiographic evidence of mechanical vessel obstruction.[15] The underlying cause of no-reflow is microvascular obstruction, which may be produced by various mechanisms. The concept of no-reflow was first described in experimental models in 1966[16] and then in the clinical setting of reperfusion after myocardial infarction in 1985.[17] No-reflow has been documented in ≥30% of patients after thrombolysis[18] or mechanical intervention for acute myocardial infarction. The prevalence is variable, ranging from 5% up to 50%, according to the methods used to assess the phenomenon and to the population under study.

A series of consistent data has clearly shown that no-reflow has a strong negative impact on outcome, negating the potential benefit of primary percutaneous coronary intervention (PCI).[19,20] Indeed, patients with no-reflow exhibit a higher prevalence of: 1) early post-infarction complications (arrhythmias, pericardial effusion, cardiac tamponade, early congestive heart failure); 2) left adverse ventricular remodeling; 3) late repeat hospital stays for heart failure; and 4) mortality.

Therefore, it is important to prevent and effectively treat the no-reflow phenomenon during PCI to achieve an optimal outcome.

2.1 Historical overview

The term no-reflow was first used by Majno and colleagues[21] in the setting of vertebral ischemia in 1967. This phenomenon was initially described by Krug *et al.*[16] during induced myocardial infarction in the canine model in 1966 and again by Kloner *et al.*[15] in 1974 in which it occurred for 90 min after temporary epicardial coronary artery occlusion followed by reperfusion. Electron microscopic examination showed severe myocardial capillary damage with loss of pinocytonic vesicles in the endothelial cells, endothelial blisters or blebs and endothelial gaps with neutrophil infiltration. Intraluminal capillary plugging by neutrophils and/or microthrombi with myocardial cell swelling was also noted. Galiuto *et al.*[22] with sequential measurements of myocardial perfusion by myocardial contrast echocardiography, have recently shown that in humans no-refow detected 24 h after successful PCI spontaneously improves over time in approximately 50% of patients. Thus, no-reflow can be categorized as sustained or reversible. Sustained no-reflow is probably the result of anatomical irreversible changes of the coronary microcirculation, whereas reversible no-reflow is the result of functional and thus, reversible, changes of the microcirculation.

In humans, no-reflow is caused by the variable combination of 4 pathogenetic components: 1) distal atherothrombotic embolization; 2) ischemic injury; 3) reperfusion injury; and 4) susceptibility of the coronary microcirculation to injury.

1. Distal embolization

Emboli of different sizes can originate from epicardial coronary thrombus and from fissured atherosclerotic plaques, in particular during primary PCI.[23] Large emboli (>200μm diameter) can obstruct pre-arterioles, causing infarctlets. Experimental observations have shown that myocardial blood flow decreases irreversibly when microspheres obstruct more than 50% of coronary capillaries.[24]

2. Ischemia-related injury

Changes in endothelial cells, visible after prolonged ischemia, are represented by endothelial protrusions and membrane-bound bodies, which often fill the capillaries up to luminal obliteration. Furthermore, large endothelial gaps with extravascular erythrocytes are common.[25]

3. Reperfusion-related injury

A massive infiltration of the coronary microcirculation by neutrophils and platelets occurs at the time of reperfusion.[25,26] Reintroduction of neutrophils in post-ischemic myocardium results in their activation, with subsequent adhesion to the endothelial surface and migration in the surrounding tissue. Activated neutrophils, in turn, release oxygen free radicals, proteolytic enzymes, and pro-inflammatory mediators that can directly cause tissue and endothelial damage. Neutrophils also form aggregates with platelets that plug capillaries, thus mechanically blocking flow.[27,28] Finally, vasoconstrictors released by damaged endothelial cells, neutrophils, and platelets contribute to sustained vasoconstriction of the coronary microcirculation.[29] Tumor necrosis factor-alpha expression is induced by reperfusion, and can impair endothelium-dependent coronary flow reserve.[30] Interleukin-1β also has recently been associated with ischemia-reperfusion injury, because interleukin-1β knockout animals exhibit marked reduction of ischemic induced inflammation.[31] Selectin expression on cell surfaces is also important for mechanical plugging of the microcirculation.[32] Finally, the balance between nitric oxide and superoxide is tipped in favor of superoxide within minutes of reperfusion of ischemic tissues, due to increased production of xanthine oxidase by neutrophils, endothelial cells, and cardiac myocytes, which leads to an exacerbation of the inflammatory state.[33]

Reperfusion might also cause irreversible injury to myocytes.[34] During ischemia there is an increase of the intracellular sodium (Na^+) content due to accumulation of hydrogen (H^+), which is exchanged by the Na^+/H^+ exchanger. The subsequent exchange of doubly charged positive calcium ion (Ca^{++}) with Na^+ by the sarcolemmal Na^+/Ca^{++} exchanger produces a calcium overload that triggers uncontrolled hypercontraction and stimulates opening of the mitochondrial permeability transition pore (m0PTP), which further enhances calcium overload. Furthermore, Na^+ extrusion trough Na^+/potassium (K^+) adenosine triphosphate (ATP)-ase is impaired and together with Ca^{++} accumulation leads to myocyte cell swelling, which contributes to subsequent rupture of the cell membrane when the extracellular osmolality is rapidly normalized by reperfusion. Of note, cyclosporine, which blocks the m-PTP, has been recently shown to reduce infarct size by 20% when administered intravenously in patients undergoing primary PCI.[35] Finally, ischemic pre-conditioning might also reduce infarct size by blockade of m-PTP.[36]

Natriuretic peptides might modulate ischemia-reperfusion injury. Atrial natriuretic peptide might suppress the rennin-angiotensin-aldosterone system and endothelin (ET)-1 that increase infarct size, microvascular obstruction, and cardiac remodeling.[37]

4. Individual predisposition of coronary microcirculation to injury

In humans, no-reflow is occasionally observed during elective procedures,[38] whereas it can be absent after primary PCI in patients with acute myocardial infarction. In particular, diabetes and hypercholesterolemia has been associated with impaired microvascular reperfusion by enhancing endothelial oxidative stress.[39,40] Pre-conditioning by using nicorandil seems to have a beneficial effect on microvascular function.[41]

2.2 Diagnosis

1. Coronary angiography

Reduced coronary flow after primary PCI (TIMI flow 0 to 2) is associated with worse outcome than normal (TIMI 3) flow, even when no significant epicardial obstruction remains.[42] More sensitive markers of tissue perfusion have now been identified and provide prognostic information beyond that of TIMI flow grade. The TIMI frame count assesses the number of angiographic frames required for the contrast medium to reach standardized distal landmarks of the coronary tree, and the myocardial blush grade (MBG) is a quantitative assessment of myocardial contrast density. The MBG is scored on a scale of 0 to 3, with higher scores indicating better perfusion. An MBG 0 to 1, suggestive of no-reflow, is observed in as high as 50% of patients with TIMI flow grade 3.[43] Taken together, angiographic no-reflow can be defined as a TIMI flow grade <3 or 3 with an MBG 0 to 1.

2. Electrocardiography

Rapid ST-segment resolution defined as a reduction of ≥50% in the ST-segment elevation index is highly specific (91%) for myocardial reperfusion (or the absence of no-reflow on myocardial contrast echocardiography) although less sensitive (77%).[44]

3. Myocardial contrast echocardiography (MCE)

Lack of intramyocardial contrast opacification is due to microvascular obstruction; thus, it represents the extent of no-reflow.[45] In the AMICI study, the extent of no-reflow at MCE was demonstrated to be the best predictor of adverse left ventricular remodeling after acute myocardial infarction, being superior to ST-segment resolution and to MBG among patients exhibiting TIMI flow grade 3.[20]

4. Cardiac magnetic resonance imaging

No-reflow can be diagnosed as: 1) lack of gadolinium enhancement during first pass; and 2) lack of gadolinium enhancement within a necrotic region, identified by late gadolinium hyperenhancement.[46]

2.3 Prevention and treatment (Figure 2)

1. Distal embolization

No specific technique is currently recommended in guidelines to prevent distal embolization during primary PCI. Direct stent implantation, by avoiding balloon-induced thrombus fragmentation and by entrapping the atherothrombus under the stent struts, has been suggested as a possible technique to reduce distal embolization in a specific subset of patients i.e. those with good distal visualization of the infarct-related artery after guidewire passage.[47]

A more promising technique is the use of thrombectomy and distal filter devices. Although distal filter devices did not improve early or late prognosis compared with standard primary PCI, thrombectomy performed with a simple manual aspiration catheter revealed improved myocardial reperfusion and significantly reduced no-reflow.[48] A recent large trial by Svilaas *et al.*[49] confirmed the improvement of reperfusion associated with manual thrombus-aspiration as compared with standard primary PCI showing a strikingly lower mortality at 12-month follow-up.[50] So, it is suggested that manual thrombus aspiration should be used in the setting of primary PCI, particularly in patients with a high thrombus burden.[51]

2. Ischemia-related injury

Strategies aimed at reducing pain onset-to-balloon time might reduce no-reflow by decreasing total ischemic time. Drugs known to reduce myocardial oxygen consumption and consequently the severity of ischemia and improve myocardial perfusion include carvedilol, fosinopril, and valsartan.[52,53]

3. Reperfusion-related injury

Intracoronary nitroglycerin is usually suggested as the first-line agent, mainly to reverse epicardial vessel spasm, even if the blood pressure is reduced. Theoretically, nitroglycerin should have little impact on arteriolar tone and hence on no-reflow since physiologically it produces little effect in the microvasculature.

Patients at high risk of no-reflow can be treated with drugs such as glycoprotein IIb/IIIa antagonists, adenosine, nicorandil, and nitroprusside aimed at counteracting endothelial, platelet, and neutrophil activation.

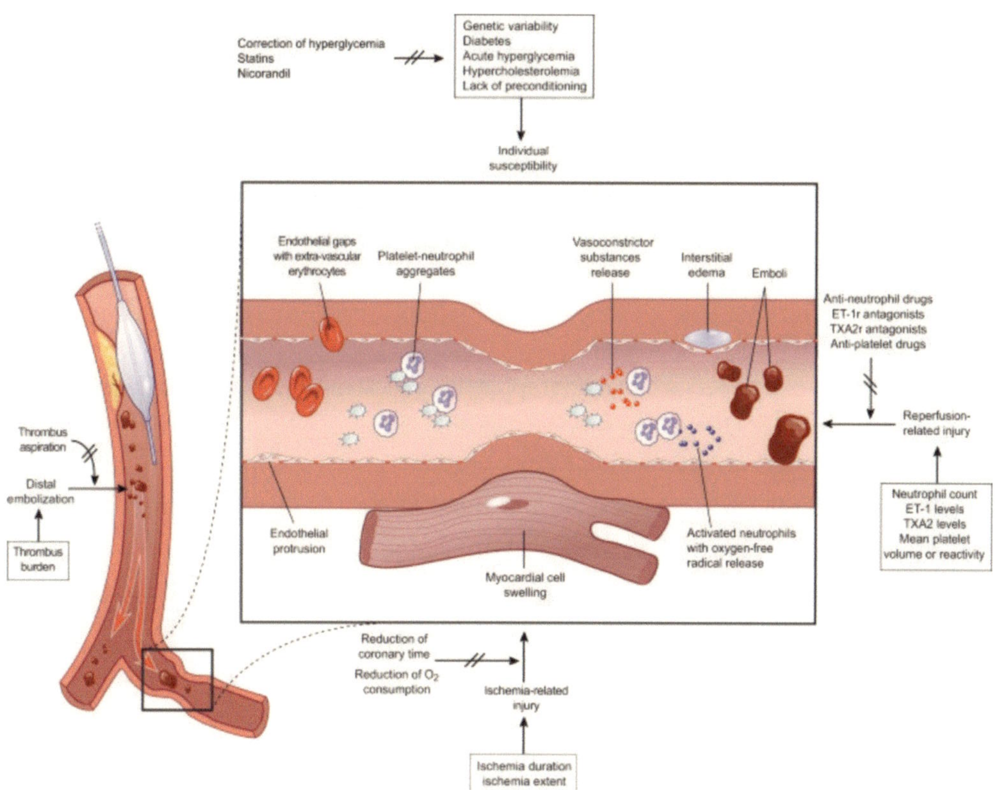

Fig. 2. Therapies of no-reflow targeted to main pathogenetic mechanisms

Among glycoprotein IIb/IIIa antagonists, abciximab has been found to improve myocardial perfusion when started during primary PCI and infused for 12 h thereafter. Interestingly, intracoronary abciximab has been proven to be superior to intravenous abciximab in patients treated by primary PCI.[54] Adenosine is an endogenous purine nucleoside that decreases arteriolar resistance and activates intracellular cardioprotective signaling pathways. Its mechanism of action may involve opening ATP-sensitive potassium channels (K_{ATP}), inhibition of neutrophil migration, prevention of superoxide generation, or blockade of coronary endothelin release. Nitroprusside is a nitric oxide donor that does not depend on intracellular metabolism to derive nitric oxide, with potent vasodilator properties. Nicorandil is a hybrid of a K_{ATP} opener and nitrate and may prevent reperfusion injury by blocking the mitochondrial permeability transition pore. Verapamil is a calcium-channel blocker that has several beneficial effects in the setting of no-reflow in addition to attenuation of microvascular spasm. Varapamil may also inhibit platelet aggregation and thrombus formation in the microvasculature and may have a direct effect on calcium flux across the sarcolemmal membrane or within intracellular compartment that could protect reversibly injuried myocytes.

3. Coronary artery perforation and cardiac tamponade

Coronary artery perforation complicating percutaneous coronary intervention (PCI) occurs in 0.1-3.0% of cases. Perforation with balloon angioplasty or stenting is rare, occurring in 0.1% of cases. However, when ablation devices, such as rotablator, directional coronary atherectomy, transluminal extraction catheter, and excimer laser, are used, the frequency is substantially higher than with balloon angioplasty or stents, occurring up to 3.0%.[55] Recently, the use of ablation devices in PCI has tended to decline. Instead, procedures for more complex lesions including calcification, severe angulation, and chronic total occlusion have increased. To treat these complex lesions, stiffer and hydrophilic wires are necessary and high pressure for balloon dilatation is needed. Increasing numbers of procedures using glycoprotein IIb/IIIa inhibitors is also contributing to the fact that coronary artery perforation still occurs.

3.1 Classification

The Ellis classification depends on angiographic findings is most widely used (table 2).[55]

Type I	Extraluminal crater without extravasation
Type II	Pericardial or myocardial blush without contrast jet extravasation
Type III	Extravasation through frank (>1 mm) perforation
Cavity	Perforation into an anatomic cavity chamber, spilling coronary sinus, etc

Table 2. Perforation Classification

3.2 Risk factors

Many factors are involved in coronary perforation during PCI. Related risk factors can be divided into patient-related, vessel-related, and procedure-related factors.[56] Patients-related factors are old age, hypertension, PCI for unstable angina or non-ST segment elevation myocardial infarction.[57] Vessel-related factors are ACC/AHA type C lesions, calcified lesions, and chronic total occlusion lesions.[3] Procedure-related factors include use of stiff hydrophilic wires, device oversizing, use of atheroablative devices. One observational study reports that 87% of perforation due to guidewires is attributed to hydrophilic wires.[58] In case of rotational atherectomy use, if lesions are eccentric, lesion length are >10cm, or lesions are very tortuous, the risk of perforation is high.

3.3 Symptoms and signs

If coronary perforation is develop, usually patients feel severe chest pain. In addition, nausea, dizziness, and vomiting can occur. The heart rate can rise suddenly, blood pressure can drop and if cardiac tamponade happens, an increase of central venous pressure with neck vein engorgement develops. Sustained ST-segment elevation or depression can be observed even though coronary balloons are deflated.

3.4 Diagnosis

The diagnosis of coronary artery perforation is not difficult by coronary angiography. If cardiac tamponade is suspected, then echocardiography is very useful. Sometimes perforation can occur 12-48 h later after PCI, if vital signs become unstable and serum hemoglobin and hematocrit levels decrease, cardiac tamponade must be suspected and urgent echocardiography should be performed.

3.5 Clinical outcomes and prognosis

Complications related to coronary artery perforation are diverse and depend on the degree of perforation. It has been reported that in cases of perforation, myocardial infarction can occurs in 13-34%, emergency coronary artery bypass graft in 11-39%, cardiac tamponade in 12-31%, and mortality in 7.6-19%.[59-61] The degree of perforation is a important marker to predict the late prognosis. Ellis classification type I perforation has a clinically good prognosis in 60% and it is rare that type II perforation has a poor prognosis. However, type III perforation reveals high major adverse events rate.[55,62]

3.6 Treatment

Generally, guidewire-related perforation does not cause grave results except with concomitant use of glycoprotein IIb/IIIa inhibitors. However, perforation due to balloon, atherectomy devices, or laser can produce hemopericardium or hemodynamic collapse.

1. Prolonged balloon inflation

The most important thing to stop bleeding is prolonged balloon inflation at the perforation site at least for 10-15 min at 2-6 atm. If bleeding does not stop, a perfusion balloon catheter can be used for 15-45 min inflated at low pressure. This prolonged balloon inflation and timely pericardiocentesis can avoid surgical treatment in patients with Ellis type I perforation.

2. Stent

In some cases, a polytetrafluoroethylene(PTFE)-covered stent is effective. Rarely, one or more conventional stent (bare metal or drug-eluting stent) implantation can be considered.

3. Pericardiocentesis

If perforation is suspected, echocardiography should be performed and if hemopericardium is confirmed, pericardiocentesis should be performed immediately. An indwelling pericardial catheter should be maintained for 6-24 h and echocardiography should repeated every 6-12 h.

4. Management of anticoagulation

When perforation occurs, anticoagulation should be maintained to prevent thrombus formation. However, if perforation happens after use of atherectomy or laser, it is recommended that protamine sulfate should be administrated intravenously in order to partially reverse the effect of heparin. If contrast leakage is sustained despite prolonged balloon inflation, repeated balloon inflation should be performed; meanwhile the dosage of protamine sulfate should increase under activated clotting time monitoring.

Glycoprotein IIb/IIIa inhibitors must be stopped. The effect of abciximab can be reversed after platelet transfusion of 6-10 units, but there are not any known antidotes for eptifibatide or tirofiban.

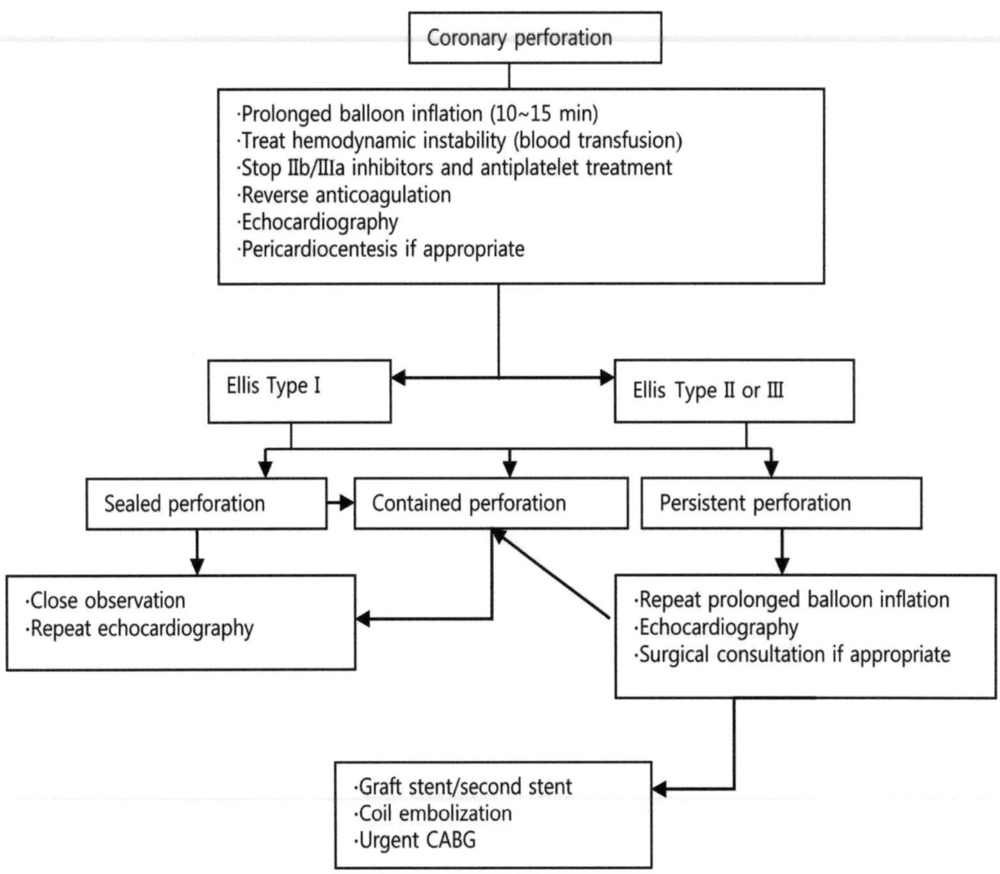

Fig. 3. Management algorithm of coronary artery perforation

5. Embolization

In case of small vessel size or distal location, limited involved myocardium, chronic total occlusion, or situation where surgery is unavailable, embolization using coils or gelfoam can successfully occlude the perforation.

6. Surgical treatment

If the perforation is severe, with hemodynamic instability or perforation is sustained despite nonsurgical management, emergency surgery is necessary.

4. Coronary dissection and acute closure

4.1 Angiographic definition

Dissection is defined as disruption of an arterial wall resulting in splitting and separation of the intimal (or subintimal) layers.

Feature	Definition
Abrupt closure	Obstruction of contrast flow (TIMI 0 or 1) in a dilated segment with previously documented anterograde flow
Ectasia	A lesion diameter greater than the reference diameter in one or more areas
Luminal irregularities	Arterial contour that has a saw-toothed pattern consisting of opacification but not fulfilling the criteria for dissection or intracoronary thrombus
Intimal flap	A discrete filling defect in apparent continuity with the arterial wall
Thrombus	Discrete, mobile angiographic filling defect with or without contrast staining
Dissection	
A	Small radiolucent area within the lumen of the vessel
B	Linear, nonpersisting extravasation of contrast material
C	Extraluminal, persisting extravasation of contrast material
D	Spiral-shaped filling defect
E	Persistent lumen defect with delayed anterograde flow
F	Filling defect accompanied by total coronary occlusion
Dissection, length(mm)	Measure end to end for type B through F dissections
Dissection, staining	Persistence of contrast within the dissection after washout of contrast material from the remaining portion of the vessel

Table 3. Standardized criteria for postprocedural lesion morphology[63,64]

4.2 Pathogenesis and incidence of coronary dissection

Intima-media cracks and medial dissection can be developed by balloon injury and if dissection involves the adventitia layer, narrowing of the lumen can occur.[65] In NHLBI classification, coronary dissection occurs in 32-41% of total balloon procedures. If the lumen narrows >50% or the length of dissection is >10mm, the risk of abrupt vessel closure increases.

In the modern PCI era, where coronary dissection can be promptly resolved by stent implantation, clinically significant dissection is reported only 1.7%. Residual dissection increases the risk of post procedure MI, emergency CABG, and stent thrombosis and mortality also increases threefold.[66]

4.3 Pathogenesis and incidence of abrupt vessel closure

Coronary balloon dilatation leads to endothelial denudation, intimal fissuring, and medial penetration and extensive damage causes obstructive dissection or intramural hematoma. When subintimal structures are exposed to the blood, then activation of platelets and thrombin formation occur. Obstructive thrombus can be formed with or without medial dissection.

An autopsy finding of patients who experienced abrupt closure within 30 days after balloon angioplasty revealed that over 50% have intimal/medial dissection flaps with or without thrombi. Cases presenting with pure thrombi without dissection was very rare.

It has been reported that the incidence of abrupt closure due to balloon angioplasty or atherectomy is 2-13.5%. About two thirds of cases of abrupt closure arise inside the catheterization laboratory and the majority occurs within the first 6 h after angioplasty. After routine stent implantation had replaced balloon angioplasty, the incidence of abrupt closure was dramatically decreased. Proper deployment technique and supportive drugs such as dual antiplatelet therapy and heparin also contribute toward the lower incidence.

4.4 Clinical manifestations of abrupt closure

Before the stent era, the incidence of abrupt closure-related mortality, myocardial infarction, and emergency CABG were 5%, 45%, and 55% respectively. However, since bailout stenting had been introduced, the incidence of emergency CABG owing to abrupt closure was reported to be 0.8%. Long term prognosis of abrupt closure in related to the increase of restenosis, 2-year mortality, myocardial infarction, and CABG. Well known predictors of abrupt closure are in Table 4.

Unstable angina
Diabetes mellitus
Female gender
Advanced age
Intraluminal thrombus
ACC/AHA score
Lesion length ≥2 luminal diameters or >10 mm
Extensive proximal tortuosity
Bend point ≥45 degrees
Branch point
Other stenoses ≥50% in same vessel
Multivessel disease
Ostial right coronary artery
Degenerated saphenous vein grafts
"Inoperable" surgical status
Collaterals originating from target vessel
Preangioplasty stenosis 90-99%

Table 4. Predictor of abrupt closure

4.5 Managements

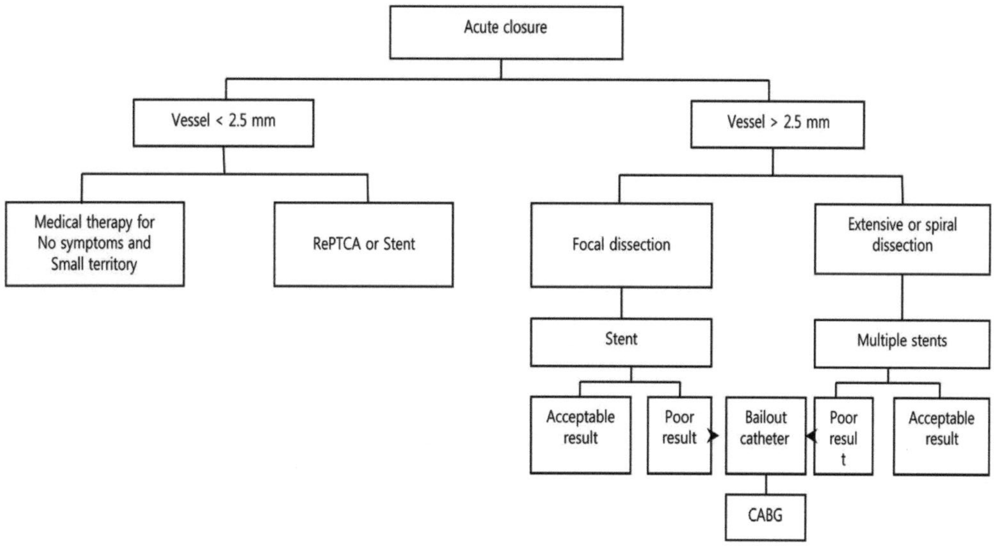

Fig. 4. Management algorithm of abrupt closure

1. Initial management

When acute chest pain is recognized, nitroglycerin 100-200mcg should be injected into the coronary artery. If activated clotting time is less than 250 sec, additional heparin should be injected. Before the stent era, a size-matched balloon was inflated for at least 5 min and sometimes perfusion balloon was used. Currently, bailout stenting is considered as the most effective tool for abrupt or threatened coronary closure. Additional balloon inflation can recover blood flow to normal. Because the effect of rescue abciximab has been reported in many clinical trials and since it reduces subacute thrombus formation, administration of glycoprotein IIb/IIIa inhibitors is recommended.

2. Coronary artery bypass graft

In cases of acute closure due to left main coronary artery injury or coronary artery perforation, installation of intra-aortic balloon counterpulsation is necessary and emergency coronary artery bypass grafting (CABG) should be considered. A long dissection which does not resolve with stenting also needs CABG.

5. Stent thrombosis

5.1 Definition

Definitions of stent thrombosis (ST) range from "angiographically proven to "clinically suspected" ST with the inclusion of myocardial infarction involving the target vessel to unexplained death (within 30 days). Although the first definition has a well-defined mechanism limited to selected patients undergoing angiography at the time of ST, there is concern for underestimation of the true incidence of ST. On the other hand, the other broader definitions include events potentially related to disease progression, life threatening arrhythmias, myocardial infarction of non-culprit lesions, and non-cardiac sudden death and therefore overestimate the true incidence. Accounting for these limitations, an academic research consortium (ARC) proposed a new standardised definition of ST (Table 5).[67] It is based on 2 principles: level of certainty that ST is underlying mechanism of the adverse event and the time of the adverse event relative to the index procedure.

ST can be classified based on the time of adverse event (Figure 5). Early ST refers to the first 30 days after stent implantation and is further stratified into acute (<24 hours) and subacute (24 hours to 30 days). Late ST is time between 1 month and 1 year. Very late ST means beyond 1 year. The rationale of this classification is to account for different pathophysiological mechanisms that may be at work at various times.

Definite ST

Definite stent thrombosis is diagnosed when either angiographic or pathological confirmation is present

Angiographic confirmation of ST*

The presence of a thrombus originating in the stent or in the segment 5 mm proximal to the stented region and at least one of the following criteria within a 48-h time window:

Acute onset of ischemic symptoms at rest (typical chest pain >20 min)

New ischemic ECG changes suggestive of acute ischemia

Typical rise and fall in cardiac biomarkers

Pathological confirmation of stent thrombosis

Evidence of recent thrombus within the stent determined at autopsy

Probable ST

Clinical definition of probable ST is diagnosed after intracoronary stenting in the following cases

Any unexplained death within the first 30 d

Regardless of the time after the index procedure, any MI that is related to documented acute ischemia in the territory of the implanted stent without angiographic confirmation of ST and in the absence of any other obvious cause

Possible ST

Clinical definition of possible ST is diagnosed with any unexplained death from 30 d after intracoronary stenting until the end of trial follow-up

*The incidental angiographic documentation of stent occlusion in the absence of clinical signs or symptoms (silent occlusion) is (for this purpose) not considered a confirmed stent thrombosis.

Table 5. Definition of ST as Proposed by the Academic Research Consortium[67]

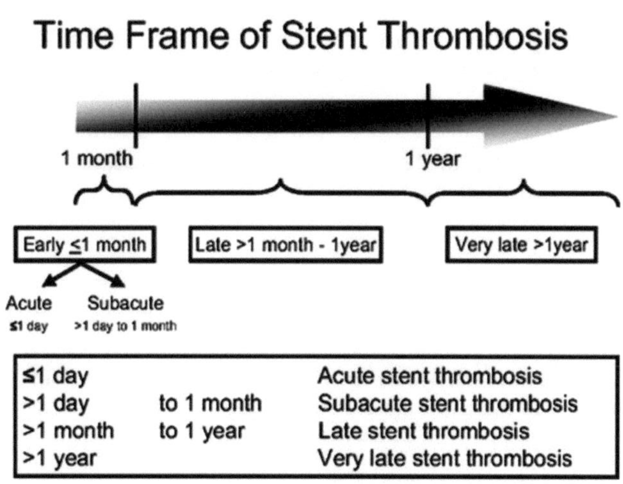

Fig. 5. Classification based on the time frame of adverse events

5.2 Incidence

In the bare metal stent (BMS) era, most of ST was early ST and very late ST was extremely rare, although several cases of late ST were reported.[73,74] Early ST is encountered with a similar or even somewhat lower frequency after drug-eluting stent (DES) compared with BMS. A meta-analysis of 6 studies comparing BMS with sirolimus-eluting stent (SES) reported that early rates of ST were 0.5% with SES and 0.6% with BMS, respectively (*P*=0.55).[68] A pooled analysis of 5 trials comparing BMS with paclitaxel-eluting stent (PES) revealed early ST was 0.5% in PES and 0.6% in BMS, respectively (*P*=0.51).[69] Although there had been some reported cases of late ST during the BMS era, this was not a clinical concern for most. According to recent a meta-analysis, no differences existed in the incidence of late ST between DES and BMS (0.2% versus 0.3%, 95% CI: 0.35-2.84; *P*=1.00).[70] In another meta-analysis of 9 trials comparing SES and PES, no significant differences were detected for up to 1 year of follow-up (Figure 6).[93]

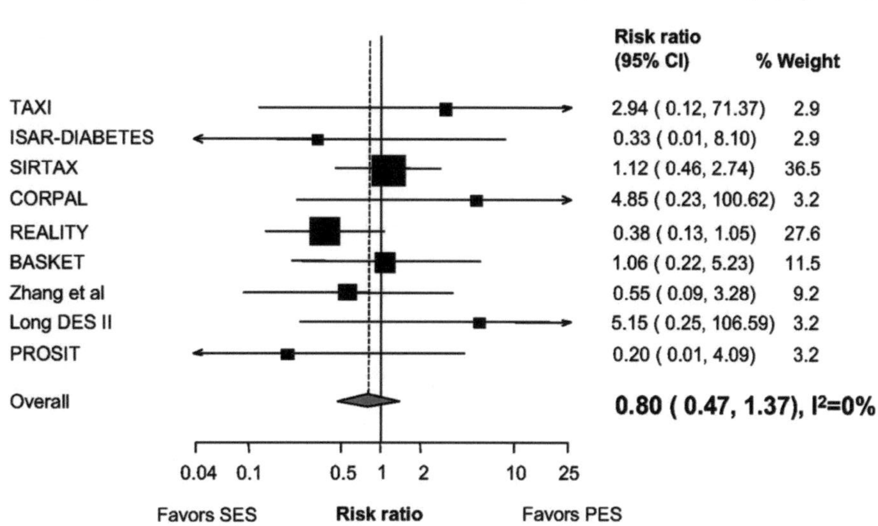

Fig. 6. Risk of ST in 9 trials directly comparing SES and PES with follow-up to 1 year.[93]

Case reports, observational studies, extended follow-up of trials comparing DES with BMS, and meta-analyses of randomized trials have corroborated that very late ST is more common with DES than BMS. Pooled analysis of 4 randomized trials comparing SES with BMS and 5 randomized trials comparing PES with BMS revealed similar rates of late ST but significantly more very late ST (0.6% versus 0% for SES versus BMS, P=0.03; 0.7% versus 0.2% for PES versus BMS, P=0.03).[72]

5.3 Clinical sequelae

The reason why ST attracts attention is that it is associated with much higher mortality compared to other complications. Moreover, ST may be responsible for late complications of MI, including heart failure, arrhythmias, or mechanical complications. The impact of ST depends upon the myocardial area at risk, its viability, the degree of instantly recruitable collaterals, and the availability of rapid reperfusion therapy. The mortality rate varies depending on the definition of ST and follow-up duration (7-45%).[73-77] Most ST patients experience myocardial infarction (>66%) with no differences between DES and BMS.[71]

5.4 Risk factors

ST is a multifactorial problem related to the stent itself, procedural factors, response to antiplatelet drugs, and lesion factors (Table 6). Many cases of early ST are caused by the procedure itself such as the presence of residual dissections or stent underexpansion. Poor response to antiplatelet drugs is also a documented cause of ST.[78] Individual or ethnic differences have been reported and it has been suggested that several genetic polymorphisms are related to this drug resistance. Discontinuation of antiplatelet drugs is one of the most important predictors of ST. Patients noncompliance is the main problem and discontinuation due to dental procedures, surgical procedures or bleeding is also an important predisposing factor for late and very late ST.[76]

5.5 Pathogenesis

1. Hypersensitivity reaction with extensive vasculitis

Virmani and colleagues[79] first described a case of local hypersensitivity reaction with extensive vasculitis of the intima, media, and adventitia consisting predominantly of lymphocytes and eosinophils in a patient suffering very late DES thrombosis. Histopathological analysis of an autopsy case revealed aneurysmal dilatation of the vessel wall within the stented segment with incomplete stent apposition and thick fibrin thrombus between the stent and the arterial wall. Most hypersensitivity cases reported to the Food and Drug administration after DES implantation were attributed to the DES itself, especially the polymer coating.

2. Delayed healing and dysfunctional endothelialization

Another possible explanation is delayed healing and endothelial dysfunction. Delayed healing manifested by persistent fibrin deposition and incomplete reendothelialization emerged as an important discriminator between BMS and DES.[80] Physiological evidence of dysfunctional endothelium comes from studies assessing vasomotion 6 months after DES implantation.[81,82] Through the use of bicycle exercise during coronary angiography, the segment proximal and distal to DES showed paradoxical vasoconstriction, whereas BMS demonstrated normal vasodilatation.

- Patient factors
    - Thickness and robustness of neointimal stent coverage
    - Drug response/interactions
    - Gene polymorphism
    - Left ventricular function
    - Acute coronary syndrome
    - Renal failure
    - Diabetes mellitus
- Antithrombotic and anticoagulation therapy
    - Coagulation activity
    - Inhibition of platelet aggregation
- Procedural factors
    - Dissection
    - Incomplete stent apposition
    - Stent expansion
- Lesion factors
    - Vessel size
    - Lesion length
    - Thrombus
    - Plaque characteristics
    - Bifurcation
- Device factors
    - Stent surface
    - Drugs
    - Polymer

Table 6. Multifactorial Origin of ST

3. Incomplete stent apposition

Incomplete stent apposition resulting from positive arterial remodeling or stent underexpansion, and penetration of the stent into a necrotic core leads to ST.

5.6 Prevention

1. Patient and lesion selection

PCI is not essential in all angina patients. The COURAGE trial, a randomization study comparing PCI and medical therapy in carefully selected patients with stable angina, revealed that there were no significant differences in mortality, acute myocardial infarction, and rehospitalization for acute coronary syndrome.[83] It is therefore appropriate to consider medical therapy to the initial treatment option in stable angina patients with relatively low risk. In determining of use of BMS or DES, the risk of restenosis, the probability of bleeding or non-cardiac surgery, and the risk of late ST should be considered. The situations that BMS can be used are as follows.

1. De novo lesions of native vessel
2. Reference diameter >3.5mm
3. Short,focal lesions
4. Patients with no diabetes mellitus
5. Non-ostial lesions

The need for non-cardiac surgical procedures may arise after recent DES implantation. ST can arise after antiplatelet therapy withdrawal, especially within 12 months after PCI. In a study of 103 stent patients undergoing noncardiac surgery, an alarming 5% mortality rate and 45% complication rate were noted.[84] It should be determined whether the surgical procedure can be postponed beyond 12 months after stenting or whether dual antiplatelet therapy can be maintained throughout the perioperative period. However if it is not possible to delay surgery beyond 12 months, balloon angioplasty or BMS implantation can be considered instead of DES implantation.

2. Antiplatelet therapy

The important of dual antiplatelet maintenance after PCI cannot be emphasized strongly enough. In a registry, 14% discontinued thienopyridine therapy within 30 days after discharge.[85] Predictors of premature thienopyridine discontinuation were older age, lower socioeconomic status, preexisting cardiovascular disease, and lack of discharge instructions or cardiac rehabilitation referral. Mortality was about 10 times higher and rehospitalization was almost twice as high in patients without thienopyridine therapy.

The optimal duration of dual antiplatelet therapy after DES implantation is not well established.

The AHA/ACC guidelines are not based upon multicenter trials. Dual antiplatelet therapy is recommended at least 1 month for BMS implantation whereas for DES implantation, adherence to a 12 month regimen is recommended.[86] It is also important that surgeons and dentists are advised not to automatically discontinue antiplatelet therapy but rather to consult first with the patient's cardiologist.

3. Technique

Attention to technical details also may improve results when PCI is performed with DES. Optimal deployment of stents by full expansion throughout their entire length should be ensured and residual dissections should be avoided. Intravascular ultrasound or optical coherence tomography is helpful to avoid stent malapposition. Multiple stenting in bifurcation lesions should be limited to only cases where really needed.

4. Development of new DES

Because the polymer coatings of DES were suspected to be responsible for some of ST, biodegradable polymers[87] and polymer-free DES[88] were developed. Another approach banks on drugs with improved healing properties such as antibodies capturing CD34+ endothelial progenitor cells[89] or antithrombotic substances[90] applied to the stent surface. Biodegradable stents, fully disintegrated in the body over a long period of time, have been recently developed.[91] The Titan-TINOX stent (Hexacath, Rueil-Malmaison, France) is made of stainless steel coated with a Titanium nitride oxide (TNO) compound. The coating minimizes the leakage of metal residues, mostly nickel, from the metal stent into the arterial wall and, to some extent, attenuates electrical conductivity. Thus, the device was designed to enhance endothelialization and decrease the rate of stent-related thrombosis and restenosis. Stent coating with TNO reduced angiographic and ultrasonic measures of restenosis compared with stainless steel control stents of otherwise identical design in the prospective, randomized, multicenter trial.[92]

6. References

[1] Chung WS, Park CS, Seung KB, et al. The incidence and clinical impact of stent strut fractures developed after drug-eluting stent implantation. Int J Cardiol 2008;125:325-331.

[2] Aoki J, Nakazawa G, Tanabe K, Hoye A, Yamamoto H, Nakayama T, et al. Incidence and clinical impact of coronary stent fracture after sirolimus-eluting stent implantation. Catheter cardiovasc Interv 2007;69:380-386.

[3] Shaikh F, Maddikunta R, Djelmami-Hani M, Solis J, Allaqaband S, Bajwa T. Stent fracture an incidental finding or a significant marker of clinical in-stent restenosis? Catheter Cardiovasc Interv 2008;71:614-618.

[4] Sianos G, Hofma S, Ligthart JM, Saia F, Hoye A, Lemos PA, et al. Stent fracture and restenosis in the drug-eluting era, Catheter Cardiovasc Interv 2004;61:111-116.

[5] Lee MS, Jurewitz D, Aragon J, Forrester J, Makkar RR, Kar S. Stent fracture associated with drug-eluting stents: clinical characteristics and implications. Catheter Cardiovasc Interv 2007;69:387-394.

[6] Makaryus AN, Lefkowitz I, Lee AD. Coronary artery stent fracture. Int J Cardiovasc Imaging 2007;23:305-309.

[7] Yang TH, Kim DI, Park SG, Seo JS, Cho HJ, Seol SH, Kim SM, Kim DK, Kim DS. Clinical characteristics of stent fracture after sirolimus-eluting stent implantation. Int J Cardiol 2009;131:212-216.

[8] Umeda H, Gochi T, Iwase M, Izawa H, Shimizu T, Ishiki R, Inagaki H, Toyama J, Yokota M, Murohara T. Frequency, predictors and outcome of stent fracture after sirolimus-eluting stent implantation. Int J Cardiol 2009;133:321-326.

[9] Nakazawa G, Finn AV, Vorpahl M, Ladich E, Kutys R, Balazs I, Kolodgie FD, Virmani R. Incidence and predictors of drug-eluting stent fracture in human coronary artery. J Am Coll Cardiol 2009;54:1924-1931.

[10] Rits J, Van Herwaarden JA, Jahrome AK, Krievins D, Moll FL. The incidence of arterial stent fractures with exclusion of coronary, aortic, and non-arterial settings. Eur J Vasc EndovascSurg 2008;36:339-345.

[11] Scheinert D, Scheinert S, Sax J, et al. Prevalence and clinical impact of stent fractures after femoropopliteal stenting. L Am Coll Cardiol 2005;45:312/315.

[12] Popma JJ, Tiroch K, Almonacid A, Cohen S, Kandzari DE, Leon MB. A qualitative and quantitative angiographic analysis of stent fracture late following sirolimus-eluting stent implantation. Am J Cardiol 2009;103:923-929.

[13] Lemos PA, Saia F, Ligthart JM, et al. Coronary restenosis after sirolimus-eluting stent implantation: morphological description and mechanistic analysis from a consecutive series of cases. Circulation 2003;108:257-60.

[14] Suziki Y, Ikeno F, Yeung AC. Drug-eluting stent distribution: a comparison between Cypher and Taxus by optical coherence tomography. J Invasive Cardiol 2006;18:111-114.

[15] Kloner RA, Ganote CE, Jennings RB. The 'no-reflow' phenomenon after temporary coronary occlusion in the dog. J Clin Invest 1974;54:1496-1508.

[16] Krug A, de Rochemont WM, Korb G. Blood supply of the myocardium after temporary coronary occlusion. Circ Res 1996;19:57-62.

[17] Schofer J, Montz R, Mathey D. Scintigraphic evidence of the 'no-reflow' phenomenon in human beings after coronary thrombolysis. J Am Coll Cardiol 1985;5:593-598.

[18] Ito H, Tomooka T, Sakai N, et al. Lack of myocardial perfusion immediately after successful thrombolysis: a predictor of poor recovery of left ventricular function in anterior myocardial infarction. Circulation 1992;85:1699-1705.

[19] Brosh D, Assali AR, Mager A, etal. Effect of no-reflow during primary percutaneous coronary intervention for acute myocardial infarction on six-month mortality. Am J Cardiol 2007;99:442-445.

[20] Galiuto L, Garramone B, Scarà A, et al., AMICI investigators. The extent of microvascular damage during myocardial contrast echocardiography is superior to other known indexes of post-infarct reperfusion in predicting left ventricular remodeling: results of the multicenter AMICI study. J Am Coll Cardiol 2008;51:552-559.

[21] Majno G, Ames A, Chaing J, Wright RL. No reflow after cerebral ischemia. Lancet 1967;2:569-570.

[22] Galiuto L, Lombardo A, Maseri A, et al. Temporal evolution and functional outcome of no-reflow: sustained and spontaneously reversible patterns following successful coronary recanalization. Heart 2003;89:731-737.

[23] Skyschally A, Leineweber K, Gres P, Haude M, Erbel R, Heusch G. Coronary microembolization. Basic Res Cardiol 2006;101:373-382.

[24] Hori M, Inoue M, Kitakaze M, Koretsune Y, et al. Role of adenosine in hyperemic response of coronary blood flow in microembolization. Am J Physiol 1986;250:H509-518.

[25] Reffelmann T, Kloner RA. The no-reflow phenomenon: a basic mechanism of myocardial ischemia and reperfusion. Basic Res Cardiol 2006;101:359-372.

[26] Tellon DM, Hausenloy DJ. Myocardial reperfusion injury. N Engl J Med 2007;357:1121-1135.

[27] Engler RL, Schmid-Schönbein GW, Pavelec RS. Leukocyte capillary plugging in myocardial ischemia and reperfusion in the dog. Am J Pathol 1983;111:98-111.

[28] Ambrosio G, Tritto I. Reperfusion injury: experimental evidence and clinical implications Am Heart J 1999;138:S69-75.

[29] Ito BR, Schmid-Schönbein G, Engler RL. Effects of leukocyte activation on myocardial vascular resistance. Blood Cells 1990;16:145-163.

[30] Lefer AM, Tsao PS, Aoki N, Palladino MA Jr. Mediation of cardioprotection by transforming growth factor-beta. Science 1990;249:61-64.

[31] Furuichi K, Wada T, Iwata Y, et al. Interleukin-1-dependent sequential chemokine expression and inflammatory cell infiltration in ischemia-reperfusion injury. Crit Care Med 2006;34:2447-2455.

[32] Chamoun F, Burne M, O'Donnell M, Rabb H. Pathophysiologic role of selectins and their ligands in ischemia reperfusion injury. Front Biosci 2000;5:E103-109.

[33] Caeden DL, Granger DN. Pathophysiology of ischemia-reperfusion injury. J Pathol 2000;190:255-266.

[34] Skyschally A, Schulz R, Heusch G. Pathophysiology of myocardial infarction: protection by ischemic pre- and postconditioning. Herz 2008;33:88-100.
[35] Piot C, Croisille P, Staat P, et al. Effect of cyclosporine on reperfusion injury in acute myocardial infarction. N Engl J Med 2008;359:473-481.
[36] Jaffe R, Charron T, Puley G, Dick A, Strauss BH. Microvascular obstruction and the no-reflow phenomenon after percutaneous coronary intervention. Circulation 2008;117:3152-3156.
[37] Mizumura T, Nithipatikom K, Gross GJ. Infarct size-reducing effect of nicorandil is mediated by the KATP channel but not by its nitrate-like properties in dogs. Cardiocasc Res 1996;32:274-285.
[38] Montalescot G, Ongen Z, Guindy R, et al., for the RIVIERA Investigators. Predictors of outcome in patients undergoing PCI. Results of the RIVIERA study. Int J Cardiol 2009;129:379-387.
[39] Collet JP, Montalescot G. The acute reperfusion management of STEMI in patients with impaired glucose tolerance and type 2 diabetes. Diabetes Vasc Dis Res 2005;2:136-143.
[40] Golino P, Maroko PR, Carew TE. The effect of acute hypercholesterolemia on myocardial infarct size and the no-reflow phenomenon during coronary occlusion-reperfusion. Circulation 1987;75:292-298.
[41] Rezkalla SH, Kloner RA. Ischemic preconditioning and preinfarction angina in the clinical arena. Nat Clin Pract Cardiovasc Med 2004;1:96-102.
[42] Morishima I, Sone T, Okumura K, Tsuboi H, Kondo J, Mukawa H, Matsui H, Toki Y, Ito T, Hayakawa T. Angiographic no-reflow phenomenon as a predictor of adverse long-term outcome in patients treated with percutaneous transluminal coronary angioplasty for first acute myocardial infarction. J Am Coll Cardiol 2000;36:1202-1209.
[43] van't Hof AW, Liem A, Suryapranata H, Hoorntje JC, de Boer MJ, Zijlstra F, Zwolle Myocardial infarction Study Group. Angiographic assessment of myocardial reperfusion in patients treated with primary angioplasty for acute myocardial infarction: myocardial blush grade. Circulation 1998;97:2302-2306.
[44] Santoro GM, Valenti R, Buonamici P, et al. Relation between ST-segment changes and myocardial perfusion evaluated by myocardial contrast echocardiography in patients with acute myocardial infarction treated by direct angioplasty. Am J Cardiol 1998;82:932-937.
[45] Iliceto S, Marangelli V, Marchese A, Amico A, Galiuto L, Rizzon P. Myocardial contrast echocardiography in acute myocardial infarction. Pathophysiological background and clinical applications. Eur Heart J 1996;17:344-353.
[46] Albert TS, Kim RJ, Judd RM. Assessment of no-reflow regions using cardiac MRI. Basic Res Cardiol 2006;101:383-390.
[47] Loubeyre C, Morice MC, Lefèvre T, Piéchaud JF, Louvard Y, Dumas P. A randomized comparison of direct stenting with conventional stent implantation in selected patients with acute myocardial infarction. J Am Coll Cardiol 2002;39:15-21.
[48] Burzotta F, Trani C, Romagnoli E, et al. Manual thrombus-aspiration improves myocardial reperfusion: the randomized evaluation of the effect of mechanical reduction of distal embolization by thrombus-aspiration in primary and rescue angioplasty (REMEDIA) trial. J Am Coll Cardiol 2005;46:371-376.
[49] Svilass T, Vlaar PJ, van der Horst IC, et al. Thrombus aspiration during primary percutaneous coronary intervention. N Engl J Med 2008;358:557-567.

[50] Vlaar PJ, Svilass T, van der Horst IC, et al. Cardiac death and reinfarction after 1 year in the Thrombus Aspiration during Percutaneous coronary intervention in Acute myocardial infarction Study (TAPAS): a 1-year follow-up study. Lancet 2008;371:1915-1920.

[51] Burzotta F, Crea F. Thrombus aspiration: a victory in the war against no reflow. Lancet 2008;371:1889-1890.

[52] Zhao J, Yang Y, You S, Cui C, Gao R. Carvedilol preserves endothelial junctions and reduces myocardial no-reflow after acute myocardial infarction and reperfusion. Int J Cardiol 2007;115:334-341.

[53] Zhao JL, Yang YJ, You SJ, et al. Pretreatment with fosinopril or valsartan reduces myocardial no-reflow after acute myocardial infarction and reperfusion. Coron Artery Dis 2006;17:463-469.

[54] Thiele H, Schindler K, Friedenberger J, et al. Intracoronary compared with intravenous bolus abciximab application in patients with ST-elevation myocardial infarction undergoing primary percutaneous coronary intervention: the randomized Leipzig immediate percutaneous coronary intervention abciximab IV versus IC in ST-elevation myocardial infarction trial. Circulation 2008;118:49-57.

[55] Ellis SG, Ajluni S, Arnold AZ, Popma JJ, Bittl JA, Eigler NL, Cowley MJ, Raymond RE, Safian RD, Whitlow PL. Increased coronary perforation in the new device era: incidence, classification, management, and outcome. Circulation 1994;90:2725-2730.

[56] Teo KK, Rogers JH, Laird JR. Use of stent grafts and coil in vessel rupture and perforation. Journal of Interventional Cardiology 2008;21:86-99.

[57] Shimony A, Zahger D, Straten MV, et al. Incidence, risk factors, management and outcomes of coronary artery perforation during percutaneous coronary intervention. Am J Cardiol 2009;104:1674-1677.

[58] Javaid A, Buch AN, Satler LF, et al. Management and outcomes of oronary artery perforation during percutaneous coronary intervention. Am J CArdiol 2006; 98:911-914.

[59] Fasseas P, Orford JL, Panetta CJ, et al. Incidence, correrates, management, and clinical outcome of coronary perforation: Analysis of 16,298 procedures. Am Heart J 2004;147:140-145.

[60] Gruberg L, Pinnow E, Flood R, et al. Incidence, management, and outcome of coronary artery perforation during percutaneous coronary intervention. Am J Cardiol 2000;86:680-682.

[61] Gunning MG, Williams IL, Jewitt DE, et al. Coronary artery perforation during percutaneous intervention: Incidence and outcome. Heart 2002;88:495-498.

[62] Lloyd W Klein, Coronary artery perforation during interventional procedures. Catheter Cardiovasc Interv 2006;68:713-717.

[63] Huber M, Mooney J, Madison J, Mooney M. Use of a morphologic classification to predict clinical outcome after dissection from coronary angioplasty. Am J Cardiol 1991;68:467-471.

[64] Smith SC, Dove JT, Jacobs AK, Kennedy JW, Kereiakes D, Kern MJ, Popma JJ, Schaff HV, Williams DO. ACC/AHA guidelines for percutaneous coronary intervention-executive summary: a report of the ACC/AHA task force on practice guidelines. Circulation 2001;103:3019-3041.

[65] Lincoff AM, Popma JJ, Ellis SG, Hacker J. Abrupt vessel closure complicating coronary angioplasty: clinical, angiographic and therapeutic profile. J AM Coll Cardiol 1992;19:926-935.

[66] Tenaglia AN, Fortin DF, Frid DJ. Long-term outcome following successful reopening of abrupt closure after coronary angioplasty. Am J Cardiol 1993;72:21-25.

[67] Cutlip DE, Windecker S, Mehran R, Boam A, Cohen DJ, Van Es GA, Steg PG, Morel MA, Mauri L, Vranckx P, McFadden E, Lansky AJ, Hamon M, Krucoff MW, Serruys P. Clinical end points in coronary stent trials. Circulation 2007;115:2344-2351.

[68] Bavry AA, Kumbhani DJ, Helton TJ, Bhatt DL. Risk of thrombosis with the use of sirolimus-eluting stents for percutaneous coronary intervention. Am J Cardiol 2005;95:1469-1472.

[69] Bavry AA, Kumbhani DJ, Helton TJ, Bhatt DL. What is the risk of stent thrombosis associated with the use of paclitaxel-eluting stents for percutaneous coronary intervention? J Am Coll Cardiol 2005;45:941-946.

[70] Moreno R, Fernandez C, Hernandez R, Alfonso F, Angiolillo DJ, Sabate M, Escaned J, Banuelos C, Fernandez-Ortiz A, Macaya C. Drug-eluting stent thrombosis. J Am Coll Cardiol 2005;45:954-959.

[71] Mauri L, Hsieh WH, Massaro JM, Ho KK, D'Agostino R, Cutlip DE. Stent thrombosis in randomized clinical trials of drug-eluting stents. N Engl J Med 2007;356:1020-1029.

[72] Stone GW, Moses JW, Ellis SG, Schofer J, Dawkins KD, Morice MC, Colombo A, Schampaert E, Grube E, Kirtane AJ, Cutlip DE, Fahy M, Pocock SJ, Mehran R, Leon MB. Safty and efficacy of sirolimus- and paclitaxel-eluting coronary stents. N Engl J Med 2007;356:998-1008.

[73] Cutlip DE, Baim DS, Ho KK, Popma JJ, Lansky AJ, Cohen DJ, Carrozza JP Jr, Chauhan MS, Rodriguez O, Kuntz RE. Stent thrombosis in the modern era. Circulation 2001;103:1967-1971.

[74] Wenaweser P, Rey C, Eberli FR, Togni M, Tuller D, Locher S, Remondino A, Seiler C, Hess OM, Meier B, Windecker S. Stent thrombosis following bare-metal stent implantation. Eur Heart J 2005;46:1180-1187.

[75] Daemon J, Wenaweser P, Tsuchida K, Abrecht L, Vaina S, Morger C, Kukreja N, Juni P, Sianos G, Hellige G, van Domburg RT, Hess OM, Boersma E, Meier B, Windecker S, Serruys PW. Early and late coronary stent thrombosis of sirolimus-eluting and paclitaxel-eluting stents in routine clinical practice. Lancet 2007;369:667-678.

[76] Iakovou I, Schmidt T, Bonizzoni E, Ge L, Sangiorgi GM, Stankovic G, Airoldi F, Chieffo A, Montorfano M, Carlino M, Michev I, Corvaja N, Briguori C, Gerckens U, Grube E, Colombo A. Incidence, predictors, and outcome of thrombosis after successful implantation of drug-eluting stents. JAMA 2005;293:2126-2130.

[77] Kuchulakanti PK, Chu WW, Torguson R, Ohlmann P, Rha SW, Clavijo LC, Kim SW, Bui A, Gevorkian N, Xue Z, Smith K, Fournadjieva J, Suddath WO, Satler LF, Pichard AD, Kent KM, Waksman R. Correlates and long-term outcomes of angiographically proven stent thrombosis with sirolimus- and paclitaxel-eluting stents. Circulation 2006;113:1108-1113.

[78] Wenaweser P, Dorffler-Melly J, Imboden K, Windecker S, Togni M, Meier B, Haeberli A, Hess OM. Stent thrombosis is associated with an impaired response to antiplatelet therapy. J Am Coll Cardiol 2005;45:1748-1752.

[79] Virmami R, Guagliumi G, Farb A, Musumeci G, Grieco N, Motta T, Mihalcsik L, Tespili M, Valsecchi O, Lolodgie FD. Localized hypersensitivity and late coronary thrombosis secondary to sirolimus-eluting stent. Circulation 2004;109:714-725.

[80] Joner M, Finn AV, Farb A, Mont EK, Kolodgie FD, Ladich E, Kutys R, Skorija K, Gold HK, Virmani R. Pathology of drug-eluting stents in humans. J Am Coll Cardiol 2006;48:193-202.

[81] Togni M, Windecker S, Cocchia R, Wenaweser P, Cook S, Billinger M, Meier B, Hess OM. Sirolimus-eluting stents associated with paradoxical coronary vasospasm. J AM Coll Cardiol 2005;46:231-236.

[82] Togni M, Raber L, Cocchia R, Wenaweser P, Cook S, Windecker S, Meier B, Hess OM. Local vascular dysfunction after coronary paclitaxel-eluting stent implantation. Int J Cardiol 2007;120:212-220.

[83] Boden WE, O'Rourke RA, Teo KK, Hartigan PM, Maron DJ, Kostuk WJ, Knudtson M, Dada M, Casperson P, Harris CL, et al. Optimal medical therapy with or without PCI for stable coronary disease. N Engl J Med 2007;356:1503-1516.

[84] Vicenzi MN, Meislitzer T, Heitzinger B, Halaj M, Fleisher LA, Metzler H. Coronary artery stenting and non-cardiac surgery. Br J Anaesth 2006;96:686-693.

[85] Spertus JA, Kettelkamp R, Vance C, Decker C, Jones PG, Rumsfeld JS, Messenger JC, Khanal S, Peterson ED, Bach RG, Krumholz HM, Cohen DJ. Prevalence, predictors, and outcomes of premature discontinuation of thienopyridine therapy after drug-eluting stent placement. Circulation 2006;113:2803-2809.

[86] Grines CL, Bonow RO, Casey DE Jr, Gardner TJ, Lockhart PB, Moliterno DJ, O'Gara P, Whitlow P. Prevention of premature discontinuation of dual antiplatelet therapy in patients with coronary artery stents: a science advisory from the AHA, ACC, Society for Cardiovascular Angiography an Interventions, American College of Surgeons, and American Dental Association, with representation from the American College of Physicians. Circulation 2007;115:813-818.

[87] Grube E, Buellesfeld L. BioMatrix Biolimus A9-eluting coronary stent. Expert Rev Med Devices. 2006;3:731-741.

[88] Scheller B, Hehrlein C, Bocksch W, Rutsch W, Haghi D, Dietz U, Bom M, Speck U. Treatment of coronary in-stent restenosis with a a paclitaxel-coated balloon catheter. N Engl J Med. 2006;355:2113-2124.

[89] Aoki J, Serruys PW, van Beusekom H, Ong AT, McFadden EP, Sianos G, van der Giessen WJ, Regar E, de Feyter PJ, Davis HR, Rowland S, Kutryk MJ. Endothelial progenitor cells capture by stents coated with antibody against CD34: the HEALING-FIM Registry. J Am Coll Cardiol 2005;45:1574-1579.

[90] Mehran R, Aymong ED, Ashby DT, Fischell T, Whiworth H Jr, Siegel R, Thomas W, Wong SC, Narasimaiah R, Lansky AJ, Leon MB. Safty of an aspirin-along regimen after intracoronary stenting with a heparin-coated stent. Circulation 2003;108:1078-1083.

[91] Abizaid A, Ribamar Costa Jr J. New drug-eluting stents : An overview on biodegradable and polymer-free next-generation stent systems. Circ Cardiovasc Interv 2010;3:384-393.

[92] Windecker S, Simon R, Lins M, Klauss V, Eberli FR, Roffi M, Pedrazzini G, Moccetti T, Wenaweser P, Togni M, Tüller D, Zbinden R, Seiler C, Mehilli J, Kastrati A, Meier B, Hess OM. Randomized comparison of a titanium-nitride-oxide-coated stent with a stainless steel stent for coronary revascularization : The TiNOX Trial. Circulation 2005;111:2617-2622.

[93] Kastrati A, Dibra A, Eberle S, Mehilli J, Suarez de Lezo J, Goy JJ, Ulm K, Schomig A. Sirolimus-eluting stents vs paclitaxel-eluting stents in patients with coronary artery disease. JAMA 2005;294:819-825.

4

Therapeutic Hypothermia in Cardiac Arrest Survivors

Roman Škulec
Emergency Medical Service of the Central Bohemian Region,
Department of Anesthesiology and Intensive Care, Charles University in Prague,
Faculty of Medicine in Hradec Kralove, University Hospital Hradec Kralove
Czech Republic

1. Introduction

In Europe, cardiac arrest is the leading cause of death. Summary data indicate that the annual incidence of out-of-hospital cardiac arrest (OHCA) treated by Emergency medical systems is 38 per 100,000 population (Atwood et al., 2005). Survival is an estimated 10 % for all initial rhythms. Return of spontaneous circulation (ROSC) is followed by the development of post-cardiac arrest syndrome (PCAS), including post-cardiac arrest brain injury. This has been identified as the main cause of death and the condition limiting a long term quality of life (Edgren et al., 1994). Therapeutic hypothermia (TH) has became a cornerstone of early post-resuscitation care in cardiac arrest survivors (Nolan et al., 2008). So far, it has been the only known post-cardiac arrest intervention which can reduce the risk of unfavourable neurological outcome and decrease mortality. After an advisory statement of the International Liaison Committee on Resuscitation endorsed the use of TH in 2003, it was recommended as a standard therapeutic procedure in cardiac arres patients in the 2005 and 2010 guidelines for resuscitation and emergency cardiac care of the European Resuscitation Council and the American Heart Association (Nolan et al., 2005; Deakin et al., 2011). Accurate and safe management during the procedure of TH is a prerequisite for achieving the optimal neuroprotective effect. Moreover, the combination of TH along with other procedures (urgent myocardial revascularization, goal-directed haemodynamic support, control of blood glucose, ventilation and seizures) improves the goal of reaching a good neurological outcome (Sunde et al., 2007). This chapter summarizes patophysiological aspects of PCAS, the evidence supporting TH and significant aspects of its practice.

2. Pathophysiology of post-cardiac arrest syndrome

The return of spontaneous circulation after severe complete whole-body ischemia is an unnatural pathophysiological state created by successful cardiopulmonary resuscitation. It is followed by a number of undesirable processes leading to the development of PCAS. The following four key clinical components of PCAS have been identified: a) post-cardiac arrest brain injury, b) post-cardiac arrest myocardial dysfunction, c) systemic ischemia/reperfusion response, and d) persistent precipitating pathology (Nolan et al., 2008). While some of the processes develop very early during cardiac arrest, others follow later on after the return of spontaneous circulation, thus allowing potential space for therapeutic intervention.

Post-cardiac arrest brain injury is the most serious condition limiting long term quality of life of cardiac arrest survivors. Figure 1 summarizes the mechanisms leading to this condition (Škulec R et al., 2009).

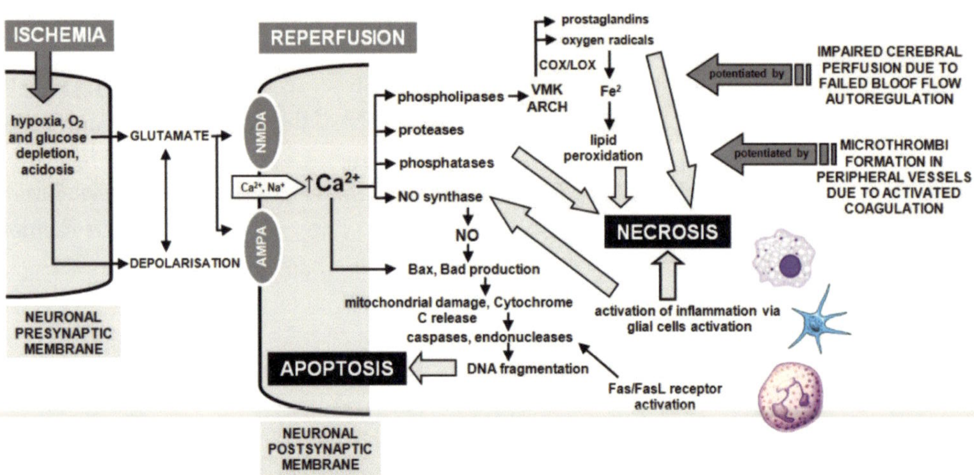

Fig. 1. Cellular and subcellular mechanisms of post-cardiac arrest brain injury.
ATP … adenosine triphosphate, NMDA … N-methyl-D-aspartate receptor, AMPA … amino-3-hydroxy-5-metylisoxazole-4-propionate receptor, NO … nitric oxide, VMK … free fatty acids, ARCH … arachidonate, COX … cyclo-oxygenase, LOX … lipo-oxygenase, DNA … deoxyribonucleotic acid.

Triggering of the glutamate neuroexcitatory cascade plays a crucial role. Cardiac arrest leads to excessive glutamate release followed by an overflow of calcium to neurons via N-methyl-D-aspartate receptor stimulation. This is a potent trigger of the metabolic and inflammatory pathways causing neuronal necrosis and apoptosis. Increased intracellular calcium pool activates phosphatases and proteases, which causes neuronal damage, phospholipases responsible for oxygen free radical formation and nitric oxide synthase activation, which enhances proinflammatory nitric oxide production. Nitric oxide also opens the apoptotic pathway via activation of proapoptotic genes of the Bcl-2 family, causing mitochondrial damage, cytochrome C release, activation of caspases and endonucleases resulting in DNA fragmentation and programmed neuronal death. Glial cell activation potentiates an undesirable proinflammatory cascade. This very complex deleterious response to global cerebral ischemia is amplified by impaired cerebral perfusion due to failed blood flow autoregulation and by microthrombi formation in small vessels due to activated coagulation (Nolan et al., 2008).

Post-cardiac arrest systolic and diastolic myocardial dysfunction is a common phenomenon of multifactorial origin. It is supposed that decreased cardiac output may contribute to the unfavourable outcome (Laver et al., 2004). Myocardial stunning has been identified as the main underlying mechanism (Laurent et al., 2002; Checchia et al., 2003). Moreover, myocardial dysfunction may be worsened through the administration of high doses of adrenaline during CPR (Tang et al., 1995). On the other hand, post-cardiac arrest myocardial stunnig is a reversible condition and can be reversed by catecholamines (Vasquez et al., 2004).

Critical whole-body ischemia during cardiac arrest, even if followed by successful reperfusion, is a very potent trigger for the whole-body immune system response. It is termed the systemic inflammatory response syndrome (SIRS) and represents a serious condition related to systemic inflammation and organ dysfunction. The underlying mechanism for development of SIRS is induced cytokine storm accompanied by activation of leucocytes and platelets, endothelial dysfunction and coagulopathy. Relative acute adrenal insufficiency may worsen the course of the disease (Hékimian et al., 2004).

Cardiac arrest does not develop on it's own but it is a complication of other underlying diseases. Persistent precipitating pathology may have a negative impact on further outcome, especially when it is a critical disease like extensive acute myocardial infarction, massive pulmonary embolism, etc.

3. Underlying mechanisms of protection by therapeutic hypothermia

Hundreds of substances have been studied to find some with clinically signifiant neuroprotective effect. However, promising pilot experimental results were always followed by further experimental or clinical failure. It is generally considered that the main reason for failure is the complexity of ischemia-reperfusion injury which can not be attenuated or reversed by a substance affecting only one specific metabolic pathway. On the other side, hypothermia is a robust non-specific intervention having an impact on all processes of ischemia reperfusion injury simultaneously.

• antiedematic effect	• anti-inflammatory effect
adjustment of cerebral blood flow to metabolic demand	supression of oxygen free radical formation
reduction of vascular permeability	decrease of intracelullar calcium
blood-brain barrier stabilizing effect	supression of nitric oxide production
• cellular protection	supression of interleukin 6 production
dna preservation from oxygen free radical-mediated damage	reduces production of matrix metalloproteinases
cell membrane stabilizing effect	supress neutrophil and microglia activation
prevention of mitochondrial dysfunction	• supression of cerebral metabolism
• antiapoptotic effect	inhibition of glutamate excessive release
inhibition of caspase activation	decrease of oxygen and glucose consumption
prevention of cytochrome c release	attenuation of thermo-pooling phenomenon

Table 1. Proposed neuroprotective mechanisms of therapeutic hypothermia.

Hypothermia reduces cerebral metabolism by 7 % for each degree Celsius reduction in Body Temperature (BT) and reduces whole-body energy demand (Erecinska et al., 2003). Other mechanisms which play a role in hypothermia-induced neuroprotection are listed in table 1 (Ostadal, 2009; Polderman, 2009; Liu & Yenari, 2007; Busto et al., 2007; Kataoka & Yanase, 1998; Globus et al., 1995; Lei et al., 1994; Xu et al., 2002; Huang et al., 1999; Fischer et al., 1999).

4. Clinical studies

Even though the idea of neuroprotection by decreasing body core temperature is not new, its implementation became sustainable in 2002, when the results of two crucial randomized clinical trials were published. Both were of similar design and reached analogical results, strongly supporting post-cardiac arrest cooling (table 2).

The European Hypothermia After Cardiac Arrest (HACA) multicenter trial has been the largest one (Hypothermia after Cardiac Arrest Study Group, 2002). A total of 275 patients who had been resuscitated from cardiac arrest due to ventricular fibrillation or pulseless ventricular tachycardia was randomised to conventional therapy or to induced mild hypothermia of 32 - 34 °C for 24 hours. In addition to a significant neuroprotective clinical effect, mortality at 6 months was 41 % in the hypothermia group, as compared with 55 % in the normothermia group (RR 0.74; CI 95% 0.58-0.95, $p<0.05$).

In the Australian study by Bernard et al, 77 patients succesfully resuscitated from cardiac arrest of presumed cardiac arrest origin, having ventricular fibrillation or pulseless ventricular tachycardia as an initial rhythm,were assigned to mild hypothermia of 32 - 34 °C for 12 hours or to standard treatment (Bernard et al., 2002). In the hypothermia group, more patients reached the favourable neurological outcome (cerebral performance category score 1 or 2) at hospital discharge than in the control group. In both studies, there was no significant diference in the frequency of adverse events.

	HYPOTHERMIA GROUP (%)	STANDARD TREATMENT GROUP (%)	RELATIVE RISK	P
	favourable neurological outcome at hospital discharge			
HACA Study Group Trial	53	36	1.50	0.006
Bernard et al.	49	26	1.75	0.052
	favourable neurological outcome at 6 months			
HACA Study Group Trial	52	36	1.44	0.009

Table 2. Outcomes of therapeutic hypothermia in randomized clinical studies.

Following this, a series of clinical studies have confirmed a positive role of TH in post-cardiac arrest care. It was also shown that a close relation of TH with other interventions such as control of blood glucose, haemodynamics, ventilation and handling of seizures can improve long term survival of patients (Sunde et al., 2007; Knafelj et al., 2007; Nolan et al, 2009).

Analyses of the registries confirmed the results of clinical studies (Oksanen et al., 2007; Arrich, 2007). Several meta-analyses have however produced inconsistent results (table 3). While Holzer et al calculated that six patients have to be treated by TH to save one more life (95% CI 4–13, p < 0,05), Nielsens meta-analysis pointed out to some gaps in the evidence (Nielsen et al., 2010). Anyway, we have still quite firm evidence compared to other commonly used procedures in intensive care medicine.

AUTHOR	TYPE OF THE ANALYSIS	NUMBER OF THE PATIENTS	DISCHARGE NEUROLOGICAL OUTCOME	6 MONTHS NEUROLOGICAL OUTCOME	HOSPITAL MORTALITY
Arrich, 2008	registry	650	TH: 45%* NO TH: 32%	-	TH: 57%* NO TH: 32%
Oksanen et al., 2007	registry	1555	-	-	TH: 44,6%
Holzer et al., 2006	metaanalysis	385	RR 1.68, 95%CI 1.29–2.07 favouring TH*	RR 1.44, 95% CI 1.11–1.76 favouring TH*	-
Nielsen et al., 2010	metaanalysis	478	RR 0.78, 95% CI 0.64-0.95 favouring TH*		RR 0.84, 95%CI 0.70-1.01 favouring TH

TH…therapeutic hypothermia, RR…relative risk, CI…confidence interval, *…p<0.05

Table 3. The results of the analyses of the registries and metaanalyses.

5. Indications and contraindications

Therapeutic hypothermia is indicated in successfully resuscitated cardiac arrest patients, persistence of coma and requirement of mechanical ventilation. While there is good evidence supporting cooling of out-of-hospital adult cardiac arrest patients presenting with ventricular fibrillation, induction in other groups of in-hospital cardiac arrest patients, such as those with non-defibrillating initial rhythm and pediatric patients is supported by lower degrees of evidence (Holzer et al., 2006; Storm et al., 2008; Don et al., 2009; Polderman et al., 2003; Biarent et al., 2010; Testori et al., 2011). Nevertheless, clinical, experimental and patophysiological data suggest that hypothermia may also have protective effects in patients other than those with ventricular fibrillation OHCA. Therefore, it may be considered reasonable to also use TH in these groups.

Experimental data suggest that TH should be started as soon as possible after ROSC. Thus, in OHCA patients, pre-hospital initiation of cooling appears to be a method of choice and this is discussed further. On the contrary, there is weak evidence of what is an acceptable delay from ROSC to start chilling. It is generally considered that it should not be delayed more than 6 hours.

There is not any general agreement on contraindications to TH and there are differences among the guidelines. However, Table 4 lists all conditions we should keep in mind.

CONTRAINDICATIONS TO THERAPEUTIC HYPOTHERMIA
• established multiple organ failure or underlying terminal illness
• pre-existing coagulopathy
• severe systemic infection
• severe active bleeding
• patient conscious after short cardiopulmonary resuscitation
• do-not-resuscitate or do-not-intubate status
• coma of origin other than cardiac arrest
• circulatory failure defined as hypotension irresponsive to volume expansion and/or vasopressoric support and/or mechanical circulatory support
• cardiac arrest of traumatic origin
• preexisting hypothermia <34 °C
• pregnancy

Table 4. Contraindications of therapeutic hypothermia.

The use of TH in children has been classified as a class IIb recommendation by pediatric guidelines 2005 and the recent guidelines have accepted this treatment in children too (Polderman et al., 2001; Losert et al., 2008). Therefore, pediatric cardiac arrest patients should not be excluded from the candidates for PTH.

6. Therapeutic hypothermia in the setting of acute myocardial infarction and PCI

Acute myocardial infarction (AMI) is the most common cause of cardiac arrest.. In a patient with cardiac arrest caused by AMI, there may arise several questions:

- What is more important and what should be prefered – TH or percutaneous coronary intervention (PCI)?
- Does TH induction interfere with the angiographic result of PCI?
- Should the patient planned for TH be treated by antithrombotics and / or thrombolytics?
- What is the impact of TH on myocardial function altered by AMI and cardiac arrest?

First, it should be noticed that successfully resuscitated cardiac arrest patient with AMI must be considered as a critically ill patient in general and not onlyanAMI patient. Therefore, PCI must not cause a delay of initiation of cooling and it is even more paramount vice versa. Performance of both procedures in parallel has been shown to be feasible and safe and PCI centers should establish TH in the catheterization laboratory as routine procedure (Koester et al., 2011). The use of common cooling methods do not interfere with the procedure of cardiac catheterisation.

Second, there is evidence, that the concomitant use of TH does not compromise angiographic results of PCI (Noc, 2010). Moreover, several studies have demonstrated, that

PCI performed during TH is not associated with an increased rate of major bleeding events (Schefold et al., 2009; Knafelj et al., 2007). It is an important issue because major bleeding has been shown to be a strong predictor of mortality in patients after PCI (Manoukian et al., 2007).

Third, it has been shown that antithrombotic and / or fibrinolytic therapy may be administered as the part of complex post-cardiac arrest care including therapeutic hypothermia. It is not a contraindication to TH and it should be used in accordance with the recent guidelines regardless of cooling (Van de Werf et al., 2008; Torbicki et al., 2008). On the other hand, most enzymatic processes in the body exhibit temperature dependency. Pilot studies presented alterations in the pharmacokinetics of many drugs used in critical care during TH. Antithrombotics are not an exclusion (table 5). Further studies are neccessary to tailor its dosage regimen for the specific conditions during TH.

AUTHOR	DRUG	EFECT OF HYPOTHERMIA ON METABOLISM
Michelson et al., 1999	aspirin	aspirin did not significantly augment hypothermia-induced platelet dysfunction in vivo
Bjelland et al., 2010	clopidogrel	in patients with hypothermia, absence of effect on day 1 after administration, with some improvement on day 3
Frelinger AL et al., 2003	glycoprotein IIb/IIIa antagonist	mild hypothermia augments eptifibatide- and tirofiban- but not abciximab-induced inhibition of platelet aggregation

Table 5. Effects of hypothermia on pharmacokinetics and pharmacodynamics of antithrombotics.

Fourth, it has been previously described that post-cardiac arrest myocardial dysfunction is a common phenomenon. In AMI patients, apart from myocardial stunning, myocardial ischemia due to coronary artery occlusion can play a role. There are several experimental and clinical data that TH does not ameliorate post-cardiac arrest myocardial dysfunction (Murphy et al, 2010; Hsu et al., 2009). Nevertheless, there is a room for further investigation. Complex hemodynamic clinical presentation of patients post-cardiac arrest can be the shock syndrome. It is a condition reflecting not only myocardial dysfunction but also systemic ischemia-reperfusion injury. A few studies have reported on the feasibility of TH in the setting of cardiogenic shock (Hovdenes et al., 2007; Skulec et al., 2008). Further investigation is needed but TH should be always considered in circulatory unstable patients who are responsive to volume expansion and/or vasopressoric support and/or mechanical circulatory support.

7. Protocol for practicing therapeutic mild hypothermia

Accurate and safe practicing of TH following a written protocol is a prerequisite for achieving optimal neuroprotective effect. Till now, only few papers summarizing practical procedural issues of the TH procedure in detail have been published (Bianchin et al., 2009; Škulec et al., 2010). Local therapeutic protocols differ from one to the other.

There are four phases of the therapeutic hypothermia protocol: cooling phase, maintenance phase, rewarming phase and period of control of normothermia (Figure 2).

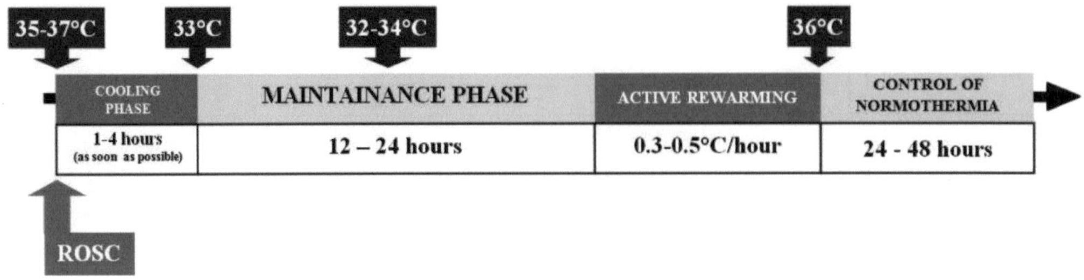

Fig. 2. The protocol for practicing therapeutic hypothermia.
ROSC...return of spontaneous circulation.

During the cooling phase, the aim is to reach the target therapeutic temperature of 33 °C as soon as possible after the return of spontaneous circulation. This is followed by BT regulation in the therapeutic range of 32 - 34 °C for 12 - 24 hours. In randomized clinical studies, both TH durations were associated with an improved outcome. It is not known, whether one protocol is better than the other or if cooling for a longer time is better. However, durations shorter than 12 hours should be avoided. It is advisable to beware of overcooling below 32 °C for its potential association with worse outcome (Merchant et al, 2006; Škulec et al., 2008). The rewarming phase is as important as the maintenance of TH. The rewarming should not be a passive but rather an active process resulting in slow and controlled reaching of normothermia with a rewarming rate of 0.1–0.33°C/hour (Seder & Van der Kloot, 2009). It can be performed by the same technique that was used for chilling. Once a BT of 36 °C is reached, normothermia should be controlled carefully for up to 48 hours since further hypothermia may worsen the outcome.

In the course of cooling, adequate sedation should be tailored for suppression of involuntary shivering. In some patients, neuromuscular blockade can be required during the cooling and maintenance phases (Hékimian et al., 2004). In the next phases, muscle paralysis should be strictly individual to avoid adverse effects of lengthy neuromuscular blockade. After rewarming, sedatives, analgesics, and muscle relaxants should be discontinued and standard intensive care should be provided. Other drugs decreasing the shivering threshold are buspirone and meperidine.

Induction of hypothermia can evoke metabolic disturbances, especially hypokalemia, hypomagnesemia, hypophosphatemia, hypocalcemia and hyperglycemia (Michelson et al., 1994; Polderman et al., 2001; Losert et al., 2008). Therefore, regular measurements are advisable. While potassium and magnesium supplementation is favourable during the maintenance phase, calcium may worsen ischemia-reperfusion injury and permissive hypocalcemia may be tolerated. However, mild hypokalemia may be tolerated to avoid excessive increase of Potassium during rewarming. Control of Glucose levels should follow conventional rather than strict targets.

Decrease of body temperature is physiologically associated with haemodynamic changes. Relative and absolute hypovolemia, bradycardia, decrease of arterial blood pressure and cardiac output are common. In general, it is impossible to distinguish these changes from those induced by cardiac arrest and the precipitating pathology. Anyhow, early goal directed therapy approach should be applied (Table 6), using standard procedures of volume expansion, vasopressor and/or inotropic support and/or mechanical circulatory support (Cvachovec et al., 2009).

mean arterial pressure (mm Hg)	65 – 100
systolic blood pressure (mm Hg)	> 100
central venous pressure (mm Hg)	8 – 12
diuresis (ml/kg/hour)	1
central venous oxygen saturation (%)	> 70

Table 6. Goals for early directed therapy in cardiac arrest survivors.

Peptic ulcer and deep vein thrombosis prophylaxis, oral care, positioning, ventilator setting assessment govern the same indications as in critically ill patients in general. There have been no publications recommending the timing and selection of suitable formulation of clinical nutrition in cardiac arrest patients. In most cases, it is initiated immediately after completion of the TH process (Škulec et al., 2010).

Monitoring the body core temperature (BT) should be continuous with a probe inserted in the pulmonary artery, rectum, urinary bladder or oesophagus. Pulmonary artery catheter is considered to be the gold standard for BT measurement but this should not be the only indication of pulmonary artery catheter insertion. In the absence of other conditions such as the need for invasive haemodynamic monitoring, an alternative approach should be used. Tympanic temperature is an acceptable for pre-hospital monitoring.

Key principles for proper practicing of TH are to keep patients deeply sedated to suppress shivering and watch for potential side effects of TH carefully.

8. Cooling methods

Currently, there is a wide range of cooling techniques available. They can be classified into two major groups - the methods inducing whole body hypothermia and the methods primarily targeted to local brain cooling (Table 7) (Škulec et al., 2009). The latter should be considered as a supplementary approach because evidence for outcome benefit has been registered only for whole body cooling.

In spite of the unproven superiority of device-based cooling techniques (endovascular catheter cooling, surface cooling via mattress or cooling pads), it is convenient for several reasons when compared with conventional approaches (surface cooling via ice-packs, cold intravenous infusion, cold gastric or urinary bladder lavage). It provides more reliable maintenance of target temperature including less indidence of overcooling, it is more friendly for nursing and allows control of BT even in the phase of controlled normothermia (Hoedemaekers et al., 2007; Škulec et al., 2009). However, it must be stressed that this does not disqualify conventional methods from routine practice. Pivotal clinical studies were based on simple surface cooling and its low cost predetermines it to serve as a starting method for new TH users (Hypothermia after Cardiac Arrest Study Group, 2002; Bernard et al., 2002).

METHOD	COOLING RATE	INCIDENCE OF OVERCOOLING	CLINICAL EVIDENCE	FINANCIAL COSTS
		WHOLE-BODY HYPOTHERMIA		
• **surface cooling**				
• **ice-packs**	+	+++	+++	€
• **water cooling mattress**	++	++	+++	€€
• **air cooling mattress**	+	+++	+	€€
• **special cooling pads**	++	++	+	€€
• **cold air flow**	?	?	-	€
• **RIVA**	+++	++	+++	€
• **cold gastric / urinary bladder lavage**	?	?	-	€
• **cold peritoneal lavage**	?	?	-	?
• **endovascular cathether cooling**	++	+	+++	€€€
• **extracorporal circuit device**	+++	?	+	€€€
		LOCAL BRAIN COOLING		
• **intranasal cooling**	+ (++ brain)	?	+++	?
• **cooling cap / helmet**	+ (++ brain)	?	+	?

RIVA...rapid intravenous administration of cold crystalloids
+...low cooling rate, incidence of overcooling or clinical evidence, +++...high cooling rate, incidence of overcooling or clinical evidence, €...low financial costs, €€€...high financial costs

Table 7. Cooling methods.

Surface cooling techniques are used most commonly. There is a variety of different modifications: simple ice-packs, more effective manufactured precooled special pads and sophisticated devices with automated feedback control of BT, chilling via gel pads or a cooling mattress (figures 3 and 4).

The method of rapid intravenous administration of cold crystalloids (RIVA) has been found efficient, simple and safe. Infusion of 15 - 30 ml/kg of 4 °C cold crystalloid (normal saline, Ringer solution, Hartmann solution) at an infusion rate >60 ml/h may induce the decrease of BT >1.4 °C (Kim et al., 2005; Kim et al., 2007; Kliegel et al., 2005; Kliegel et al., 2007; Virkkunen et al., 2004; Kämäräinen et al., 2008; Bernard & Rosalion, 2008; Bruel et al., 2008; Polderman et al., 2005; Vanden Hoek et al., 2004). However, additional cooling techniques are necessary for TH maintainance (Kliegel et al., 2007).

Endovascular catheter cooling is a highly sophisticated method of invasive cooling with a cooling rate 1.0 - 1.5 °C/h (Škulec et al., 2009). It is performed by inserting the cooling catheter into the inferior vena cava using the femoral approach. Circulation of cold normal saline through the catheter is directed by an extracorporeal unit to reach a satisfactory cooling rate and an excellent temperature stability of the patient (figure 5) (Hoedemaekers et al., 2007).

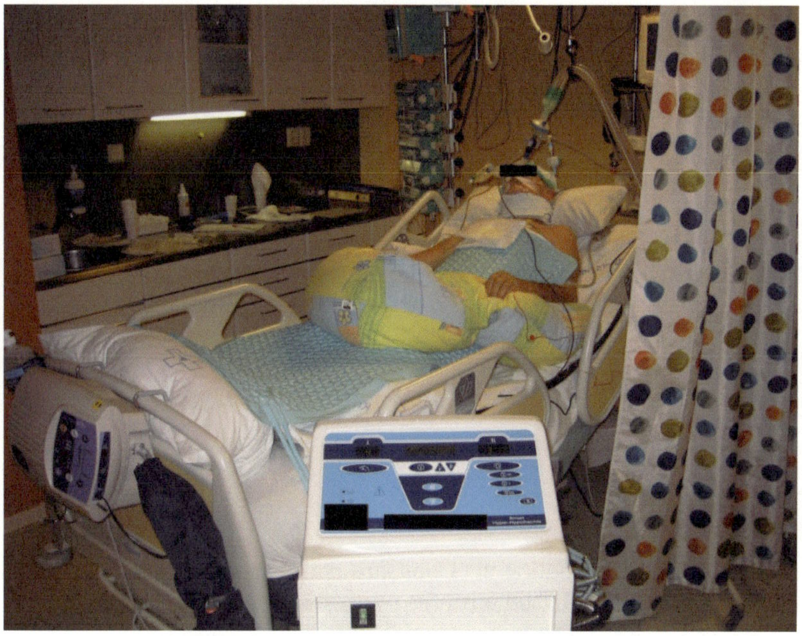

Fig. 3. Watter cooling mattress system Blanketrol III, Cincinnati Sub-Zero Products, Inc., Cincinnati, USA. Published with the permission of P. Telekes, M.D., Cardiac Center, Liberec Hospital, Czech republic.

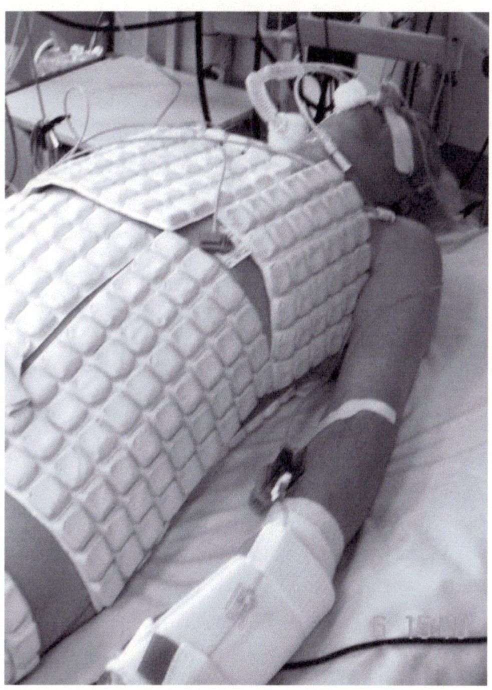

Fig. 4. Highly effective cooling pads EMCOOLS pad, EMCOOLS, Emergency Medical Cooling Systems AG, Vienna, Austria, with the permission.

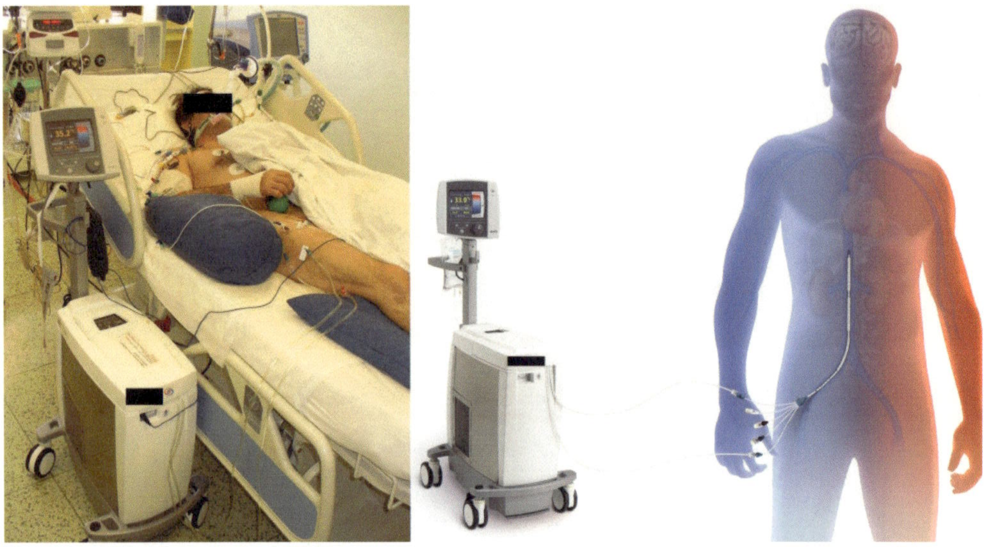

Fig. 5. Endovascular catheter cooling via CoolGard 3000TM and Icy femoral cathether TM, Alsius Corp., Irvine, USA. Published with the permission of P. Ostadal, M.D., PhD., Department of Cardiology, Na Homolce Hospital, Czech republic.

It can be used also for controlling normothermia after the rewarming phase and guide the patients through the whole early post-resuscitation period. Cooling efficacy and safety was documented not only for cardiac arrest patients but also for patients with traumatic brain injury, stroke and acute myocardial infarction (Diringer et al., 2004; Schmutzhard et al., 2002; Lyden et al., 2005; Guluma et al., 2008; Georgiadis et al., 2001; Keller et al., 2003; De Georgia et al., 2004; Dixon et al., 2002; Kandzari et al., 2004; Stone et al., 2006). Dixon et al. randomized 42 patients with AMI to primary PCI with or without endovascular cooling (target core temperature 33 degrees C) for 3 hours after reperfusion. Reduction of infarct size ws not identifyed but the study confirmed the safety of endovascular cooling as an adjunct to primary PCI. Kandzari et al. reached similar results in a nonrandomized study of 18 patients.

Intranasal cooling is a new and safe method to easily cool down the brain. It is a very simple method with minimal burdening of the staff (Castrén et al., 2010). Like RIVA, it is convenient for the rapid induction of TH and suitable for pre-hospital care and emergency medicine departments.

There are many other experimental thermoregulatory methods. Some of them, like cardiopulmonary bypass, femorocarotic bypass with extracorporeal cooling of blood, peritoneal cooling or total liquid ventilation cooling are too invasive and/or complicated in comparison with the current effective techniques (Reed et al., 2002; Mori et al., 2001; Hong et al., 2002; Xiao et al., 1995). The others are just in the beginning of their development and perhaps represent the future. On the gate of science-fiction stands the possibility of pharmacological induction of hibernation. Hibernation is a behavioural, physiological, and molecular adaptation exhibited by diverse mammalian species to withstand protracted periods or seasons of insufficient or unpredictable food availability (Kelly, 2007). Distribution of this process amongst different species argues that hibernation genes required for hibernation are common to all mammals (Srere et al., 1992). Such capacity to profoundly decrease the metabolic demand of organs and tissues has the potential to translate into a novel approach to prevention of ischemia-reperfusion injury. Neurotensin and its analogies are studied as potential triggers of this process (Schneider et al., 2006).

9. Side effects of cooling

TH treatment may be associated with adverse events (Table 8) (Polderman et al., 2009; Skulec et al., 2008; Nielsen et al., 2009). These are related to the cooling device or caused by hypothermia itself. While the former are rare, the latter are quite common. However, we should keep in mind the fact that some of them are physiological responses to hypothermia rather than avderse events.

	FREQUENCY (%)
pneumonia	40 - 50
any arrhythmias	33
recurrence of cardiac arrest	7 - 11
metabolic disturbances	
sustained hyperglycaemia >8 mmol/l	37
hypokalaemia <3 mmol/l	18
hypomagnesaemia	18
hypophosphataemia	19
hyperamylasaemia	12
seizures	24
major bleeding	3 - 6
sepsis	4

Table 8. Adverse effects of therapeutic hypothermia (Nielsen et al., 2009).

Often, it is not possible to distinguish whether the event is caused by hypothermia or by post-cardiac arrest syndrome itself. This is especially the case of post-cardiac arrest shock syndrome. It may affect as much as 18 - 50% of cardiac arrest patients. Although TH induces cold diuresis, hypovolemia, bradycardia and decrease of cardiac output, post-cardiac arrest myocardial dysfunction and precipitating pathology arises independently of TH and all must be treated together. It was shown that TH does not worsen the course of the disease even in the presence of shock syndrome (Škulec et al., 2008). Pneumonia, cardiac arrhythmias, metabolite disturbances and seizures have been identified as the most common adverse events of cooling.

Recently, Nielsen et al analyzed a set of 765 patients and identified that sustained hyperglycaemia and seizures are associated with increased mortality while other adverse events are not (Nielsen et al., 2011). Randomized clinical studies showed comparable incidence of adverse events except for pneumonia and sepsis, which exhibited a trend of increased appearance in cooled patients (Hypothermia after Cardiac Arrest Study Group, 2002; Bernard et al., 2002).

Device related adverse events depend on the cooling method. Surface cooling may be complicated by frostbite, the RIVA method may lead to volume overload and pulmonary oedema, endovascular catheter cooling may be complicated by deep venous thrombosis (Škulec et al., 2009). The occurance of these can be minimalized by proper and careful practicing of TH.

10. Complex post-cardiac arrest intensive care

An intensivist should be aware of the fact that TH is not a self-salvable technique after cardiac arrest. Care must be contextualized to the complex neuroprotective and cardioprotective post-cardiac arrest support. The main components are:

- therapeutic hypothermia,
- urgent coronary angiography and PCI if indicated,
- control of blood glucose,
- early haemodynamic goal-directed therapy,
- control of normoventilation,
- control of seizures.

It has been shown by Sunde et al that a transition from the conventional passive approach to the standardised active treatment protocol including all mentioned items can improve prognosis of the patients (Sunde et al., 2007). Further studies have confirmed this observation (Škulec et al., 2008; Tømte et al., 2011; Werling et al., 2007). Thus, it is of major importance to consider every cardiac arrest patient as to be like any other critically ill patient requiring complex, active and protocolized therapy, beyond the scope of isolated TH procedure.

The most sophisticated component of such approach is the ensurance of availability of immediate coronary angiography and PCI. At present, the discussion is held whether all OHCA patients should be transfered to cardiac arrest centers with PCI facility or not. To answer this question needs further studies. Nevertheless, all patients with supposed cardiac origin of cardiac arrest are candidates of such approach and those with ST elevation acute myocardial infarction undoubtly.

There is an association between post-cardiac arrest hyperglycaemia and poor neurological outcome. However, tight glucose control (4.5 - 6.0 mmol/l) should not be practiced after cardiac arrest because of the increased risk of hypoglycaemia. Blood glucose should be maintained at ≤10mmol/l (Padkin, 2009; Deakin et al., 2010).

Early haemodynamic goal-directed therapy has been shown to improve prognosis of patients with severe sepsis and septic shock (Rivers et al., 2001). There is limited evidence that this approach can be also benefitial to cardiac arrest survivors (Gaieski et al., 2009). Reasonable goals are listed in table 4.

Several reasons make control of normoventilation an important part of post-cardiac arrest care. Firstly, while during cardiopulmonary resuscitation we should maintain FIO_2 of 1.0, it is not the setting for post-cardiac arrest care. There is a body of preclinical evidence that hyperoxia may worsen neuronal ischemia-reperfusion injury by augmenting oxidative stress (Balan et al., 2006). On this basis, it is recommended to eliminate hypoxia but unnecessary hyperoxia should be avoided. This can be achieved by adjusting the FiO_2 to produce an arterial oxygen saturation of 94 - 96% (Nolan et al., 2008). Secondly, in brain-injured patients, cerebral vasoconstriction caused by hyperventilation may induce cerebral ischaemia (Coles et al., 2007). Hyperventilation also decrease cardiac output via increased intrathoracic pressure (Aufderheide & Lurie, 2004). On the other hand, hypoventilation may cause hypoxia and hypercapnia could increase intracranial pressure and cause acidosis. Therefore, ventilation should be adjusted to achieve normocapnia and should be monitored by regular measurement of arterial blood gas values (Nolan et al., 2008).

Seizures and/or myoclonus occur in 10–40% of succesfully resuscitated comatose cardiac arrest patients. It increases oxygen demand dramaticaly and may aggravate neurological injury (Ingvar, 1986). It should be treated after the first event and followed by maintainance therapy. Drugs of choice are benzodiazepines, phenytoin, sodium valproate, propofol, or a barbiturate (Nolan et al., 2008). Preventive treatment has not been studied yet.

Treatment of other conditions like adrenal dysfunction, organ dysfunctions and infection therapy do not differ from common practice in critically ill patients.

11. Pre-hospital cooling

It has been recommended that the target therapeutic temperature should be reached as soon as possible (Safar, 2002). In successfully resuscitated out-of-hospital cardiac arrest (OHCA) patients, pre-hospital initiation of cooling appears to be the method of choice. However, initiation of cooling in the field is not a simple shift of in-hospital procedure to pre-hospital area. A pre-hospital emergency team frequently operates in demanding conditions and is engaged in the process of cardiopulmonary resuscitation, early post-cardiac arrest stabilisation and decision on transport direction. Therefore, pre-hospital cooling calls for a very simple, efficient and safe cooling method and its usage should not cause a transport delay. A background of regional hospitals practicing TH is essential to ensure cooling continuity.

A few studies demonstrating the efficacy and safety of this strategy, predominantly for the RIVA method, have been published (Kim et al., 2007; Kämäräinen et al., 2008). When performed properly, it can decrease BT by >1.4 °C during transport. Moreover, a dose of 10 - 20 ml/kg of cold normal saline can contribute to hemodynamic stabilization. In addition, this way of cooling exhibits an excelent safety profile with minimal risk of volume overload. Considering its simplicity and low costs, the RIVA method is the first choice for pre-hospital cooling (Figure 6).

A major barrier for a wide recommendation of pre-hospital cooling in successfully resuscitated OHCA patients is the absence of clear evidence of the outcome benefit. Apparently, improved survival is not related to pre-hospital hypothermia itself but to the close coupling of PTH with its in-hospital continuation (Škulec et al., 2010; Castrén et al., 2010). In any case, a large randomized trial is required.

Considering the pros and cons, at present, in the setting of proper collaboration of the emergency medical service and the target in-hospital facility, it is justifiable to implement prehospital cooling even in the absence of unambiguous evidence to support this practice.

Other possibilities suitable for pre-hospital cooling include surface cooling via manufactured cooling pads and intanasal local brain cooling.

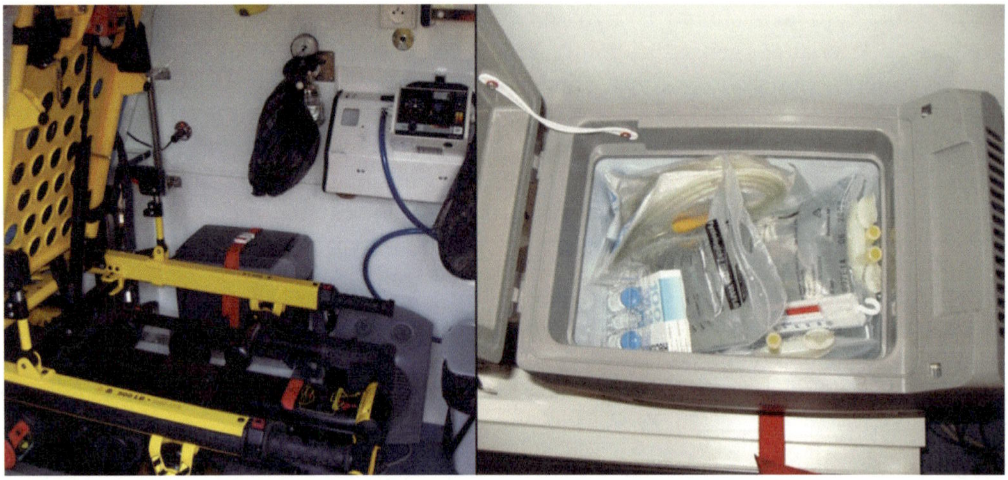

Fig. 6. Refrigerator in the ambulance car with supply of cold saline.

12. Worldwide implementation of therapeutic hypothermia

Nine years have elapsed since randomized clinical studies allowing the use of TH were published. During this period, in-hospital TH utilisation has varied from 8 to 95 % in different countries until now (figure 7) (Škulec et al., 2010).

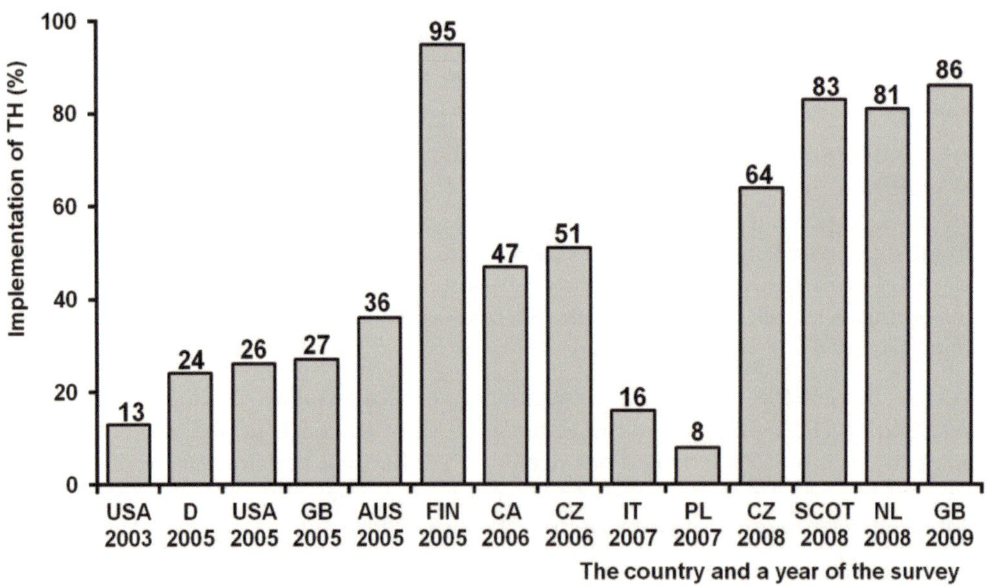

Fig. 7. TH implementation in different countries in the last years.
USA…United States of America, D…Germany, GB…Great Britain, AUS…Australia, FIN…Finland, CA…Canada, CZ…Czech republic, PL…Poland, SCOT…Scotland, NL…Netherlands, TH…therapeutic mild hypothermia

More or less, implementation has increased over the years. Nevertheless, there are a lot of challenges and room for improvement. Firstly, effort should be focused on enhancing the frequency of TH application in every ICU. Secondly, unavailability of cooling techniques should not be a barrier for TH implementation, it is reliable to start with low-cost simple conventional cooling methods (RIVA, surface cooling). Thirdly, growth of TH implementation has to progress hand in hand with the quality of provided care. The method must be protocol-guided, respecting clear indications and contraindications and applying complex neuroprotective and cardioprotective post-cardiac arrest care.

13. Alternative thermoregulation strategies in cardiac arrest survivors

There are two alternative thermoregulation neuroprotective strategies other than post-cardiac arrest cooling: intra-arrest cooling and a principle of emergency preservation and resuscitation (also called suspended reanimation).

Animals experiments showed that early intra-arrest initiation of cooling resulted in significantly better neurological outcome than cooling after return of spontaneous circulation (Abella et al., 2004; Kuboyama et al., 1993). This concept was also evaluated in a few clinical studies. RIVA method was very effective but clinical outcome was inconclusive (Kämäräinen et al., 2008; Bruel et al., 2008). More promising seems to be the method of intranasal cooling. The recent PRINCE study revealed its safety, effectivity and suggested outcome improvement (Castrén et al., 2010). A large outcome trial is ongoing. Nevertheless, it must be stressed that intra-arrest cooling intervenes in standard cardiopulmonary resuscitation while cooling after return of spontaneous circulation does not. Therefore, inta-arrest cooling should be reserved only for clinical studies, until the clinical benefit is clearly proved.

Emergency preservation and resuscitation is a novel approach supposed to treat victims of exsanguination cardiac arrest. Management is to be as follows: a cold aortic flush is used to induce deep hypothermic preservation in the field followed by transport to hospital facility for emergent surgical treatment and delayed resuscitation with cardiopulmonary bypass (Drabek, 2007). This approach has been tested in animal experiments and stands at door of clinical studies.

14. References

Abella BS, Zhao D, Alvarado J, Hamann K, Vanden Hoek TL, Becker LB. (2004). Intra-arrest cooling improves outcomes in a murine cardiac arrest model. *Circulation*,109:2786-2791.

Arrich, J. (2007). European Resuscitation Council Hypothermia After Cardiac Arrest Registry Study Group. Clinical application of mild therapeutic hypothermia after cardiac arrest. *Crit Care Med*,35:1041–1047.

Atwood C, Eisenberg MS, Herlitz J, Rea TD. (2005). Incidence of EMS-treated out-of-hospital cardiac arrest in Europe. *Resuscitation*,67:75-80.

Aufderheide TP, Lurie KG. (2004). Death by hyperventilation: a common and life-threatening problem during cardiopulmonary resuscitation. *Crit Care Med*,32:S345-S351.

Balan IS, Fiskum G, Hazelton J, Cotto-Cumba C, Rosenthal RE. (2006). Oximetry-guided reoxygenation improves neurological outcome after experimental cardiac arrest. *Stroke*,37:3008–3013.

Bernard SA, Gray TW, Buist MD, Jones BM, Silvester W, Gutteridge G, Smith K. (2002). Treatment of comatose survivors of out-of-hospital cardiac arrest with induced hypothermia. *N Engl J Med*,346: 557-563.

Bernard SA, Rosalion A. (2008). Therapeutic hypothermia induced during cardiopulmonary resuscitation using large-volume, ice-cold intravenous fluid. *Resuscitation*,76: 311-313.

Bianchin A, Pellizzato N, Martano L, Castioni CA. (2009). Therapeutic hypothermia in Italian intensive care units: a national survey. *Minerva Anestesiol*,75:357-362.

Biarent D, Bingham R, Eich C, López-Herce J, Maconochie I, Rodríguez-Núñez A, Rajka T, Zideman D. (2010). European Resuscitation Council Guidelines for Resuscitation 2010 Section 6. Paediatric life support. *Resuscitation*,81:1364-1388.

Bjelland TW, Hjertner Ø, Klepstad P, Kaisen K, Dale O, Haugen BO. (2010). Antiplatelet effect of clopidogrel is reduced in patients treated with therapeutic hypothermia after cardiac arrest. *Resuscitation*,81:1627-1631.

Bruel C, Parienti JJ, Marie W, Arrot X, Daubin C, Du Cheyron D, Massetti M, Charbonneau P. (2008). Mild hypothermia during advanced life support: a preliminary study in out-of-hospital cardiac arrest. *Crit Care*,12: R31.

Busto R, Globus MY, Dietrich WD, Martinez E, Valdés I, Ginsberg MD. (1989). Effect of mild hypothermia on ischemia-induced release of neurotransmitters and free fatty acids in rat brain. *Stroke*,20:904-910.

Castrén M, Nordberg P, Svensson L, Taccone F, Vincent JL, Desruelles D, Eichwede F, Mols P, Schwab T, Vergnion M, Storm C, Pesenti A, Pachl J, Guérisse F, Elste T, Roessler M, Fritz H, Durnez P, Busch HJ, Inderbitzen B, Barbut D. (2010). Intra-arrest transnasal evaporative cooling: a randomized, prehospital, multicenter study (PRINCE: Pre-ROSC IntraNasal Cooling Effectiveness). *Circulation*,122:729-736.

Checchia PA, Sehra R, Moynihan J, Daher N, Tang W, Weil MH. (2003). Myocardial injury in children following resuscitation after cardiac arrest. *Resuscitation*,57:131-137.

Coles JP, Fryer TD, Coleman MR, Smielewski P, Gupta AK, Minhas PS, Aigbirhio F, Chatfield DA, Williams GB, Boniface S, Carpenter TA, Clark JC, Pickard JD, Menon DK. (2007). Hyperventilation following head injury: effect on ischemic burden and cerebral oxidative metabolism. *Crit Care Med*,35:568–578.

Cvachovec, K., Černý, V., Dostál, P, et al.; Czech Society of Anaesthesiology and Intensive Care Medicine CLS JEP, Czech Society of Intensive Medicine CLS JEP, Czech Society for Emergency and Disaster Medicine CLS JEP. (2009). Consensual statement for the application of therapeutic hypothermia. *Anest Intenziv Med*,20:221-224.

De Georgia MA, Krieger DW, Abou-Chebl A, Devlin TG, Jauss M, Davis SM, Koroshetz WJ, Rordorf G, Warach S. (2004). Cooling for Acute Ischemic Brain Damage (COOL AID): a feasibility trial of endovascular cooling. *Neurology*,63: 312-317.

Deakin CD, Nolan JP, Soar J, Sunde K, Koster RW, Smith GB, Perkins GD. (2010). European Resuscitation Council Guidelines for Resuscitation 2010 Section 4. Adult advanced life support. *Resuscitation*,81:1305-1352.

Diringer MN, Neurocritical Care Fever Reduction Trial Group. (2004). Treatment of fever in the neurologic intensive care unit with a catheter-based heat exchange system. *Crit Care Med*,32:559-564.

Dixon SR, Whitbourn RJ, Dae MW, Grube E, Sherman W, Schaer GL, Jenkins JS, Baim DS, Gibbons RJ, Kuntz RE, Popma JJ, Nguyen TT, O'Neill WW. (2002). Induction of mild systemic hypothermia with endovascular cooling during primary percutaneous coronary intervention for acute myocardial infarction. *J Am Coll Cardiol*,40: 1928-1934.

Don CW, Longstreth WT Jr, Maynard C, Olsufka M, Nichol G, Ray T, Kupchik N, Deem S, Copass MK, Cobb LA, Kim F. (2009). Active surface cooling protokol to induce mild therapeutic hypothermia after out-of-hospital cardiac arrest: a retrospective before-and-after comparison in a single hospital. *Crit Care Med*,37:3062–3069.

Drabek T. (2007). Emergency Preservation and Resuscitation - new hope for traumatic cardiac arrest victims. *Anest Intenziv Med*,18: 351–356.

Edgren E, Hedstrand U, Kelsey S, Sutton-Tyrrell K, Safar P. (1994). Assessment of neurological prognosis in comatose survivors of cardiac arrest. BRCT I Study Group. *Lancet*,343:1055-1059.

Erecinska M, Thoresen M, Silver IA. (2003). Effects of hypothermia on energy metabolism in Mammalian central nervous system. *J Cereb Blood Flow Metab*,23:513-530.

Frelinger AL 3rd, Furman MI, Barnard MR, Krueger LA, Dae MW, Michelson AD. (2003). Combined effects of mild hypothermia and glycoprotein IIb/IIIa antagonists on platelet-platelet and leukocyte-platelet aggregation. *Am J Cardiol*,92:1099-1101.

Fischer S, Renz D, Wiesnet M, Schaper W, Karliczek GF. (1999). Hypothermia abolishes hypoxia-induced hyperpermeability in brain microvessel endothelial cells. *Brain Res Mol Brain Res*,74:135–144.

Gaieski DF, Band RA, Abella BS, Neumar RW, Fuchs BD, Kolansky DM, Merchant RM, Carr BG, Becker LB, Maguire C, Klair A, Hylton J, Goyal M. (2009). Early goal-directed hemodynamic optimization combined with therapeutic hypothermia in comatose survivors of out-of-hospital cardiac arrest. *Resuscitation*,80:418-424.

Georgiadis D, Schwarz S, Kollmar R, Schwab S. (2001). Endovascular cooling for moderate hypothermia in patients with acute stroke: first results of a novel approach. *Stroke*,32:2550-2553.

Globus MY, Busto R, Lin B, Schnippering H, Ginsberg MD. (1995). Detection of free radical activity during transient global ischemia and recirculation: effects of intraischemic brain temperature modulation. *J Neurochem*,65:1250-1256.

Guluma KZ, Oh H, Yu SW, Meyer BC, Rapp K, Lyden PD. (2008). Effect of endovascular hypothermia on acute ischemic edema: morphometric analysis of the ICTuS trial. *Neurocrit Care*,8:42-47.

Hékimian G, Baugnon T, Thuong M, Monchi M, Dabbane H, Jaby D, Rhaoui A, Laurent I, Moret G, Fraisse F, Adrie C. (2004). Cortisol levels and adrenal reserve after successful cardiac arrest resuscitation. *Shock*,22:116-119.

Hoedemaekers CW, Ezzahti M, Gerritsen A, van der Hoeven JG. (2007). Comparison of cooling methods to induce and maintain normo–and hypothermia in intensive care unit patients: a prospective intervention study. *Crit Care*,11:R91-R94.

Holzer M, Müllner M, Sterz F, Robak O, Kliegel A, Losert H, Sodeck G, Uray T, Zeiner A, Laggner AN. (2006). Efficacy and safety of endovascular cooling after cardiac arrest: cohort study and Bayesian approach. *Stroke*,37:1792–1797.

Holzer M, Bernard SA, Hachimi-Idrissi S, Roine RO, Sterz F, Müllner M; Collaborative Group on Induced Hypothermia for Neuroprotection After Cardiac Arrest. (2005). Hypothermia for neuroprotection after cardiac arrest: systematic review and individual patient data meta-analysis. *Crit Care Med*,33:414-418.

Hong SB, Koh Y, Shim TS, Lee SD, Kim WS, Kim DS, Kim WD, Lim CM. (2002). Physiologic characteristics of cold perfluorocarbon-induced hypothermia during partial liquid ventilation in normal rabbits. *Anesth Analg*,94: 157–162.

Hovdenes J, Laake JH, Aaberge L, Haugaa H, Bugge JF. (2007). Therapeutic hypothermia after out-of-hospital cardiac arrest: experiences with patients treated with percutaneous coronary intervention and cardiogenic shock. *Acta Anaesthesiol Scand*,51:137-142.

Hsu CY, Huang CH, Chang WT, Chen HW, Cheng HJ, Tsai MS, Wang TD, Yen ZS, Lee CC, Chen SC, Chen WJ. (2009). Cardioprotective effect of therapeutic hypothermia for postresuscitation myocardial dysfunction. *Shock*,32:210-216.

Huang ZG, Xue D, Preston E, Karbalai H, Buchan AM. (1999). Biphasic opening of the blood-brain barrier following transient focal ischemia: effects of hypothermia. *Can J Neurol Sci*,26:298–304.

Hypothermia after Cardiac Arrest Study Group. (2002). Mild therapeutic hypothermia to improve the neurologic outcome after cardiac arrest. *N Engl J Med*,346: 549-556.

Ingvar M. (1986). Cerebral blood flow and metabolic rate during seizures. Relationship to epileptic brain damage. *Ann NY Acad Sci*,462:194–206.

Kämäräinen A, Virkkunen I, Tenhunen J, Yli-Hankala A, Silfvast T. (2008). Prehospital induction of therapeutic hypothermia during CPR: a pilot study. *Resuscitation*,76:360-363.

Kandzari DE, Chu A, Brodie BR, Stuckey TA, Hermiller JB, Vetrovec GW, Hannan KL, Krucoff MW, Christenson RH, Gibbons RJ, Sigmon KN, Garg J, Hasselblad V, Collins K, Harrington RA, Berger PB, Chronos NA, Hochman JS, Califf RM. (2004). Feasibility of endovascular cooling as an adjunct to primary percutaneous coronary intervention (results of the LOWTEMP pilot study). *Am J Cardiol*,93:636-639.

Kataoka K, Yanase H. (1998). Mild hypothermia--a revived countermeasure against ischemic neuronal damages. *Neurosci Res*,32:103-117.

Keller E, Imhof HG, Gasser S, Terzic A, Yonekawa Y. (2003). Endovascular cooling with heat exchange catheters: a new method to induce and maintain hypothermia. *Intensive Care Med*,29:939-943.

Kelly LD. (2007). Central nervous system regulation of mammalian hibernation: implications for metabolic suppression and ischemia tolerance. *Journal of Neurochemistry*,102,1713–1726.

Kim F, Olsufka M, Carlbom D, Deem S, Longstreth WT Jr, Hanrahan M, Maynard C, Copass MK, Cobb LA. (2005). Pilot study of rapid infusion of 2 L of 4 degrees C normal saline for induction of mild hypothermia in hospitalized, comatose survivors of out-of-hospital cardiac arrest. *Circulation*,112: 715-719.

Kim F, Olsufka M, Longstreth WT Jr, Maynard C, Carlbom D, Deem S, Kudenchuk P, Copass MK, Cobb LA. (2007). Pilot randomized clinical trial of prehospital induction of mild hypothermia in out-of-hospital cardiac arrest patients with a rapid infusion of 4 degrees C normal saline. *Circulation*,115: 3064-3070.

Kliegel A, Losert H, Sterz F, Kliegel M, Holzer M, Uray T, Domanovits H. (2005). Cold simple intravenous infusions preceding special endovascular cooling for faster induction of mild hypothermia after cardiac arrest-a feasibility study. *Resuscitation*,64: 347-351.

Kliegel A, Janata A, Wandaller C, Uray T, Spiel A, Losert H, Kliegel M, Holzer M, Haugk M, Sterz F, Laggner AN. (2007). Cold infusions alone are effective for induction of therapeutic hypothermia but do not keep patients cool after cardiac arrest. *Resuscitation*, 73: 46-53.

Knafelj R, Radsel P, Ploj T, Noc M. (2007). Primary percutaneous coronary intervention and mild induced hypothermia in comatose survivors of ventricular fibrillation with ST-elevation acute myocardial infarction. *Resuscitation*,74:227-234.

Koester R, Kaehler J, Barmeyer A, Müllerleile K, Priefler M, Soeffker G, Braune S, Nierhaus A, Meinertz T, Kluge S. (2011). Coronary angiography and intervention during hypothermia can be performed safely without cardiac arrhythmia or vasospasm. *Clin Res Cardiol*,Jun 21.

Kuboyama K, Safar P, Radovsky A, Tisherman SA, Stezoski SW, Alexander H. (1993). Delay in cooling negates the beneficial effect of mild resuscitative cerebral hypothermia after cardiac arrest in dogs: a prospective, randomized study. *Crit Care Med*,21:1348-1358.

Laurent I, Monchi M, Chiche JD, Joly LM, Spaulding C, Bourgeois B, Cariou A, Rozenberg A, Carli P, Weber S, Dhainaut JF. (2002). Reversible myocardial dysfunction in survivors of out-of-hospital cardiac arrest. *J Am Coll Cardiol*,40:2110-2116.

Laver S, Farrow C, Turner D, Nolan J. (2004). Mode of death after admission to an intensive care unit following cardiac arrest. *Intensive Care Med*,30:2126-2128.

Lei B, Tan X, Cai H, Xu Q, Guo Q. (1994). Effect of moderate hypothermia on lipid peroxidation in canine brain tissue after cardiac arrest and resuscitation. *Stroke*,25:147-152.

Liu L, Yenari MA. (2007). Therapeutic hypothermia: neuroprotective mechanisms. *Front Biosci*,12:816-825.

Losert H, Sterz F, Roine RO, Holzer M, Martens P, Cerchiari E, Tiainen M, Müllner M, Laggner AN, Herkner H, Bischof MG. (2008). Strict normoglycaemic blood glucose levels in the therapeutic management of patients within 12h after cardiac arrest might not be necessary. *Resuscitation*,76:214-220.

Lyden PD, Allgren RL, Ng K, Akins P, Meyer B, Al-Sanani F, Lutsep H, Dobak J, Matsubara BS, Zivin J. (2005). Intravascular Cooling in the Treatment of Stroke (ICTuS): early clinical experience. *J Stroke Cerebrovasc Dis*,14: 107-114.

Manoukian SV, Feit F, Mehran R, Voeltz MD, Ebrahimi R, Hamon M, Dangas GD, Lincoff AM, White HD, Moses JW, King SB 3rd, Ohman EM, Stone GW. (2007). Impact of major bleeding on 30-day mortality and clinical outcomes in patients with acute coronary syndromes: an analysis from the ACUITY Trial. *J Am Coll Cardiol*,49:1362-1368.

Merchant RM, Abella BS, Peberdy MA, Soar J, Ong ME, Schmidt GA, Becker LB, Vanden Hoek TL. (2006). Therapeutic hypothermia after cardiac arrest: unintentional overcooling is common using ice packs and conventional cooling blankets. *Crit Care Med*,34(12 Suppl):S490-S494.

Michelson AD, MacGregor H, Barnard MR, Kestin AS, Rohrer MJ, Valeri CR. (1994). Reversible inhibition of human platelet activation by hypothermia in vivo and in vitro. *Thromb Haemost*,71:633-640.

Mori K, Saito J, Kurata Y, Takeyama Y, Itoh Y, Kaneko M, Asai Y, Renzi FP, Dickson EW. (2001). Rapid development of brain hypothermia using femoral-carotid bypass. *Acad Emerg Med*,8:303–308.

Murphy MC, Callaway C, Guyette F, Rittenberger J. (2010). Hypothermia Does Not Ameliorate Post-Cardiac Arrest Myocardial Dysfunction. *Circulation*, 122(Suppl):A235.

Noc M. (2010). Hypothermia during percutaneous coronary intervention in comatose survivors of cardiac arrest. *Signa vitae*,5(Suppl. 1):13-16.

Nielsen N, Hovdenes J, Nilsson F, Rubertsson S, Stammet P, Sunde K, Valsson F, Wanscher M, Friberg H; Hypothermia Network. (2009). Outcome, timing and adverse events in therapeutic hypothermia after out-of-hospital cardiac arrest. *Acta Anaesthesiol Scand*,53:926-934.

Nielsen N, Friberg H, Gluud C, Herlitz J, Wetterslev J. (2010). Hypothermia after cardiac arrest should be further evaluated-A systematic review of randomised trials with meta-analysis and trial sequential analysis. *Int J Cardiol*,Jun 29.

Nielsen N, Sunde K, Hovdenes J, Riker RR, Rubertsson S, Stammet P, Nilsson F, Friberg H; Hypothermia Network. (2011). Adverse events and their relation to mortality in out-of-hospital cardiac arrest patients treated with therapeutic hypothermia. *Crit Care Med*,39:57-64.

Nolan JP, Deakin CD, Soar J, Böttiger BW, Smith G, European Resuscitation Council (2005). European Resuscitation Council guidelines for resuscitation 2005. Section 4. Adult advanced life support. *Resuscitation*,67(Suppl 1):S39-S86.

Nolan JP, Neumar RW, Adrie C, Aibiki M, Berg RA, Böttiger BW, Callaway C, Clark RS, Geocadin RG, Jauch EC, Kern KB, Laurent I, Longstreth WT, Merchant RM, Morley P, Morrison LJ, Nadkarni V, Peberdy MA, Rivers EP, Rodriguez-Nunez A, Sellke FW, Spaulding C, Sunde K, Hoek TV. (2008). Post-cardiac arrest syndrome: Epidemiology, pathophysiology, treatment, and prognostication. A Scientific Statement from the International Liaison Committee on Resuscitation; the American Heart Association Emergency Cardiovascular Care Committee; the Council on Cardiovascular Surgery and Anesthesia; the Council on Cardiopulmonary, Perioperative, and Critical Care; the Council on Clinical Cardiology; the Council on Stroke. *Resuscitation*,79:350-379.

Oksanen T, Pettilä V, Hynynen M, Varpula T; Intensium Consortium study group. (2007). Therapeutic hypothermia after cardiac arrest: implementation and outcome in Finnish intensive care units. *Acta Anaesthesiol Scand*,51:866–871.

Ostadal P. (2009). Ischemia-reperfusion injury following cardiac arrest and protective effects of hypothermia. *Kardiol Rev*,11:11-15.

Padkin A. (2009). Glucose control after cardiac arrest. *Resuscitation*,80:611–612.

Polderman KH, Peerdeman SM, Girbes AR. (2001). Hypophosphatemia and hypomagnesemia induced by cooling in patients with severe head injury. *J Neurosurg*, 94:697-705.

Polderman KH, Sterz F, van Zanten ARH. (2003). Induced hypothermia improves neurological outcome in asystolic patients with out-of hospital cardiac arrest. *Circulation*,108: IV-58I.

Polderman KH, Rijnsburger ER, Peerdeman SM, Girbes AR. (2005). Induction of hypothermia in patients with various types of neurologic injury with use of large volumes of ice-cold intravenous fluid. *Crit Care Med*,33:2744-2751.

Polderman KH. (2009). Mechanisms of action, physiological effects, and complications of hypothermia. *Crit Care Med*,37(7 Suppl):S186-S202.

Reed C, Clark D. Heat Exchangem and hypothermia. Cardiopulmonary Perfusion. Texas: Texas Medical Press 2002:272- 278.

Rivers E, Nguyen B, Havstad S, Ressler J, Muzzin A, Knoblich B; Early Goal-Directed Therapy Collaborative Group. (2001). Early goal-directed therapy in the treatment of severe sepsis and septic shock. *N Engl J Med*,345:1368-1377.

Safar P, Behringer W, Böttiger BW, Sterz F. (2002). Cerebral resuscitation potentials for cardiac arrest. *Crit Care Med*,30: S140-S144.

Schefold JC, Storm C, Joerres A, Hasper D. (2009). Mild therapeutic hypothermia after cardiac arrest and the risk of bleeding in patients with acute myocardial infarction. *Int J Cardiol*,132:387-391.

Schmutzhard E, Engelhardt K, Beer R, Brössner G, Pfausler B, Spiss H, Unterberger I, Kampfl A. (2002). Safety and efficacy of a novel intravascular cooling device to control body temperature in neurologic intensive care patients: a prospective pilot study. *Crit Care Med*,30:2481–2488.

Schneider A, Popp E, Böttiger BW. (2006). Regulated hypothermia after cardiac arrest. A glimpse into the future. Anaesthesist,55:1247-1254.

Seder DB, Van der Kloot TE. (2009). Methods of cooling: practical aspects of therapeutic temperature management. *Crit Care Med*,37(7 Suppl):S211-S222.

Srere H K, Wang LC, Martin SL. (1992). Central role for differential gene expression in mammalian hibernation. *Proc Natl Acad Sci USA*,89:7119–7123.

Stone GW, Dixon SR, Foster M. (2006). Abstract 3794: Systemic Hypothermia to Prevent Contrast Nephropathy: the COOL RCN Pilot Trial 2006; 114: II_811-II_812.

Storm C, Steffen I, Schefold JC, Krueger A, Oppert M, Jörres A, Hasper D. (2008). Mild therapeutic hypothermia shortens intensive care unit stay of survivors after out-of-hospital cardiac arrest compared to historical controls. *Crit Care*,12:R78.

Sunde K, Pytte M, Jacobsen D, Mangschau A, Jensen LP, Smedsrud C, Draegni T, Steen PA. (2007). Implementation of a standardised treatment protocol for post resuscitation care after out-of-hospital cardiac arrest. *Resuscitation*,73:29–39.

Škulec R, Kovarnik T, Dostalova G, Kolar J, Linhart A. (2008). Induction of mild hypothermia in cardiac arrest survivors presenting with cardiogenic shock syndrome. Acta Anaesthesiol Scand,52:188-194.

Škulec R, Kovárník T, Bělohlávek J, Dostálová G, Kolár J, Linhart A, Seblová J. (2008). Overcooling during mild hypothermia in cardiac arrest survivors-phenomenon we should keep in mind. *Vnitr Lek*,54:609-614.

Škulec R, Truhlář A, Knor J, Šeblová J, Černý V. (2010). The practice of therapeutic mild hypothermia in cardiac arrest survivors in the Czech republic. *Minerva Anestesiol*,76:617-623.

Škulec R, Truhlář A, Šeblová J, Dostál P, Černý V. (2010). Pre-hospital cooling of patients following cardiac arrest is effective using even low volumes of cold saline. *Crit Care*,14:R231.

Škulec R, Truhlář A, Šeblová J, Knor, J, Dostál P, Černý V. (2010). In-hospital use of therapeutic mild hypothermia in cardiac arrest survivors. *Anest Intenziv Med*,21:317-323.

Tang W, Weil MH, Sun S, Noc M, Yang L, Gazmuri RJ. (1995). Epinephrine increases the severity of postresuscitation myocardial dysfunction. *Circulation*,92:3089-3093.

Testori C, Sterz F, Behringer W, Haugk M, Uray T, Zeiner A, Janata A, Arrich J, Holzer M, Losert H. (2011). Mild therapeutic hypothermia is associated with favourable outcome in patients after cardiac arrest with non-shockable rhythms. *Resuscitation*,Jun 12.

Tømte O, Andersen GO, Jacobsen D, Drægni T, Auestad B, Sunde K. (2011). Strong and weak aspects of an established post-resuscitation treatment protocol-A five-year observational study. *Resuscitation*,May 14.

Torbicki A, Perrier A, Konstantinides S, Agnelli G, Galiè N, Pruszczyk P, Bengel F, Brady AJ, Ferreira D, Janssens U, Klepetko W, Mayer E, Remy-Jardin M, Bassand JP; ESC Committee for Practice Guidelines (CPG). (2008). Guidelines on the diagnosis and management of acute pulmonary embolism: the Task Force for the Diagnosis and management of Acute Pulmonary Embolism of the European Society of Cardiology (ESC). *Eur Heart J*,29:2276-2315.

Van den Broek MP, Groenendaal F, Egberts AC, Rademaker CM. (2010). Effects of hypothermia on pharmacokinetics and pharmacodynamics: a systematic review of preclinical and clinical studies. *Clin Pharmacokinet*,49:277-294.

Van de Werf F, Bax J, Betriu A, Blomstrom-Lundqvist C, Crea F, Falk V, Filippatos G, Fox K, Huber K, Kastrati A, Rosengren A, Steg PG, Tubaro M, Verheugt F, Weidinger F, Weis M; ESC Committee for Practice Guidelines (CPG), Vahanian A, Camm J, De Caterina R, Dean V, Dickstein K, Filippatos G, Funck-Brentano C, Hellemans I, Kristensen SD, McGregor K, Sechtem U, Silber S, Tendera M, Widimsky P, Zamorano JL, Silber S, Aguirre FV, Al-Attar N, Alegria E, Andreotti F, Benzer W, Breithardt O, Danchin N, Di Mario C, Dudek D, Gulba D, Halvorsen S, Kaufmann P, Kornowski R, Lip GY, Rutten F. (2008). Management of acute myocardial infarction in patients presenting with persistent ST-segment elevation: the Task Force on the Management of ST-Segment Elevation Acute Myocardial Infarction of the European Society of Cardiology. *Eur Heart J*,29:2909–2945.

Vanden Hoek TL, Kasza KE, Beiser DG, Abella BS, Franklin JE, Oras JJ, Alvarado JP, Anderson T, Son H, Wardrip CL, Zhao D, Wang H, Becker LB. (2004). Induced hypothermia by central venous infusion: saline ice slurry versus chilled saline. *Crit Care Med*,32:S425-S431.

Vasquez A, Kern KB, Hilwig RW, Heidenreich J, Berg RA, Ewy GA. (2004). Optimal dosing of dobutamine for treating post-resuscitation left ventricular dysfunction. *Resuscitation*,61:199-207.

Virkkunen I, Yli-Hankala A, Silfvast T. (2004). Induction of therapeutic hypothermia after cardiac arrest in prehospital patients using ice-cold Ringer's solution: a pilot study. *Resuscitation*,62:299-302.

Werling M, Thorén AB, Axelsson C, Herlitz J. (2007). Treatment and outcome in post-resuscitation care after out-of-hospital cardiac arrest when a modern therapeutic approach was introduced. *Resuscitation*,73:40-45.

Xiao F, Safar P, Alexander H. (1995). Peritoneal cooling for mild cerebral hypothermia after cardiac arrest in dogs. *Resuscitation*,30:51–59.

Xu L, Yenari MA, Steinberg GK, Giffard RG. (2002). Mild hypothermia reduces apoptosis of mouse neurons in vitro early in the cascade. *J Cereb Blood Flow Metab*,22:21–28.

5

Percutaneous Intervention Post Coronary Artery Graft Surgery in Patients with Saphenous Vein Graft Disease – State of the Art

R. Ernesto Oqueli
Ballarat Health Services, Victoria
Australia

1. Introduction

The success of coronary artery bypass grafting, although the gold standard for the treatment of multivessel coronary artery disease is limited by poor long-term vein graft patency. Despite the superiority of arterial graft patency over that of vein grafts, the multivessel nature of coronary artery disease and ready availability of saphenous veins still result in its use in over 70% of coronary artery bypass graft procedures (Murphy & Angelini, 2004). These thin walled grafts promptly begin to fail with intimal hyperplasia, thrombosis and progressive atherosclerosis when exposed to an abrupt increase in wall stress imparted by systemic arterial pressure (Hiscock et al., 2007).

Recurrent ischaemia in patients who have had previous saphenous bypass surgery occurs not only because of attrition of the saphenous vein grafts but also because of progression of coronary artery disease in the native coronary arteries (de Feyter et al., 1993).

During the first year after bypass surgery up to 15% of venous grafts occlude, between 1 and 6 years the graft attrition rate is 1% to 2% per year, and between 6 and 10 years it is 4% per year. By 10 years after surgery only 60% of vein grafts are patent and only 50% of patent vein grafts are free of significant stenosis. In addition, native coronary artery disease progresses in approximately 5% of patients annually (Motwani & Topol, 1998).

Reflecting this graft and native vessel attrition, angina recurs in up to 20% of patients during the first year after saphenous vein grafting and in approximately 4% of patients annually during the ensuing 5 years (Motwani & Topol 1998).

Angiographic studies have shown that 70% to 80% of bypass surgery patients who present with acute coronary syndrome have their culprit lesion located in the saphenous vein graft (Pregowski J et al., 2005).

Further revascularisation, either reoperative bypass surgery or percutaneous intervention, is required in approximately 4% of patients by 5 years, 19% of patients by 10 years, and 31% of patients by 12 years after initial bypass surgery.

Both surgical and percutaneous forms of repeat revascularisation have considerable limitations. As compared with initial surgery, reoperation carries a higher mortality rate (3%

to 7%) with a high rate of perioperative myocardial infarction (4% to 11.5%). Coronary atheroembolism from diseased vein grafts is a major cause of the morbidity and mortality associated with reoperation. Redo surgery is also associated with less complete relief of angina and with reduction in saphenous vein graft patency as compared with initial bypass surgery. As increasing numbers of patients undergo second and third reoperations, the perioperative morbidity and mortality escalates further and the clinical benefit diminishes (Motwani & Topol, 1998). Thus, currently percutaneous coronary intervention is the preferred treatment for saphenous vein graft lesions (Vermeersh et al., 2006).

Percutaneous treatment of soft and friable, degenerated saphenous vein graft lesions provides unique challenges to the interventionalist due to the tendency for distal embolisation to result in slow or no-reflow phenomena with peri-procedural myocardial infarction and the relatively frequent association of superimposed thrombus on critical graft stenoses. This has sprawled a number of pharmaceutical and device-based approaches that may afford distal protection during percutaneous intervention. Nonetheless, there remains a disappointingly high long-term recurrence rate due to restenosis and the emergence of new lesions resulting in target vessel failure (Hiscock et al., 2007).

2. Mechanisms of saphenous vein graft ischaemia

The mechanisms of saphenous vein graft related ischaemia vary with the time that has elapsed since the surgery.

Early, 1-year and late graft failure may be due to thrombosis, fibrointimal hyperplasia and atherosclerosis respectively. There is general agreement that vein graft atherosclerosis differs from arterial lesions in terms of temporal and histological changes. Vein graft atherosclerosis is more rapid, with diffuse concentric changes and a less noticeable fibrous cap, making venous plaques more vulnerable to rupture and subsequent thrombus formation (Hassantash et al., 2008).

2.1 Early postoperative ischaemia (<1month)

The most common cause of ischaemia within hours or days of surgery is acute vein graft thrombosis (60%) (Nguyen T et al., 2004), possibly attributed to harvesting and handling of the vein, to failure of surgical techniques at sites of anastomosis such as surgical failure to carry the graft distal to obstructive points indicated by angiography (Vlodaver & Edwards, 1973) or to poor distal runoff due to severely diseased native arteries (de Feyter et al., 1993). Other causes are incomplete surgical revascularisation (10%), kinked grafts, and focal stenosis distal to the insertion site and at the proximal or distal anastomotic sites, spasm or injury, insertion of graft to a vein causing AV fistulae, or bypass of the wrong vessel. The patients at increased risk for early postoperative ischaemia include those undergoing technically demanding minimally invasive and "off bypass" techniques. (Nguyen T et al., 2004)

2.2 Early postoperative ischaemia (1 month -1 year)

Recurrent angina between 1 month and 1 year after the surgery is most often due to perianastomotic stenosis, graft occlusion or mid saphenous vein graft stenosis from fibrointimal hyperplasia (Nguyen T et al., 2004). These occlusions are predominantly focal, not associated with diffuse vein graft disease, and usually the thrombotic component of the occlusion is not extensive (de Feyter et al., 1993). Recurrence of angina at about 3 months postoperatively is highly suggestive of a distal graft anastomotic lesion and should, in most cases lead to evaluation for percutaneous coronary intervention. (Nguyen T et al., 2004)

2.3 Late postoperative ischaemia (>3 years after surgery)

At this stage, the most common cause of ischaemia is due to formation in vein grafts of new atherosclerotic plaque, which contains foam cells, cholesterol crystals, blood elements, and necrotic debris as in native vessels, however, these plaques have less fibrocollagenous tissue and calcification, so they are softer, more friable, of larger size, and frequently associated with thrombus. (Nguyen T et al., 2004)

3. Selection of revascularisation strategy in patients who experience recurrence of ischaemia after coronary artery bypass surgery

The optimal revascularization strategy in patients with symptomatic multivessel coronary artery disease and previous coronary artery bypass grafting remains unknown.

Brener et al evaluated 2191 consecutive patients with previous coronary artery bypass graft surgery undergoing isolated, non-emergency multivessel revascularization (1487 with reoperation and 704 with percutaneous coronary intervention) between 1 January 1995 and 31 December 2000. The analysis concentrated on the independent predictors of the revascularization method, as well as on long-term mortality and its predictors, after calculating a propensity score for the method of revascularization.

These authors concluded that in the absence of a dedicated, randomized controlled trial to guide multivessel revascularization in post-coronary artery bypass graft patients, clinical practice appears to favour reoperation over percutaneous coronary intervention for patients at higher risk, with fewer functional grafts, more chronic total occlusions, and impaired systolic function, whereas percutaneous coronary intervention is favoured in those with patent left internal mammary artery and amenable anatomy.

In their study long-term mortality was mostly affected by age and ejection fraction, while the choice of revascularization had a modest impact. Percutaneous coronary intervention appeared to be related to a slight excess in long-term mortality (despite better 30-day outcome) compared with reoperation, an effect markedly attenuated by risk adjustment.

The effect of drug-eluting stents, higher success in percutaneous recanalization of chronic total occlusions and improvements in surgical techniques and overall medical care needs to be evaluated prospectively, particularly in high-risk subsets defined by advanced age and systolic dysfunction, before a definitive recommendation can be made for this important segment of the coronary artery disease population (Brener et al., 2006).

4. Balloon angioplasty for the treatment of saphenous vein graft disease

Percutaneous treatment of saphenous vein grafts was attempted in the early days of balloon angioplasty.

4.1 Initial results of balloon angioplasty of saphenous vein bypass grafts

In carefully selected patients the initial success rate of balloon angioplasty for saphenous vein grafts varied from 75% to 94%, with a combined overall success rate of 88%. The initial success rate was dependent on the site of dilatation. The overall combined initial result of dilatation of the proximal site was 87%, of the graft body 94% and of the distal site 90%.

The procedure related death rate was <1%, the myocardial infarction rate was approximately 4% and the need for coronary bypass surgery was <2%. These results reflected the careful selection of patients and probably the exclusion of complex lesions (de Feyter et al., 1993).

4.2 Restenosis after successful balloon angioplasty of saphenous vein bypass grafts

The restenosis rate was also dependent on the site of dilatation within the graft. Ostial or very proximal graft lesions had very high restenosis rate (58% on average), the restenosis rate of the body of the graft was 52% and the restenosis rate in the distal anastomotic part of the graft was 28%. The overall combined restenosis rate was 42%(de Feyter et al., 1993).

It was suggested that the interval to restenosis after angioplasty of a saphenous vein graft was longer than the usual 6 months interval after angioplasty in native coronary arteries. In a series published by Douglas, the restenosis rate was 32% at six months, but it rose to 43%, 61% and 64% after 6-12 months, 1-5 years, and 5 years respectively. (Douglas, 1994). The reason for this late pattern according to some authors, could be the larger reference diameter, which means more time would be required to reach a minimum luminal diameter small enough to yield clinical findings. (Hong et al., 2000; Lozano et al., 2005)

4.3 Long term outcome after balloon angioplasty of saphenous vein bypass grafts

The 5-year follow-up was poor, and although 74% of the patients were still alive, only 26% were event free with no myocardial infarction or repeat revascularisation (de Feyter, 2003). The interval between balloon angioplasty and bypass surgery was a significant predictor for 5 year-event free survival.

4.4 Risk factors predictive of unfavourable outcome after balloon angioplasty of saphenous vein bypass grafts

Several variables predictive of unfavourable outcome after balloon angioplasty of saphenous vein graft were identified.

Factors that predicted a poor initial result included 1) diffuseness of saphenous vein graft disease; 2) attempted angioplasty of stenoses in grafts more than 4 to 6 years old; 3) chronic totally occluded grafts; and 4) the presence of intravein graft thrombus. The presence of one or more of those variables was associated with a high frequency of major complications, often due to embolization of friable material into the coronary circulation or the occurrence of abrupt occlusion with thrombosis formation.

Variables predictive of late restenosis after balloon angioplasty of saphenous vein grafts included 1) lesions in old (more than 36 months) grafts; 2) multiple lesions, diffuse graft disease and total occlusion; 3) small diameter (<2.2 mm) of the grafted coronary artery; 4) length of stenosis grater than 10mm; and 5) dilation of lesion at the proximal site and body of the graft (de Feyter et al., 1993).

Some authors advocated the use of aggressive adjunctive pharmacotherapy with intravenous and intracoronary heparin, urokinase, nitroglycerin, oral aspirin, calcium channel blocking agents and Coumadin for patients undergoing balloon angioplasty of saphenous vein grafts (Morrison et al., 1994).

Balloon angioplasty of saphenous vein grafts is a palliative procedure, not a long-term solution in patients with previous coronary bypass graft surgery. The high restenosis rate is a serious limitation of balloon angioplasty (de Feyter et al., 1993).

5. Bare metal stents in the treatment of saphenous vein grafts

Given the limitations of balloon angioplasty for the treatment of saphenous vein graft disease stent implantation was suggested as an alternative therapeutic approach.

Initial observational studies with balloon-expandable stent implantation in saphenous vein graft lesions had claimed a high procedural success rate, low early complication rate, and more favourable long-term outcome than previously reported for balloon angioplasty alone (Hanekamp et al., 2003).

The SAVED (Saphenous Vein De Novo) trial was the first multicentre, prospective, randomized trial of saphenous vein graft stenting. This study compared the placement of Palmaz-Schatz stents (Johnson & Johnson Interventional Systems, Warren, N.J.) with standard balloon angioplasty in 220 patients with relatively focal de-novo lesions in aortocoronary-venous bypass grafts. The primary angiographic end point of this trial was restenosis, defined as stenosis of 50% or more of the luminal diameter at follow-up.

Patients assigned to stenting had a higher rate of procedural efficacy, defined as a reduction in stenosis to less than 50% of the vessel diameter without a major cardiac complication (92% versus 69%, $P<0.001$). Bleeding and vascular complications were significantly more common in the stent group (17 % versus 5%, $P<0.01$) probably related to the intense anticoagulation protocol used in this trial. Patients in the stent group had a larger mean increase in luminal diameter immediately after the procedure (1.92 ± 0.3 mm versus 1.21 ± 0.37 mm) and a greater mean net gain in luminal diameter at six months (0.85 ± 0.96 mm versus 0.54 ± 0.91 mm). The rate of event free survival (freedom from death, myocardial infarction, repeated bypass surgery and revascularisation of the target lesion) at 240 days was significantly greater for patients assigned to stenting than for patients assigned to balloon angioplasty (73% versus 58%, $P=0.03$). When the results were analysed according to intention-to-treat principles, restenosis was found in 37% of the patients in the stent group and in 46% of the patients in the angioplasty group, $p=0.24$ (Savage et al., 1997).

These authors concluded that as compared with conventional angioplasty, stent placement in new vein-graft lesions was associated with better initial angiographic results and higher rates of procedural success. Although the luminal diameter at six months was larger in the stent group, there was no significant difference in the rate of restenosis. However, major cardiac events occurred less frequently in the stent group (Savage et al., 1997).

The SAVED trial used aspirin in combination with dypiridamole and warfarin therapy post stent implantation, instead of thienopiridines.

The Venestent study was a prospective, randomised, multicenter study that compared balloon angioplasty versus elective Wiktor I stent (Medtronic, Minneapolis, MN) implantation using thienopyridines in 150 patients with de novo lesions in the body of a saphenous vein graft. Diffusely diseased grafts, ostial and restenotic lesions, total occlusions and grafts with angiographic evidence of thrombus were excluded. The primary end point of this study was the binary angiographic restenosis rate at 6-month follow-up. Restenosis was defined as diameter stenosis of more than 50%.

Seventy-three patients were randomised to balloon angioplasty and 77 patients to stent implantation. In 17 patients randomised to balloon angioplasty, a bailout stent was implanted, corresponding with a crossover rate of 23.3%.

The angiographic and the procedural success rates were comparable for the balloon and the stent group (97.3% versus 98.7% and 89.0% versus 89.6%, respectively). No difference was present between the balloon group and the stent group with respect to in-hospital major adverse cardiac events (9.6% versus 10.4%). The angiographic restenosis rate at 6-month follow-up was 32.8% in the balloon group and 19.1% in the stent group, $p = 0.069$. At one year follow-up, target vessel revascularisation rate was 31.4% versus 14.5%, $P < 0.05$; and event-free survival was 60.0% versus 76.3%, $P < 0.05$, for the balloon and the stent group, respectively.

The authors of this study concluded that elective stent implantation in de novo saphenous vein graft lesions was associated with a significantly lower target vessel revascularisation rate and a significant higher event-free survival at 1year follow-up as compared to balloon angioplasty (Hanekamp et al., 2003). Although the difference in restenosis rate between both groups was not statistically significant; a strong trend in favour of stenting was suggested.

As compared with balloon angioplasty elective stent implantation in selected de novo saphenous vein graft stenosis is associated with better initial angiographic results, higher rates of procedural success, lower target vessel revascularisation rate and significant higher event-free survival. It is important to note however, that the results of bare metal stents in saphenous vein grafts are less favourable than those in native vessels, with restenosis rates exceeding 30% (Savage et al., 1997; Silber et al., 2005).

6. Direct stenting in saphenous vein grafts

Lesions located in saphenous vein grafts have different characteristics to those located in native vessels with greater cellular and less fibrotic components, more necrotic debris, cholesterol, thrombi and foamy cells. Thus, one of the greatest restrictions to stent implantation with predilatation is the risk of distal embolisation, with a high incidence of peri-procedural myocardial infarction (Lozano et al., 2005).

Direct stenting is defined as stent deployment without predilation with balloon or preparation via atherectomy. Direct stenting was introduced as a strategy of percutaneous coronary revascularisation in native vessels and was equivalent or was associated with better results when compared with balloon angioplasty followed by stenting (Leborgne et al., 2003). Direct stenting was also proposed as a strategy to reduce complications during the treatment of acute myocardial infarction, by reducing the distal embolization rate and the no-reflow phenomenon (Leborgne et al., 2003). Because saphenous vein graft lesions are more friable, the beneficial impact of direct stenting might be amplified in saphenous vein grafts compared to native arteries (Leborgne et al., 2003).

Distal embolization and CK elevation remain a common complication after percutaneous treatment of saphenous vein grafts. The postulated mechanisms by which direct stenting minimizes distal embolisation in saphenous vein graft intervention is that by direct stenting the stent acts as scaffold to trap the friable tissue of the plaque before inflation of a balloon and reduce its fragmentation (Leborgne et al., 2003).

In a retrospective assessment of 527 consecutive patients treated with stent implantation for saphenous vein graft stenosis, 170 patients with 229 lesions were treated with direct stenting and 357 patients with 443 lesions were treated with conventional stenting (stent deployment preceded by balloon predilation). Procedural success was high and results were similar between the 2 groups with the same rate of combined major in-hospital complications (death, Q-wave myocardial infarction, and emergent coronary artery bypass surgery). However, the maximum CK-MB elevation postprocedure (9.5 ± 18.1 versus 19.6 ± 47.8 mg/dl, $P < 0.001$), CK-MB elevation > 4 times the upper normal value (13.6% versus 23.0 %, $P = 0.012$), and non-Q wave myocardial infarction (10.7% versus 18.4%, $P = 0.024$) were much lower in the direct stenting group. At one year, the composite end point of death, Q wave myocardial infarction, and target lesion revascularisation was significantly lower in the direct stenting group (21.5%) versus the conventional stent group (34.3%), $p = 0.021$ (Leborgne et al., 2003).

In another retrospective study involving 117 consecutive patients who underwent stenting for at least 1 lesion located in saphenous vein grafts, 71 patients with 83 lesions had been treated with direct stenting and 46 patients with 54 lesions with stenting preceded by balloon predilatation. No differences were found between both groups regarding the success of the procedure. The distal embolisation rate was significantly higher in the predilatation group with a trend toward a greater frequency of periprocedural myocardial infarction. Median follow-up time was 36.1 months. No differences were found in long-term mortality between the two groups (Lozano et al., 2005).

Direct stenting seems to be actually the best approach for treating saphenous vein graft stenosis when it is technically feasible. This strategy may be especially useful when a distal protection device cannot be used (Leborgne et al., 2003).

7. Covered stents for the treatment of saphenous vein grafts

Despite the fact that stents have improved the outcome of percutaneous intervention of obstructed vein grafts, prognosis of patients undergoing this procedure is still poor. Targets to improve intervention in saphenous vein grafts are to inhibit distal embolisation of atherosclerotic debris and to reduce the restenosis rate, which is elevated, compared with native vessels (Stone et al., 2011). These targets provided the rationale to propose the use of a membrane-covered stent as a new option for the treatment of saphenous vein grafts.

Initial experiences using the JOSTENT coronary stent graft (Jomed GmbH, Rangendingen, Germany) were promising when used in saphenous vein grafts (Elsner et al., 1999).

The JOSTENT stent-graft consists of a distensible polytetrafluoroethylene (PTFE) membrane sandwiched between two 316L stainless steel slotted tube, balloon-expandable stents. This device is currently available as the GraftMaster (Abbott Vascular, Santa Clara, California) for treatment of life-threatening coronary perforations (Figure 1).

Hypothetical benefits of elective use of the JOSTENT PTFE stent-graft in saphenous vein grafts included reduced periprocedural myocardial infarction (by trapping potentially embolic degenerated atherosclerotic debris behind the PTFE membrane) and decreased restenosis (by serving as a barrier isolating the lumen from smooth muscle cell proliferation, migration, and extracellular matrix production arising from the media) (Stone et al., 2011).

Results of a German multicenter registry suggested that the PTFE-membrane-covered stent appeared to be a safe and efficient treatment strategy for obstructed vein grafts with restenosis rates of about 17% (Baldus et al., 2000). Several prospective, randomised, multicenter trials were then conducted to compare the JOSTENT stent-graft with different conventional stents in patients undergoing percutaneous coronary intervention of obstructed saphenous vein grafts.

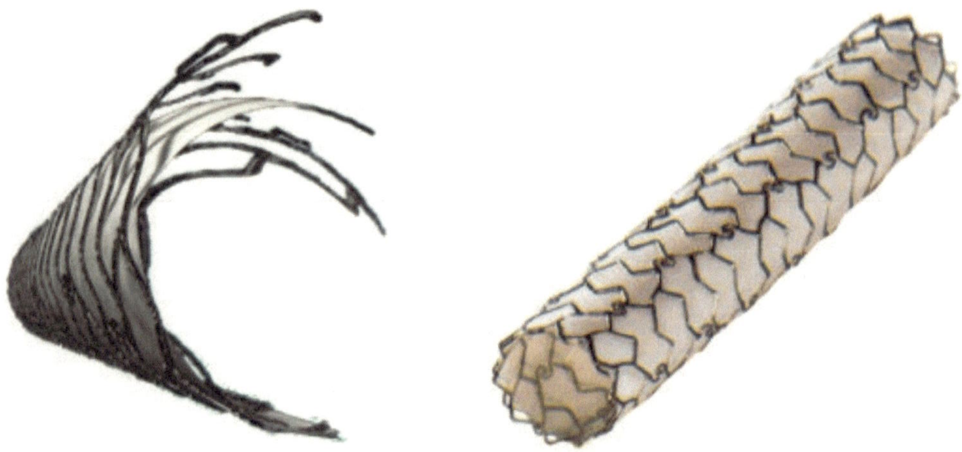

Fig. 1. Image of the GraftMaster polytetrafluoroethylene membrane covered stent. Courtesy of Abbott Vascular.

The STING (STents IN Grafts) trial was a prospective, multicenter study that included a total of 211 patients who were randomly assigned to receive either a Jostent Flex coronary stent or a JOSTENT stent-graft for the treatment of de novo lesions in saphenous vein grafts with a lesion length between 5 and 45 mm and a reference diameter between 3.0 and 5.0 mm. Patients were pretreated with aspirin (100 mg per day). Ticlopidine (500 mg per day) or clopidogrel (75 mg per day) were started after loading doses at the day of the procedure and continued for three months.

The primary end point was binary restenosis rate at six months by core lab quantitative coronary angiography.

Postprocedural minimal luminal diameter was comparable between the two groups. Periprocedural events during the intervention were similar between groups.

At follow-up, there were no statistically significant differences in minimal luminal diameter or percent stenosis between the groups. With respect to the primary end point restenosis rate at six months, there was also no significant difference between the Flex (20%) and the Stentgraft groups (29%), p=0.15. The restenosis rate in both groups was lower in this study than in other contemporary studies involving vein graft stenting, probably related to patient selection. There was a nonsignificant trend toward a higher late occlusion rate in the Stentgraft group (7% versus 16%, p= 0.069) at follow-up. After a mean observation period of 14 months, cumulative event rates (death, myocardial infarction, or target lesion revascularisation were comparable in the two groups (31% versus 31%, p = 0.93) (Schächinger et al., 2003). The outcome of the stent graft group in this study was worse than the expectations.

The RECOVERS (Randomized Evaluation of polytetrafluoroethylene COVERed stent in Saphenous vein grafts) trial was a prospective, multicenter trial that randomized 301 patients with saphenous vein graft lesions to either the polytetrafluoroethylene-covered JOSTENT stent-graft or the JoFlex stent. Angiographic and procedural success rates were similar between the 2 groups (97.4% versus 97.9% and 87.3% versus 93.8%, respectively). The incidence of 30-day of major adverse cardiac events was higher in the JOSTENT stent-graft group (10.9% versus 4.1%, p = 0.047) and was mainly attributed to myocardial infarction (10.3% versus 3.4%, p = 0.037). The primary end point, the restenosis rate at 6-month follow-up, was similar between the two groups (24.2% versus 24.8%, p =0.237). Although the 6-month non Q-wave myocardial infarction rate was higher in the stent-graft group (12.8% versus 4.1%, p =0.013), the cumulative major adverse cardiac event rate was not different (23.1% versus 15.9%, p=0.153). This study also failed to demonstrate a beneficial effect of the JOSTENT stent-graft for saphenous vein graft treatment (Stankovic et al., 2003).

The prior Trials of the JOSTENT stent-graft did not mandate high-pressure implantation or prolonged dual antiplatelet therapy, measures that might be necessary to mechanically optimize the implant and facilitate endothelialisation without thrombosis. Moreover, they were limited by short-term follow-up.

The BARRICADE (Barrier Approach to restenosis: Restrict Intima to Curtail Adverse Events) trial was a prospective, multicenter study that included 243 patients that were randomised to the JOSTENT versus any bare-metal stent.

JOSTENT post-dilation to ≥ 18 atmospheres was mandated to overcome limitations of prior studies, as was the use of dual antiplatelet therapy for ≥ 8 months, and all patients were followed for a total duration of 5 years.

The primary end point of in-lesion binary restenosis at 8 months was not statistically different between the groups and occurred in 31.8% of lesions treated with the JOSTENT versus 28.4% of lesions treated with bare-metal stents (relative risk: 1.12, 95% confidence interval: 0.72 to 1.75, p = 0.63).

At 9 months, the major secondary end point of target vessel failure (death, myocardial infarction, or clinically driven target vessel revascularisation) occurred in 32.2% of patients treated with the JOSTENT versus 22.1% of patients treated with bare metal stents (hazard ratio: 1.54, 95% CI: 0.94 to 2.53, $p = 0.08$). During long-term follow-up, significantly more events accrued in the JOSTENT arm such that by 5 years target vessel failure had occurred in 68.3% of JOSTENT patients versus 51.8% of bare metal stent patients (hazard ratio: 1.59, 95% CI: 1.13 to 2.23, $p = 0.007$). Although there were no statistically significant differences between the 2 stent types in the rates of myocardial infarction or stent thrombosis, target vessel occlusion was noted more frequently in the JOSTENT arm during long-term follow-up. This study was designed to overcome several potentially important limitations from prior randomised trials of the JOSTENT stent-graft in diseased saphenous vein grafts, despite this stent-grafts had a grater failure rate when used for this application than bare metal stents (Stone et al., 2011).

Covered stents showed a tendency toward a higher rate of total occlusions at follow-up. It has been speculated that a postponed re-endothelialisation or enhanced thrombogenicity of the PTFE membrane might predispose for late thrombotic occlusions. However, the clinical course of most documented late occlusions was surprisingly benign, with only a few cases associated with a myocardial infarction. The fact that late occlusions >150 days were not associated with myocardial infarction might indicate that progressively proliferating restenosis, rather than acute thrombosis, might be the mechanism of late occlusion in these patients (Schächinger et al., 2003)

The Symbiot self expanding polytetrafluoroethylene covered stent (Boston Scientific Corporation, Natick, MA) was developed to reduce the potential for acute and long term complications associated with percutaneous intervention in degenerated saphenous vein conduits. The Symbiot™ covered stent system consists of a self-expanding, nitinol, multi-segmented stent encased within a thin (13μm), porous, polytetrafluoroethylene polymer membrane designed to maintain cellular viability of the adjacent tissue.

Two nonrandomized registries were conducted with the Symbiot stent. Symbiot I enrolled 25 patients. Of the 16 patients with angiographic follow-up at 6 months, the mean percent diameter stenosis was 18.8 ± 28.6%, and 19% had in-stent binary restenosis (unpublished data, Boston Scientific corporation).

Symbiot II, which enrolled 77 patients (58 with angiographic follow-up), demonstrated excellent outcome for the Symbiot stent with a mean percent diameter stenosis of 26.1 ± 20.9%, an in-stent binary restenosis rate of 7.0%, and an overall major adverse cardiac event rate of 14.3% at 6 months. These two studies demonstrated promising results but were limited by the absence of an active control group for comparison and small sample size.

The Symbiot III trial was designed to evaluate the clinical and angiographic outcomes of the Symbiot covered stent versus bare metal stents for the treatment of saphenous vein graft disease. The Symbiot III trial was a prospective randomized trial of 400 patients, with 201 patients in the Symbiot covered stent group and 199 in the bare metal stent group. Randomization was stratified based on the intended use of embolic protection devices and glycoprotein IIb/IIIa inhibitors. The primary endpoint of the study was percent diameter stenosis at 8 months, as measured by quantitative coronary angiography. Secondary endpoints included major adverse cardiac events, consisting of cardiac death, myocardial infarction, and target vessel revascularization. In-hospital and 30-day overall major adverse event rates were comparable between groups. At 8 months, percent diameter stenosis was comparable between groups (30.9% Symbiot, 31.9% bare metal stent, $p=0.80$). Although the rates of binary restenosis in the stented segment were similar (29.1% Symbiot, 21.9% bare metal stent, $p=0.17$), more patients in the Symbiot group had binary restenosis at the proximal edge (9.0% Symbiot, 1.8% bare metal stent, $p=0.0211$). Overall major adverse cardiac event rates at 8 months were comparable for both groups, with 30.6% of Symbiot patients and 26.6% of bare metal stents patients experiencing major adverse cardiac events ($p=0.43$).

This study failed to show an advantage for the Symbiot stent in the treatment of degenerated saphenous vein grafts. These authors concluded that the polytetrafluoroethylene covering does not appear to act as a barrier to reduce neointimal hyperplasia (Turco et al., 2006).

The hypothesis that covered stents for the treatment of saphenous vein grafts may reduce periprocedural myocardial infarction and decrease restenosis seems to have been invalidated. Covered stents should be reserved for life-threatening perforations of the coronary vasculature (Lansky et al., 2006; Stone et al., 2011).

8. Drug eluting stents in the treatment of saphenous vein graft disease

In recent times, drug-eluting stents have become the leading device for the treatment of native coronary artery disease, because of the reduction in the incidence of restenosis, target lesion revascularisation, and target vessel revascularisation compared with bare metal stents (Michishita, 2011). Drug-eluting stents were developed to remove the incidence of restenosis and target lesion revascularisation only, but it has been hypothesised that drug eluting stents can improve the mortality and myocardial infarction rates, compared with bare metal stents, because their effect on reducing restenosis is remarkable and because restenosis after bare metal stent implantation could manifest as acute coronary syndrome in some patients. In real-world nonrandomised observational studies with large numbers of patients, but with a potential for selection bias and residual confounding, use of drug-eluting stents in native coronary arteries has been associated with reduced mortality and myocardial infarction rates (Michishita, 2011). In randomized controlled trials, no significant differences have been observed in the long-term mortality or myocardial infarction rate after the use of drug-eluting stents or bare metal stents in native coronary arteries for either off-label or on-label indications (Michishita, 2011).

Although drug-eluting stents have been a major advance in interventional cardiology, evidence for using these devices does not exist for all types of lesions or for all subsets of patients. One area where data have been lacking is the indication of diseased aortocoronary saphenous vein grafts (Bittl, 2009). Lesions in saphenous vein grafts have been poorly represented if not totally excluded in pivotal drug-eluting stent trials. However, this lesion subset represents a consistent proportion of lesions in which percutaneous procedures are performed, up to 10% to 15%in most centres (Baim, 2003 & Vermeersch et al., 2007).

The current limited evidence of drug eluting stent use in saphenous vein graft intervention comes mainly from a few small but well performed mechanistic randomised trials, multiple larger observational studies and more recently from several meta-analysis that have included evidence from these randomised trials and observational studies.

8.1 Randomized trials

The RRISC (Reduction of Restenosis In Saphenous vein grafts with Cypher sirolimus-eluting stent) trial was a randomised, double blind, non-industry sponsored trial performed in a single centre. Patients with one or more "de novo" target lesions localized in ore or more diseased saphenous vein grafts with a reference vessel diameter > 2.5 and < 4.0 mm were allocated randomly to treatment with Cypher Sirolimus-eluting stent or BX-Velocity bare metal stent (both from Cordis, Johnson & Johnson, Warren, New Jersey). Direct stenting was promoted. Clopidogrel was administered for 2 months in all patients. All were scheduled to undergo six-month coronary angiography.

A total of 75 patients with 96 lesions localized in 80 diseased saphenous vein grafts were included: 38 patients received 60 Sirolimus-eluting stents for 47 lesions, whereas 37 patients received 54 bare metal stents for 49 lesions. Distal protection devices were used in more than 80% of the lesions treated.

The six-month in-stent late lumen loss (primary end point of the study) was significantly reduced in Sirolimus-eluting stents (0.38 ± 0.51 mm versus 0.79 ± 0.66 mm in bare metal stents, $p = 0.001$). Binary in-stent and in-segment restenosis were reduced in the Sirolimus-eluting stents, 11.3% versus 30.6% (relative risk 0.37; 95% confidence interval 0.15 to 0.97, $p = 0.024$) and 13.6% versus 32.6% (relative risk 0.42: 95% confidence interval 0.18 to 0.97, $p = 0.031$), respectively. The pattern of restenosis was different between both groups. After Sirolimus-eluting stent implantation, most restenosis were focal (83.3%) whereas after bare metal stent implantation most restenosis (62.5%) had a non-focal pattern.

Target lesion and vessel revascularisation rates (all ischaemia-driven percutaneous interventions) were significantly reduced in the Sirolimus-eluting stent group, 5.3% versus 21.6% (relative risk 0.24; 95% confidence interval 0.05 to 1.0, $p = 0.047$) and 5.3% versus 27% (relative risk 0.19; 95% confidence interval 0.05 to 0.83, $p = 0.012$) respectively. Death and myocardial infarction rates were not different between groups.

The RRISC Trial suggested a benefit for Sirolimus-eluting stents over bare metal stents in diseased saphenous vein grafts mainly for a reduced revascularisation procedure rate at a follow-up of 6 months. The small sample size of this study made it underpowered for major clinical outcomes (Vermeersch et al., 2006).

Great focus has recently been put on the evaluation of long-term follow-up of drug-eluting stents in native coronary arteries, mainly after publication of original and meta-analytical studies showing a possible increase in "hard" adverse events, specifically very late stent thrombosis, after drug-eluting stent deployment with respect to bare metal stents (Vermeersch et al., 2007).

Due to the lack in long-term data in patients with saphenous vein graft lesions and to offer additional information to the debate on safety of Sirolimus-eluting stents, the investigators of the RRISC trial performed a clinical follow-up evaluation of the 75 patients enrolled in the RRISC trial up to 3 years, focusing specifically on all-cause mortality and was published as the DELAYED RRISC (Death and Events at Long-term follow-up AnalYsis: Extended Duration of the Reduction of Restenosis In Saphenous vein grafts with Cypher stent) trial. The new post-hoc main end point of this secondary long-term follow-up analysis was all-cause mortality.

Death occurred in 11 patients (7 cardiac, of which one was caused by a very late stent thrombosis and 3 were sudden) after Sirolimus-eluting stent (29% [95% confidence limits 17% to 45%]) versus 0 after bare metal stents (0% [0% to 9%]) with an absolute difference of 29% (95% confidence interval 14% to 45%, $p < 0.001$). The overall rate of definite angiographically documented stent thrombosis was 5% in the Sirolimus-eluting stent group (2 of 38, both very late) versus 0% in the bare metal stent group ($p=0.49$), whereas the rate of any possible stent thrombosis was 13% (5 of 38, 2 late and 3 very late) after Sirolimus-eluting stents versus 0% after bare metal stents (Fischer exact test 2-sided p value = 0.054; log rank test = 0.022). The rates of myocardial infarction and target vessel revascularisation were not different; 18% and 34% after Sirolimus-eluting stents, respectively, versus 5% and 38% after bare metal stents, respectively ($p = 0.15$ and $p = 0.74$, respectively).

In this extended post hoc analysis of the RRISC trial, patients treated with Sirolimus-eluting stents showed a significant increase in total mortality and the benefits of Sirolimus-eluting stents in terms of reduced revascularisation procedures shown at 6 months (Vermeersch et al., 2006) was no longer evident up to 3 years, suggesting that in saphenous vein grafts there can be a potential late catch-up phenomenon leading to a lack of benefit of Sirolimus-eluting stents over bare metal stents in reduction of clinical restenosis (Vermeersch et al., 2007).

This study had several major limitations. First, the sample size of patients was small, thus the results could be underpowered to appropriately address specific questions and can be prone to type I and type II statistical error. Second, the recommended duration of double antiplatelet therapy was only mandatory for at least 2 months in this study. Recent evidence has shown that double antiplatelet therapy should be recommended in all patients receiving drug-eluting stents for at least 12 months (Grines et al., 2007). Therefore, it cannot be excluded that some of the events described in the DELAYED RRISC study could be explained by "premature" discontinuation of dual antiplatelet therapy. Third, this study presented a secondary post-hoc analysis; thus, the main end point (death) was not prespecified at the moment of the beginning of the trial (which was powered for a 6-month difference in angiographic late loss analysis). The authors of this study concluded that given that the observations seen in this secondary post hoc analysis may have arisen from the play of chance or other clinical factors unrelated to stent type, further studies were required before conclusions could be made about the safety or harm of using Sirolimus-eluting stents for saphenous vein graft lesions (Vermeersch et al., 2007).

The SOS (Stenting Of Saphenous Vein Grafts) Trial was a randomised, controlled multicenter, prospective trial. Patients with one or more de novo or restenotic lesions in a saphenous vein graft that were between 2.5 and 4.0 mm in diameter were randomised to a polymer-based paclitaxel-eluting stent (Taxus, Boston Scientific, Natick, Massachusetts) or a bare metal stent with similar design (Express2, Boston Scientific).

Eighty patients with 112 lesions in 88 saphenous vein grafts were randomised to receive a paclitaxel-eluting stent (41 patients, 45 grafts, 57 lesions) or to receive a bare metal stent (39 patients, 43 grafts, 55 lesions).

The primary end point of the study was binary angiographic restenosis/lesion, defined as a stenosis of $\geq 50\%$ of the minimal luminal diameter in the target saphenous vein graft segment at 12-month angiographic follow-up. The use of embolic protection devices and intravascular ultrasound were strongly encouraged. Aspirin was administered indefinitely after stenting. Clopidogrel was initially recommended for 6 months after paclitaxel-eluting stent placement and for at least one month after bare metal stent placement. Since December 2006 (patients were enrolled between 2005 and 2007), a minimum of one year of clopidogrel was recommended after paclitaxel-eluting stent placement. Primary stenting was used in most lesions. Procedural success was achieved in 96% of the patients.

Binary angiographic restenosis occurred in 51% of the bare metal stent-treated lesions versus 9% of the paclitaxel-eluting stent-treated lesions (relative risk: 0.18; 95% confidence interval: 0.07 to 0.48, $p < 0.0001$). During a median follow-up of 1.5 years the paclitaxel-eluting stent patients had less target lesion revascularisation (28% versus 5%, hazard ratio: 0.38; 95% confidence interval: 0.15 to 0.74, $p = 0.003$) and less target vessel failure defined as the composite end point of cardiac death, myocardial infarction and target vessel revascularisation (46% versus 22%, hazard ratio 0.65; 95% confidence interval: 0.42 to 0.96, $p = 0.03$). There were trends toward fewer myocardial infarctions (31% versus 15%, hazard ratio: 0.67; 95% confidence interval: 0.40 to 1.08, $p = 0.10$) and less target vessel revascularisation (31% versus 15%, hazard ratio: 0.66; 95% confidence interval: 0.39 to 1.05, $p =0.08$) in paclitaxel eluting stent patients (Brilakis et al., 2009). An important finding of this 80-patient study was that all-cause mortality was similar between the 2 groups at a median follow-up of 1.5 years (Bittl, 2009; Brilakis et al., 2009). This study was limited by the relatively small number of patients and was underpowered to detect differences in clinical outcome (Brilakis et al., 2009).

In summary, the use of paclitaxel-eluting stents in saphenous vein graft lesions in the SOS trial was associated with lower rates of angiographic restenosis and target vessel failure than bare metal stents. The median follow-up of patients in this trial was 1.5 years; it is unknown whether the outcomes would change with longer-term follow-up.

The ISAR-CABG (Is Drug-Eluting Stenting Associated with Improved Results in Coronary Artery Bypass Grafts) trial randomized 610 patients with de novo lesions in saphenous vein grafts to receive either a drug-eluting stent (n=303) or a bare metal stent (n=307). Patients in the drug-eluting sent group received a paclitaxel-eluting, sirolimus-eluting, or bio-absorbable polymer sirolimus-eluting stent. The average age of the saphenous vein grafts was 13 years. The primary endpoint was a composite of major adverse cardiac events (death, myocardial infarction, or target lesion revascularization at 1-year follow-up).

At one-year post intervention the incidence of major adverse cardiac events was reduced by 35% in the drug-eluting stent cohort compared to the bare metal stent group (15.4% versus 22.1%, $p = 0.03$). The difference was almost entirely driven by a nearly 50% relative reduction in the risk of target lesion revascularization (7.2% versus 13.1%, $p= 0.02$). There were no statistically significant differences in the individual rates of death or myocardial infarction (Mehilli et al., 2011).

Two ongoing trials are comparing drug-eluting stents with bare metal stents in saphenous vein grafts; the BASKETSAVAGE (Basel Stent Kosten Effektivitäts Trial-Saphenous Venous Graft Angioplasty Using Glycoprotein IIb/IIIa Receptor Inhibitors and Drug-Eluting Stents) (NCT00595647); and the Veterans Affairs Cooperative Study # 571, DIVA (Drug-Eluting Stents Versus Bare Metal Stents in Saphenous Vein Graft Angioplasty) trials (NCT01121224) (Lee et al., 2011).

The results of randomised trials of drug-eluting stents in saphenous vein grafts can not be extrapolated to large saphenous vein grafts (with a reference vessel diameter > 4.0 mm) or to totally occluded vein grafts because they were excluded from randomisation in those studies.

8.2 Meta-analysis

Several meta-analysis including evidence from randomised trials and observational studies that compared the use of drug-eluting stents versus bare metal stents in the percutaneous treatment of saphenous vein graft disease have been published.

A meta-analysis by Lupi et al included 23 studies comparing drug-eluting stents versus bare metal stents enrolling a total of 7,090 patients with saphenous vein graft disease. Three of the 23 studies included in this meta-analysis were randomised controlled trials and the remaining 20 were non-randomised studies. These authors included in their meta-analysis randomised and/or non-randomised studies, studies reporting clinical outcomes as overall death and/or acute myocardial infarction and/or target vessel revascularisation and studies with follow-up period longer than 6 months.

Patients treated by drug-eluting stents showed lower overall mortality rates with marginal statistical significance compared with those treated by bare metal stents (odds ratio, 0.63; confidence interval, 0.40-0.99; $p = 0.05$; 7.0% versus 15.3% respectively). Subgroup analysis revealed a difference in the outcome between randomised and non-randomised studies. In particular, a survival benefit following drug eluting stent implantation was observed in non-randomised studies (odds ratio, 0.57; confidence interval, 0.36-0.90; $p=0.02$), but not in randomised controlled trials (odds ratio, 2.23; confidence interval, 0.15-32.35; $p=0.56$).

Patients treated by drug-eluting stents showed no benefit in myocardial infarction rates compared with bare metal stent treated patients (odds ratio, 0.92; confidence interval, 0.64-1.33; $p = 0.7$; 6.7% versus 6.8% respectively). Prespecified separate analysis for randomised and non-randomised studies yielded similar results.

In patients treated by drug-eluting stents a strong significant reduction of target vessel revascularisation compared with bare metal stent-treated patients was observed (odds ratio, 0.53; confidence interval, 0.39-0.72; $p < 0.0001$; 12.3% versus 18.8%). Drug-eluting stent advantage was comparable and statistically significant for both randomised and non-randomised studies. The prespecified meta-regression analysis showed an advantage for drug-eluting stents in diabetic patients ($p = 0.03$) and in percutaneous graft intervention performed with embolic protection devices ($p = 0.04$); reduction of target vessel revascularisation with dug-eluting stent use was directly proportional to saphenous vein graft age ($p = 0.005$).

This meta-analysis supports the use of drug-eluting stents to reduce target vessel revascularisation in patients with saphenous vein graft disease. However, in this patient population, clear benefits from the use of drug-eluting stents in the reduction of death and myocardial infarction were not observed (Lupi et al., 2011).

Another recent and large meta-analysis by Hakeem et al included 2 randomised trials, one subgroup analysis from a randomised trial and 26 observational studies comparing drug-eluting stents with bare metal stents for saphenous vein graft lesions comprising a total of

7,994 patients (4,187 patients in the drug-eluting stent arm and 3,807 patients in the bare metal stent group). This meta-analysis reaffirmed the benefit of drug-eluting stents over bare metal stents in major adverse cardiac event reduction, which was primarily driven by lower revascularisation rates in the drug-eluting stent group. The observed drug-eluting stent benefit was largely based on the outcome of observational studies. Pooled analysis of all studies in this meta-analysis showed a mortality benefit associated with the use of drug-eluting stents. However, for studies with 12 and 24 months of follow-up, there was no difference with respect to mortality between drug-eluting stents and bare metal stents. Hence, long-term use of drug-eluting stents was not associated with an increased risk of death. Target vessel revascularisation was 12% in drug-eluting stents compared with 17% in bare metal stents, with risk ratio of 0.71 (0.59, 0.85), $p = 0.0002$. This effect was sustained in studies with > 12 and > 24 months follow-up. This study observed a significant reduction in the risk of myocardial infarction with the use of drug-eluting stents compared with bare metal stents. Although there was no statistically significant difference in the incidence of stent thrombosis, there was a trend towards increased stent thrombosis in the bare metal stent group (1% in drug-eluting stents and 1.7% in bare metal stents with a risk ratio of 0.63 [0.36 - 1.11] $p= 0.11$). According to this authors, the use of drug-eluting stents in saphenous vein grafts appears to be safe both in the short term and long term as demonstrated primarily in observational nonrandomised studies.

Target vessel revascularization is the only outcome with consistent benefit from drug-eluting stent versus bare metal stents in saphenous vein grafts in both randomised and observational data. While patients undergoing saphenous vein graft percutaneous intervention are at higher baseline risk, this "negative result" on myocardial infarction and death is consistent with the overall experience. Meta-analysis of all drug-eluting stent versus bare metal stent randomized controlled trials (n = 22 studies with 9740 patients) yields no significant reduction in death [OR = 0.97 (0.81 - 1.15)] or myocardial infarction [OR = 0.94 (0.78 - 1.13)] in those randomly assigned to drug eluting stents (Hillegass, 2011). There is clear-cut target vessel revascularisation benefit of drug-eluting stents in largely native vessels [OR = 0.45 (0.37 - 0.54), $p < 0.001$]. Interestingly, the point estimate for reduction in target vessel revascularisation with drug-eluting stents in saphenous vein grafts is similar to native vessels. Over the longer term of 2 years, however, we remain with limited proof of a prolonged saphenous vein graft patency advantage with drug-eluting stents versus bare metal stents in well-controlled trials (Hillegass, 2011).

9. No-reflow phenomenon a major complication during percutaneous intervention of saphenous vein grafts

Distal embolisation of atheroemboli is a well-known consequence of saphenous vein grafts intervention and may result in diminished blood flow to the distal vascular bed resulting in peri-procedural ischaemia and infarction. This appropriately named "no-reflow" phenomenon occurs as a result of distal embolisation of atheroembolic debris (Carter et al., 2007). No-reflow is defined as the failure to restore normal coronary antegrade flow despite appropriate treatment of a coronary obstruction in the absence of dissection, thrombus formation or vessel closure.

The cause of no-reflow is complex and multifactorial. Various mechanisms like alpha-adrenergic vascular constriction, local increase in angiotensin II receptor density, neutrophils activation and interaction with endothelium, distal embolisation of plaque and/or thrombus, local release of vasoconstrictor substances have been thought to be among many causes of no-reflow (Habibzadeh et al., 2011).

As expected, no-reflow is associated with worse clinical outcomes including post-procedural myocardial infarction (17.7% versus 3.5%in patients with and without no-reflow, respectively) and death (7.4% versus 2%).

Various techniques, both interventional and pharmacological, have been used in the treatment of no-reflow. Covered stents, as already discussed, were thought to inhibit distal embolisation by sequestering friable atheroemboli; however, this hypothesis seems to have been invalidated. Clinical trials of the routine use of glycoprotein IIb/IIIa receptor blockers during percutaneous intervention of saphenous vein grafts have shown no benefit for the reduction of major adverse cardiac events (Carter et al., 2007). A pooled analysis of 5 randomised intravenous glycoprotein IIb/IIIa inhibitor trials assessed the outcomes of graft interventions at 30 days and 6 months. The study population consisted of 13,158 patients undergoing percutaneous treatment of native coronary arteries and 627 patients treated for by pass graft disease. Treatment assignment and complete follow-up data were available for 605 patients with graft intervention (96.5%). Among them 389 patients were randomised to IIb/IIIa integrin blockade (abciximab in 51% of cases and eptifibatide in 49% of cases) and 216 patients were allocated to placebo. The incidence of death myocardial infarction or urgent revascularization at 30 days was 16.5% among patients allocated to glycoprotein IIb/IIIa inhibitors and 12.6% among those receiving placebo (odds ratio 1.38; 96% confidence interval, 0.85 to 2.24; $p = 0.18$). At six months, the combined event rate of death, myocardial infarction or revascularisation was 39.4% and 32.7% (hazards ratio 1.29; 95% confidence interval, 0.97 to 1.72; $p = 0.07$), respectively. The incidence of major bleeding was 6.8% among graft percutaneous intervention patients randomised to platelet glycoprotein IIb/IIIa inhibitors and 1.4% among those allocated to placebo ($p = 0.004$). The corresponding incidences of minor bleeding were 14.9% versus 8.1% ($p = 0.016$) respectively. Accordingly, no benefit from IIb/IIIa integrin blockade was detected in terms of individual or combined end points either at 30 days or at 6 months in patients undergoing saphenous vein graft interventions. From a safety perspective, adjunctive glycoprotein IIb/IIIa receptor inhibition was associated with an increased incidence of major and minor bleedings (Roffi et al., 2002). The authors of this analysis stated that additional studies were needed to define whether the use of platelet glycoprotein IIb/IIIa receptor inhibitors in conjunction with embolic protection devices might improve outcomes. According to them profound platelet inhibition may have complementary beneficial effect in particular when associated with filter devices. In this regard, whereas the filter offers mechanical protection from larger particles, glycoprotein IIb/IIIa inhibitors could exert their beneficial effect on the microvasculature jeopardized from microparticles that escape the filters. In addition, the use of potent platelet inhibition may allow for reduced filter pore size by preventing filter thrombosis, thereby increasing filter efficiency (Roffi et al., 2002).

The SAFER and FIRE trials established the safety an efficacy of balloon occlusion/aspiration (GuardWire) and filter-based (FilterWire) protection devices as useful adjuncts during saphenous vein grafts intervention. In both trials the use of glycoprotein IIb/IIIa inhibitors was at the discretion of the investigator, with randomisation stratified by intention to use glycoprotein IIb/IIIa blockade so that roughly equal numbers of patients in each arm would be treated with glycoprotein IIb/IIIa inhibitors. In the SAFER trial patients pre-selected for IIb/IIIa treatment in both the GuardWire assigned and control (unprotected) arms had higher rates of major adverse cardiac events than those not treated with glycoprotein IIb/IIIa inhibitors; this observation is most likely due to selection of a higher-risk cohort to receive IIb/IIIa antagonists.

Jonas et al., studied the FIRE trial database to examine whether glycoprotein IIb/IIIa blockers would interact differently with the FilterWire EX and the GuardWire embolic protection devices. The principal findings of their report were that patients pre-selected for glycoprotein IIb/IIIa inhibitor therapy manifested higher risk baseline characteristics, greater procedural complexity and correspondingly higher overall 30-day major adverse cardiac event rates. They also had higher bleeding risk and required more transfusions. Among patients randomised to distal embolic protection with the GuardWire, major adverse cardiac events were higher with glycoprotein IIb/IIIa inhibitors than without. In contrast among patients randomised to the FilterWire, major adverse cardiac events were not higher with glycoprotein IIb/IIIa inhibitors than without. Glycoprotein IIb/IIIa inhibitor therapy was associated with superior FilterWire (but not GuardWire) performance, including better preservation of flow through the filter, reduced procedural ischaemia and reduced occurrence of abrupt closure, no reflow, or distal embolization (Jonas et al., 2005).

Intracoronary calcium channel blockers and the vasodilators adenosine and nitroprusside are commonly used in the treatment of no-reflow. Unfortunately this therapy is usually employed once the phenomenon has occurred (Carter et al., 2007).

Nitroprusside is a direct donor of nitric oxide that is a potent vasodilator in the resistance arteriolar circulation and plays a significant role in the control of coronary blood flow through the microcirculation. In a retrospective analysis of 20 percutaneous coronary interventions including 9 (45%) in saphenous vein grafts, intracoronary nitroprusside administered for no-reflow (median injection dose 200 μg) led to a rapid improvement in both angiographic flow ($p<0.01$ compared with pretreatment angiogram) and blood flow velocity ($p<0.01$ compared with pretreatment angiogram). No significant hypotension or other adverse clinical events were associated with nitroprusside administration (Hillegass, 2001).

Adenosine inhibits platelet activation, impedes platelet aggregation, and is a potent arteriolar dilator that has been shown to reduce the incidence of no-reflow following percutaneous coronary intervention in native vessels, and reverse but not prevent no-reflow in degenerated saphenous vein grafts. Intracoronary adenosine has an extremely short half-life and duration of action, and thus requires repetitive dosing during percutaneous coronary intervention (Fischell, 2008). In a small study, 8 patients who experienced 9 no-reflow and 2 slow flow events complicating saphenous vein graft interventions were treated with the rapid and repeated injection of adenosine (average of 12.1 ± 3.4 boluses of adenosine per event, with 3-4 saline 3-ml flushes following each adenosine syringe bolus). All 11 no-reflow/slow-flow events were substantially improved within 7 minutes of treatment. Angiographically normal flow (TIMI 3) was achieved in 10 of 11 events (91%). These authors hypothesized that the combination of microvascular (arteriolar) vasodilatation by adenosine combined with forceful mechanical flushing of embolic debris out of the target vascular bed may act synergistically to reverse the no-reflow process (Fischell, 1998).

Intracoronary nicardipine has been shown to be the most potent vasodilator used for no-reflow prevention. Intragraft administration of nicardipine can cause longer vasodilation with a lower risk of serious systemic side effects compared to intracoronary diltiazem or verapamil infusion.

In 2007, Fischell et al reported some promising results with the use of intracoronary nicardipine to prevent no-reflow without distal mechanical protection in saphenous vein graft intervention. They evaluated 83 saphenous vein grafts interventions involving 68 consecutive patients. All saphenous vein grafts lesions underwent successful stent placement. All patients received 200-300 μg of intragraft nicardipine (10-15 μg/ ml of normal saline) injected via the guiding catheter immediately prior to stenting (Habibzadeh et al., 2011). These authors showed favourable results with reduction in major adverse cardiac events comparable to that of the early distal protection trials (Carter et al., 2007).

Despite the increasing use of pharmacologic means to prevent no-reflow, distal embolic protection remains a vital component of therapy (Carter et al, 2007). It is of note; however, that despite the use of protection devices, significant no-reflow can occur during saphenous vein graft intervention. The no-reflow phenomenon might be predominantly caused by microvascular spasm and not directly by mechanical obstruction from distal embolisation (Habibzadeh et al., 2011). A combination of intragraft administration of nicardipine together with the use of protection devices has not been studied but appears to be logical, with significant potential to reduce the occurrence of no-reflow compared to each preventive measure alone (Habibzadeh et al., 2011).

10. Embolic protection devices during saphenous vein graft interventions

There are two types of embolic protection devices: balloon occlusion-aspiration (proximal or distal) and filter devices. These systems have different characteristics and to date none has demonstrated enough advantages over the other mechanism to be ideally recommended universally (Morís et al., 2009).

10.1 Distal balloon occlusion devices

The Guard-Wire (Medtronic, Minneapolis, MN) temporary occlusion-aspiration system, consist of a wire with a central lumen that inflates an elastomeric balloon at the distal tip of the wire. The lesion is crossed with the Guard-Wire. Once the balloon is inflated (2.5 to 5.0 mm or 3.0 to 6.0 mm in diameter) with diluted contrast using an adaptor device, it occludes flow distal to the target lesion. The procedure (angioplasty and stenting) is then performed over the Guard-Wire shaft instead of using a standard angioplasty guidewire. Liberated plaque and thrombotic debris trapped proximal to the balloon are then aspirated through a 5 French monorail Export aspiration catheter. The balloon is then deflated with restoration of antegrade flow (Figure 2).

The SAFER (Saphenous vein graft Angioplasty Free of Emboli Randomized) trial enrolled 801 patients with signs of myocardial ischemia resulting from a target lesion > 50% diameter stenosis located in the mid-portion of a saphenous vein graft, with a reference vessel diameter between 3 and 6 mm. Four hundred and six patients were randomized to stent placement over the shaft of the distal protection device and 395 were assigned to stent placement over a conventional angioplasty guidewire (control group). There was a 6.9% absolute (42% relative) reduction in the 30-day primary end point - a composite of death, myocardial infarction, emergency bypass, or target lesion revascularisation - 9.6% for GuardWire patients versus 16.5% for control patients; $p = 0.004$. The reduction in major adverse cardiac events was driven by a reduction in myocardial infarction of all magnitudes (8.6% versus 14.7%, $p= 0.008$). In addition, rates of TIMI grade 3 flow were higher for the GuardWire arm (98%) compared with the control arm (95%; $p = 0.04$) and the incidence of clinically evident no-reflow was reduced (3% versus 9%; $p = 0.001$). A per-protocol analysis on the patients with technically successful use of the GuardWire (90.1%) showed an even lower incidence of myocardial infarction (7.9%) and no-reflow phenomenon (2.4%). The rates of the primary end point and no-reflow in patients with technical failure of Guard-wire arm were similar to the control arm (Baim et al., 2002).

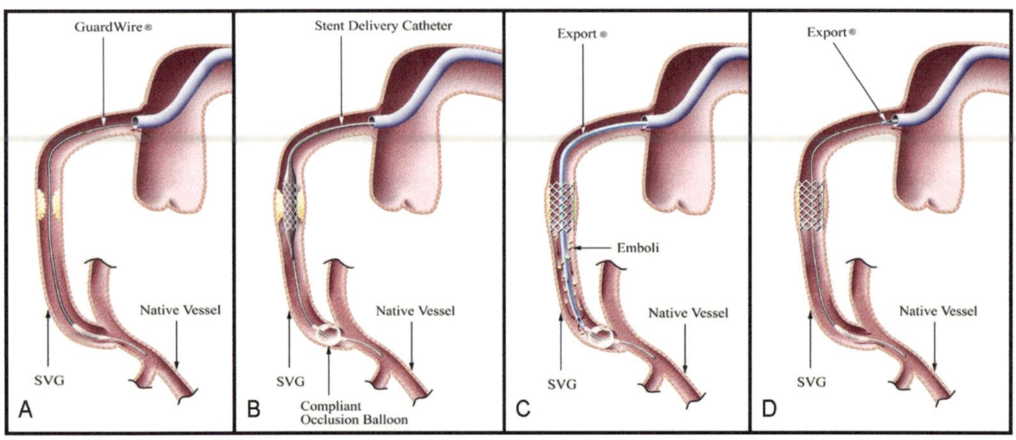

Fig. 2. Diagram of the GuardWire temporary occlusion and aspiration system. A) The lesion is crossed with the GuardWire. The distal occlusion balloon is positioned proximal to anastomosis. The stent/balloon is advanced to the tip of the guide catheter. B) The compliant occlusion balloon at the GuardWire tip is inflated to occlude flow before the stent is deployed. C) After stent deployment, an Export catheter is advanced over the GuardWire and aspiration is performed to remove the stagnant column of blood with suspended embolic debris. D) The GuardWire balloon is deflated to restore antegrade blood flow. Courtesy of Medtronic.

A morphometric and histological analysis of aspirated debris in the SAFE (Saphenous Vein Graft Angioplasty Free of Emboli) trial, using the GuardWire, showed grossly visible red and/or yellow debris extracted from 91% of the patients (Figure 3). Scanning electron microscopy documented particles ranging from 17 to 807 µm in diameter, with 81% of the aspirated particle size smaller than 96 microns (Grube et al., 2020). This is of particular consideration when one considers that the FilterWire (Boston Scientific, Natic, MA) has an 80 µm diameter pore size (Carter et al., 2007).

Despite these results there are some disadvantages with the use of these devices. The resulting absence of antegrade flow during balloon inflation may result in distal ischaemia, which is poorly tolerated by some patients. Sixty one percent of patients in the SAFE trial developed angina during balloon inflation; however, in no patient was ischaemia so severe as to prompt premature deflation of the occlusion balloon. Additionally, balloon-induced injury may occur if they are not used carefully and it is difficult to get adequate imaging during the procedure while the distal vessel is occluded (Morís et al., 2009).

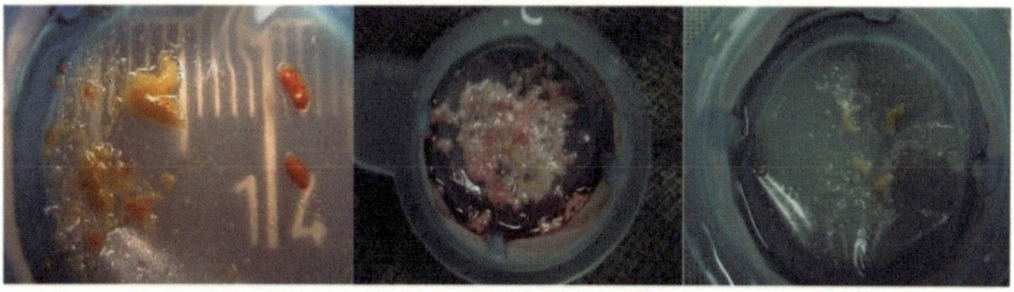

Fig. 3. Aspirated debris from a saphenous vein graft. Courtesy of Medtronic.

A second-generation distal balloon occlusion device, TriActiv (Kensey Nash Corp., Exton, PA), has 4 principal components: a balloon guidewire consisting of a 0.014" hypotube with a carbon dioxide–inflated compliant occlusion balloon on the wire (balloon diameter 3-5 mm), a modified syringe filled with sterile carbon dioxide used to inflate the occlusion balloon, a 4F side-attachable flush catheter, and a drive console with mechanical pumps for infusion and extraction. The lesion is crossed with the balloon guidewire and the occlusion balloon is positioned at least 20 mm beyond the distal edge of the target lesion. The occlusion balloon is inflated with carbon dioxide. A stent is delivered over the Balloon Guidewire and deployed at the lesion. The flush catheter is advanced over the balloon guidewire and saline is infused via holes in the distal end. Extraction of fluid and debris is performed through the guiding catheter. The occlusion balloon is deflated and flow is restored (Carrozza et al., 2005a).

The PRIDE (Protection During Saphenous Vein Graft Intervention to Prevent Distal Embolization) study was a prospective randomized trial, which enrolled patients with coronary ischemia and lesions in saphenous vein grafts in two cohorts. Cohort I randomized patients to protection with the TriActiv System versus percutaneous coronary intervention without embolic protection, to demonstrate superiority of the TriActiv System compared with an "unprotected" group. Given the small number of patients in Cohort I, meaningful conclusions regarding the superiority of TriActiv to saphenous vein graft intervention without embolic protection could not be made.

Cohort II randomized 631 patients to embolic protection with the TriActiv System or control group (Guardwire System [Medtronic] or Filterwire EX [Boston Scientific]) to establish non-inferiority to other distal protection devices. The incidence of major adverse cardiac events at 30 days was 11.2% for the TriActiv group and 10.1% for the control group (relative risk = 1.1%; 95% confidence interval 0.67 to 1.76; $p = 0.65$; $p = 0.02$ for non-inferiority). Safety and efficacy end points were similar between groups except that patients randomized to the TriActiv System had more hemorrhagic complications (10.9% vs. 5.4%; $p = 0.01$). Patients in the TriActiv group were more likely to require blood transfusion. Sub-group analysis indicated that the higher rate of transfusion in the TriActiv cohort was associated with an early design of the haemostatic valve in combination with 8-F guiding catheters. The

TriActiv System was shown to be not inferior to approved embolic protection devices for the treatment of diseased saphenous vein grafts (Carrozza et al., 2005b).

10.2 Proximal balloon occlusion devices

The Proxis Embolic Protection System (St. Jude Medical, Maple Grove, Minnesota) is a unique single-operator catheter that is deployed proximal to the target lesion before crossing. Inflation of the sealing balloon interrupts antegrade flow during the period of lesion intervention. Stagnated blood and emboli liberated during intervention is then retrieved by gentle aspiration or via ancillary flushing of the vessel (Figure 4).

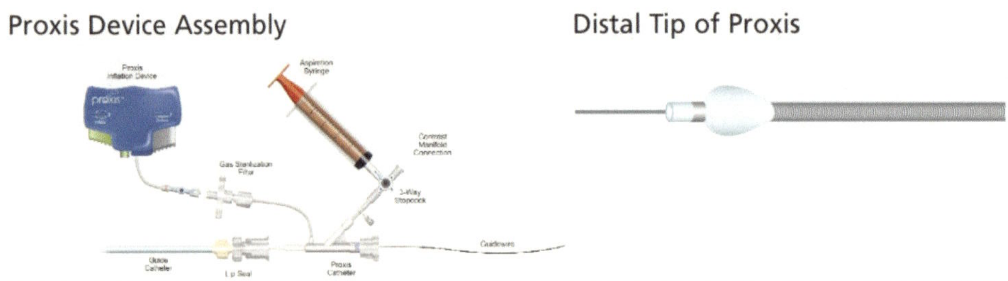

	REORDER NUMBER	VESSEL COMPATIBILITY	SHEATH ID	TOTAL LENGTH	GUIDE CATHETER COMPATIBILITY	GUIDEWIRE COMPATIBILITY
7F	0981-012	3.0-5.0 mm	0.059" (1.50 mm)	126 cm	7F ≥ 0.078	0.014

Fig. 4. Image of the Proxis embolic protection system. Courtesy of St. Jude Medical.

The PROXIMAL (Proximal Protection During Saphenous Vein Graft Intervention) trial was a multicenter prospective randomized trial, which compared 2 treatment strategies in a noninferiority format. Patients with saphenous vein graft stenosis were randomized to 1 of 2 treatment strategies: a current-care control arm (distal embolic protection device with FilterWire or GuardWire whenever possible, and no embolic protection when not) or a test arm (proximal protection with the Proxis system whenever possible and distal embolic protection when anatomy precluded proximal protection).

A total of 594 patients undergoing stenting of 639 saphenous vein grafts were prospectively randomized. The primary composite end point of death, myocardial infarction, or target vessel revascularization at 30 days by intention to treat analysis occurred in 10.0% of control and 9.2% of test patients; difference = -0.8% (95% confidence interval [CI] -5.5% to 4.0%); p for noninferiority= 0.0061. In device specific analysis, this composite end point occurred in 11.7% of distal protection patients and 7.1% of proximal protection patients (difference = -4.6% [95% CI -9.6% to 0.3%]; p for superiority = 0.10, p for noninferiority = 0.001). Finally, in the subset of patients with lesions amenable to treatment with either proximal or distal protection devices (n = 410), the primary composite end point occurred in 12.2% of distal protection patients and 7.4% of proximal protection patients; p for superiority = 0.14, p for noninferiority = 0.001.

This study concluded that using proximal embolic protection whenever possible during treatment of diseased saphenous vein grafts produced outcomes similar to those with distal embolic protection (Mauri et al., 2007).

Unfortunately, this device also has limitations: there is no antegrade flow with the subsequent possibility of myocardial ischaemia during the procedure, its utilization is more complex than the distal filters and they can not be used in ostial disease (Morís et al., 2009).

10.3 Filter devices

Distal embolic filter devices maintain distal perfusion and allow injection of contrast medium during PCI while trapping most particulate debris. The advantages are that they preserve antegrade flow, contrast imaging is possible throughout the procedure and they are very simple to use. However, they are associated with limitations such as the fact that may not be able to capture all the debris, it may also be difficult to evaluate retrieval of the debris during the procedure, delivery catheters may cause embolization before filter deployment and the possibility of snagging of the retrieval sheath on the stent (Morís et al., 2009).

The FilterWire EZ (Boston Scientific) consists of a distal polyurethane filter with a 110 µm pore size mounted on a 0.014-inch guidewire. The latest version has a 100 µm pore size. The system consists of a protection wire, a delivery sheath, a retrieval sheath and accessories (Figures 5 and 6). When deployed, the protection wire's filter bag is designed to capture and recover emboli that may be released during the procedure. The protection wire is used as the primary guidewire during the procedure. The floppy tip of the protection wire and the filter loop are radiopaque to enable visual guidance during placement. At the completion of the procedure, the filter is captured using the retrieval sheath and then removed from the patient (Figure 7). The loop of the device is designed to appose vessels ranging from 3.5 to 5.5 mm.

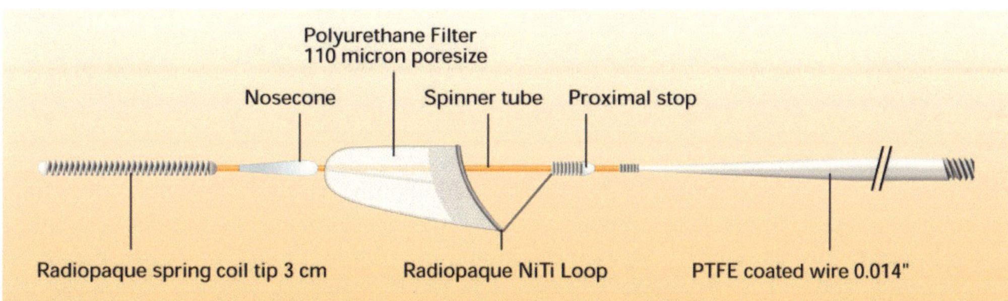

Fig. 5. Image of the FilterWire EZ. Courtesy of Boston Scientific.

The FIRE (FilterWire EX Randomized Evaluation) trial was a multicenter randomized trial designed to evaluate the safety and efficacy of distal microcirculatory protection with the FilterWire EX compared with the GuardWire balloon occlusion and aspiration device during percutaneous intervention of diseased saphenous vein grafts. Six hundred and fifty one patients undergoing stent implantation in 682 de novo lesions in saphenous vein grafts with a reference diameter between 3.5 to 5.5 mm were randomized. Device success (defined as the ability to deliver, deploy and retract a device at and from the target location for FilterWire and the ability to deliver a device to the target, obtain distal occlusion and perform aspiration without loss of occlusion attributable to leak or rupture for GuardWire) was 95.5% and 97.2% with the FilterWire EX and GuardWire, respectively ($p = 0.25$).

Postprocedural measures of epicardial flow, angiographic complications and the extent of myonecrosis were similar between the 2 groups. The primary end point of the study, the composite occurrence of major adverse cardiac events, including death, myocardial infarction or target vessel revascularization at 30-days occurred in 9.9% of FilterWire EX patients and 11.6% of GuardWire patients (difference [95% confidence interval] = -1.7% [-6.4%, 3.1%]; p for superiority = 0.53, p for noninferiority = 0.0008). This was driven primarily by non-Q wave myocardial infarction. Although exploratory subgroup analyses demonstrated a possible benefit of the FilterWire EX compared with the GuardWire in smaller vessels and eccentric lesions, the mechanistic explanation for these observations is uncertain, and these findings may be attributable to chance. It is important to note that, event rates were very low in both groups when only one stent was implanted or the total length of stents was limited. Conversely, the longer the lesion and the greater the number and length of stents implanted, the higher the event rate with both protection devices. Periprocedural adverse event rates were also increased in thrombotic lesions and degenerated vein grafts (Stone et al., 2003). By 6 months, the outcomes of the FIRE trial showed similar major adverse cardiac event increases to 19.3% in the FilterWire EX and to 21.9% in the GuardWire groups (p= 0.44) (Halkin et al., 2006).

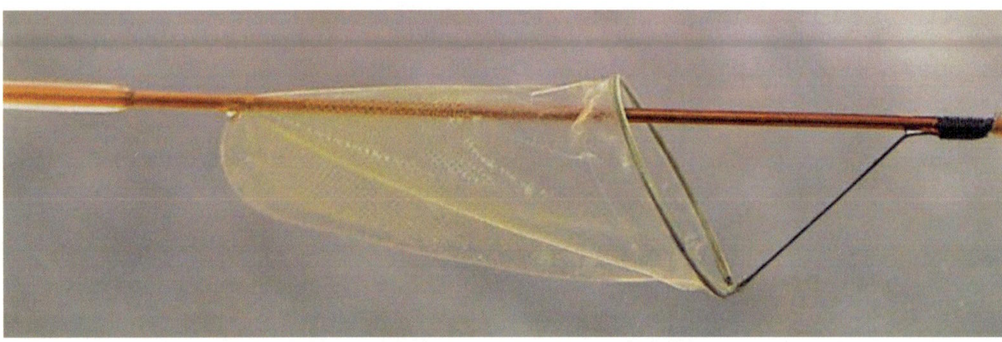

Fig. 6. Image of the FilterWire EZ. Courtesy of Boston Scientific.

The SpiderRX embolic protection device (eV3, Plymouth, MN) is a nitinol mesh filter system. One major innovation of this filter is the ability to cross the lesion with a conventional 0.014-inch guidewire, then deploying the filter via monorail delivery catheter (Carter et al., 2007). This device was assessed in the Spider trial, which randomized 732 patients to saphenous vein intervention using either the Spider device or a control arm of distal protection with the GuardWire or the FilterWire. Major adverse cardiac event rates were statistically similar between both groups after 30 days. Compared with controls, the SpiderRX showed non-inferiority in terms of all secondary end points, including device success, in-hospital major adverse cardiac events, clinical success and procedural success (Carter et al., 2007 & White, 2006).

One concern regarding the use of filter based systems versus balloon occlusion systems has been the functional limitations of the pore size and retrieved particulate debris. This concern however, has not been substantiated by the outcomes of the clinical trials. In fact, one analysis of retrieved particles using a filter device and the GuardWire showed retrieval of particles well less than 100 µm. It is possible that deposition of platelets and debris reduces the functional pore size (Carter et al., 2007).

Although, as has been mentioned above, none of these devices has demonstrated more efficacy than others in a randomized trial, some recommendations can be made based on anatomical considerations and tolerance of absence of antegrade flow: distal occlusion may be the preferred choice in cases of proximal disease with high plaque or thrombus burden; filters may be proposed in cases of poor tolerance for ischaemia or single remaining grafts without distal disease and proximal occlusion devices would be indicated in grafts with distal disease, especially in relatively straight vessels (Morís et al., 2009).

Distal protection devices have been shown to enhance procedural success rates, reduce the occurrence of no reflow, and prevent large as well as small periprocedural infarctions; the former of which is clearly prognostically relevant. These results thus support the general recommendation for routine use of distal protection devices during saphenous vein graft intervention when possible. However, it should be recognised that the long-term course after intervention in diseased saphenous vein grafts is not benign even when distal protection is used. Periprocedural major adverse events still occur in approximately 10% of patients, and the rates of death, myocardial infarction and repeat revascularisation procedures are relatively high compared with percutaneous coronary interventions in native coronary arteries, due not only to restenosis at the target site but also to disease progression in sites remote from that of the index intervention. These observations underscore the need for intensive post-discharge surveillance and secondary prevention measures in this population (Halkin et al., 2006).

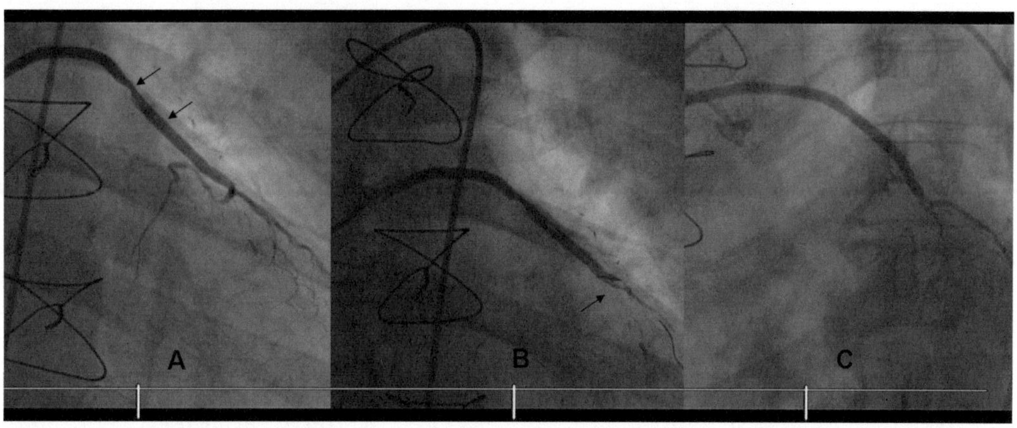

Fig. 7. Percutaneous intervention in a saphenous vein graft using a FilterWire embolic protection device. A) Saphenous vein graft stenosis with superimposed thrombus (arrows). B) Particulate debris trapped within the FilterWire embolic protection device (arrow). C) End result after removing the FilterWire.

11. Conclusions

Saphenous vein graft disease represents the "Achilles heel" of coronary artery bypass surgery interventions, due to the high failure rate of saphenous vein grafts (Lupi et al., 2011).

Stenosed saphenous vein grafts can be treated by percutaneous intervention or a second coronary artery bypass surgery; however, a repeated bypass surgery is burdened by a higher risk of death and provides less symptomatic improvement (Lupi et al., 2011).

Attempts at percutaneous revascularisation in saphenous vein graft lesions with balloon angioplasty were limited by a relatively low procedural success rate and a high incidence of angiographic recurrence.

Stent implantation in patients with focal saphenous vein graft lesions improved procedural success and clinical outcome compared with balloon angioplasty. However, even with the use of stents treatment of saphenous vein graft lesions is associated with a high incidence of acute complications, principally distal embolisation and periprocedural myocardial infarction, because of the more friable atherosclerotic or thrombotic components of the saphenous vein graft lesions (Stankovic et al., 2003). Besides, the results of bare metal stents in saphenous vein grafts are less favourable than those in native vessels, with restenosis rates exceeding 30% (Savage et al., 1997; Silber et al., 2005). In fact some authors recommend carrying out percutaneous coronary intervention in native vessels whenever possible even when there is complete obstruction or to consider the possibility of new revascularisation surgery rather than percutaneous saphenous vein graft intervention (Lozano et al., 2005).

In an attempt to improve the outcome of intervention in stenotic vein grafts, several approaches and adjunctive pharmacological regimens have been studied, but with the exception of distal protection devices, none showed a clear benefit in reducing the incidence of distal embolisation, especially in complex lesions (Stankovic et al., 2003). However, despite the existence of successful proximal and distal filters and balloons, 30-day major adverse cardiac event rates still hover between 8% and 10%. A logical approach to assess a potential reduction in the incidence of no-reflow phenomenon and its deleterious consequences would be to conduct prospective, randomised, controlled trials assessing the combination of distal filter protection devices, glycoprotein IIb/IIIa inhibitors and pre-treatment with intra-graft administration of vasodilators, particularly nicardipine.

Drug-eluting stents have been shown to reduce restenosis in many lesion types and clinical syndromes. However, there is a paucity of prospective data on drug-eluting stents in saphenous vein graft intervention (Brilakis et al., 2009). Most meta-analysis of randomised trials and observational studies comparing drug-eluting stents and bare metal stents in saphenous vein graft percutaneous intervention suggest that drug-eluting stent use in saphenous vein graft is safe and reduces target vessel revascularisation.

Patients with previous coronary artery bypass graft surgery suffer from diffuse atherosclerosis of native coronary arteries as well as rapid saphenous vein graft degeneration, thus the benefit from drug-eluting stents could be largely diluted by acute coronary syndromes arising from other previously untreated coronary lesions (Lupi et al., 2011).

In addition, it is well established that the long-term prognosis of patients with diseased saphenous vein grafts is mainly impacted by progression of disease in the nonintervened saphenous vein grafts segments (Ellis et al., 1997 & Keeley et al., 2001).

Large, prospective, multicenter, randomised-controlled clinical trials that use a clinical rather than angiographic end point are needed to confirm the beneficial role of drug-eluting stents in saphenous vein graft lesions (Brilakis & Berger, 2008). Additionally, longer-term follow-up of at least 3 to 5 years is essential for randomised trials involving the use of drug-eluting stents in saphenous vein grafts to address two potentially harmful events. First, the possibility of late restenosis catch-up with drug-eluting stents in saphenous vein graft disease, considering their higher restenosis rate and more delayed restenosis process than in native vessels. Second, the possible risk of late stent thrombosis, which has been already shown for native coronary arteries (Mc Fadden et al., 2004; & Ong et al., 2005), in a potentially favourable milieu such as that in saphenous vein graft disease.

12. References

Baim D.S.; Wahr, D.; George B.; Leon, M.B.; Greenberg, J.; Cutlip, D.E.; Kaya, U.; Popma, J.J.; Ho, K.K.L. & Kuntz. R.E. (2002). On behalf of the Saphenous vein graft Angioplasty Free of Emboli Randomized (SAFER) trial investigators. Randomized Trial of a Distal Embolic Protection Device During Percutaneous Intervention of Saphenous Vein Aorto-Coronary Bypass Grafts*Circulation*, Vol 105, No. 11, (March 2002), pp. 1285-1290.

Baim, D. (2003). Percutaneous treatment of saphenous vein graft disease: the ongoing challenge. *J Am Coll Cardiol*, Vol 42, No. 8 (October 2003), pp. 1370-1372.

Baldus, S.; Köster, R.; Elsner, M.; Walter, D.H.; Arnold, R.; Auch-Schwelk, W.; Berger, J.; Rau, M.; Meinertz, T.; Zeiher, A.M. & Hamm, C.W. (2000). Treatment of aortocoronary vein graft lesion with membrane-covered stents: a multicenter surveillance trial. *Circulation*, Vol 102, No.17, (October 2000), pp. 2024-2027.

Bittl, J.A. (2009). Drug-eluting stents for saphenous vein graft lesions. The limits of evidence. *J Am Coll Cardiol*, Vol 53, No. 11, (March 2009), pp. 929-930.

Brener, S.J.; Lytle, B.W.; Casserly, I.P.; Ellis, S.G.; Topol, E.J. & Lauer, M.S. (2006). Predictors of revascularization method and long-term outcome of percutaneous coronary intervention or repeat coronary bypass surgery in patients with multivessel coronary disease and previous coronary bypass surgery. *Eur Heart J*, Vol. 27, No. 4, (February 2006), pp. 413–418.

Brilakis, E.S. & Berger, P.B. (2008). Should bare metal or drug-eluting stents be used during PCI of saphenous vein graft lesions: waiting for Godot?. *Catheter Cardiovasc Interv.* Vol. 72, No 6, (November 2008), pp. 815-818.

Brilakis, E.S.; Lichtenwalter, C.; de Lemos, J.A.; Roesle, M.; Obel, O.; Haagen, D.; Saeed, B.; Gadiparthi, C.; Bissett, J.K.; Sachdeva, R.; Voudris, V.V.; Karyofillis, P.; Kar, B.; Rossen, J.; Fasseas, P.; Berger, P. & Banerjee, S. A Randomized Controlled Trial of a Paclitaxel-Eluting Stent Versus a Similar Bare-Metal Stent in Saphenous Vein Graft Lesions: The SOS (Stenting Of Saphenous Vein Grafts) Trial. *J Am Coll Cardiol*, Vol. 53, No. 11, (March 2009), pp. 919-928.

Carrozza, J.P.; Caussin, C.; Braden, G.; Braun, P.; Hansell, F.; Fatzinger, R.; Walters, G.; Kussmaul, W. & Breall, J. for the TriActiv Pilot Study Investigators. (2005 a). Embolic protection during saphenous vein graft intervention using a second-generation balloon protection device: Results from the combined US and European pilot study of the TriActiv Balloon Protected Flush Extraction System. *Am Heart J*, Vol. 149, No. 6, (June 2005), pp. 1136.e1-1136.e7.

Carrozza, J.P.; Mumma, M.; Breall, J.A.; Fernandez, A.; Heyman, E. & Metzger, C. for the PRIDE Study Investigators (2005 b). Randomized Evaluation of the TriActiv Balloon-Protection Flush and Extraction System for the Treatment of Saphenous Vein Graft Disease. *J Am Coll Cardiol*, Vol. 46, No. 9, (November 2005), pp. 1677-83.

Carter, L.; Golzar, J.A.; Cavendish, J.J. & Dixon, S. R. (2007). Embolic protection of saphenous vein graft percutaneous interventions. *J Interven Cardiol*, Vol 20 No 5, (October 2007), pp. 351-358.

de Feyter, PJ.; van Suylen, RJ.; de Jaegere, PPT.; Topol, EJ. & Serruys PW. (1993). Balloon Angioplasty for the Treatment of Lesions in Saphenous vein Bypass Grafts. *J Am Coll Cardiol* 1993; Vol 21, No. 7, (June 1993), pp. 1539-1549.

de Feyter, P.J. (2003). Percutaneous Treatment of Saphenous Vein Bypass Graft Obstructions. A Continuing Obstinate Problem. *Circulation* 2003, Vol 107, No. 18, (May 2003), pp. 2284-2286.

Douglas, J.S. Jr. (1994). Percutaneous approaches to recurrent myocardial ischemia in patients with prior surgical revascularization. *Semin Thorac Cardiovasc Surg*, Vol. 6, No. 2, (April 1994) pp. 98-108.

Ellis, S.G.; Brener, S.J.; DeLuca, S.; Murat Tuzcu, E.; Raymond, R.E.; Whitlow, P.L. & Topol, E.J. (1997). Late myocardial ischemic events after saphenous vein graft intervention importance of initially "nonsignificant" vein graft lesions. *Am J Cardiol*, Vol. 79, No. 11, (June 1997), pp. 1460-1464.

Elsner, M.; Auch-Schwelk, W.; Britten, M.; Walter, D.H.; Schächinger, V. & Zeiher, A.M. (1999). Coronary stent grafts covered by a polytetrafluoroethylene membrane. *Am J Cardiol*, Vol. 84, No. 3, (August 1999), pp. 335-338.

Fischell, T. A.; Carter, A. J.; Foster M.T.; Hempsall, K.; DeVries, J.; Kim, D.H. & Kloostra A. (1998) Reversal of "no-reflow" during vein graft stenting using high velocity boluses of intracoronary adenosine. *Cathet. Cardiovasc. Diagn. Vol.45, No.4, (December 1998), pp.360-365.*

Fischell, T.A. (2008). Pharmaceutical interventions for the management of no-reflow. *J Invasive Cardiol. Vol. 20, No. 7, (July 2008), pp. 374-9.*

Grines, C.L.; Bonow, R.O.; Casey Jr, D.E.; Gardner, T.J.; Lockhart, P.B.; Moliterno, D.J.; O'Gara, P. & Whitlow. P. (2007). Prevention of Premature Discontinuation of Dual Antiplatelet Therapy in Patients With Coronary Artery Stents: A Science Advisory From the American Heart Association, American College of Cardiology, Society for Cardiovascular Angiography and Interventions, American College of Surgeons, and American Dental Association, With Representation From the American College of Physicians. *J Am Coll Cardiol*, Vol. 49, No. 6, (February 2007), pp. 734-739.

Grube, E.; Schofer, J.; Webb, J.; Schuler, G.; Colombo, A.; Sievert, H.; Gerkens, U. & Stone, G.W. (2002). For the Saphenous Vein Graft Angioplsty Free of Emboli (SAFE) Trial study group. Evaluation of a balloon occlusion and aspiration system for protection from distal embolisation during stenting in saphenous vein grafts. *Am J Cardiol*, Vol. 89, No. 8, (April 2002), pp. 941-945.

Habibzadeh, M.R.; Thai, H. & Movahed, M.R. (2011). Prophilactic intragraft injection of nicardipine prior to saphenous vein graft percutaneous intervention for the prevention of no-reflow: a review and comparison to protection devices. *J Invasive Cardiol*, Vol. 23, No. 5, (May 2001), pp. 2002-206.

Hakeem, A.; Helmy, T.; Munsif, S.; Bhatti, S.; Mazraeshahi, R.; Cilingiroglu, M.; Effat, M.; Leesar, M. & Arif, I. (2011). Safety and efficacy of drug eluting stents compared with bare metal stents for saphenous vein graft interventions: A comprehensive meta=analysis of randomised trials and observational studies comprising 7,994 patients. *Catheter Cardiovasc Interv*, Vol. 77, No. 3, (February 2011), pp. 343-355.

Halkin, A.; Masud, A.Z.; Rogers, C.; Hermiller, J.; Feldman, R.; Hall, P.; Haber, R.H.; Cambier, P.A.; Caputo, R.P.; Turco, M.; Kovach, R.; Brodie, B.; Hermann, H.C.; Kuntz, R.E.; Popma, J.J.; Ramee, S.; Cox, D.A.; Mehran, R. & Stone, G. (2006). Six-month outcomes after percutaneous intervention for lesions in aortocoronary saphenous vein grafts using distal protection devices: Results from the FIRE trial. *Am Heart J*. Vol. 151, No. 4, (April 2006), pp. 915.e1-915. e7.

Hanekamp, C.E.E.; Koolen, J.; den Heijer, P.; Schalij, M.J.; Piek, J.J.; Bar, F.W.H.M.; Scheerder I.D.; Bonnier, H.J.R.M. & Piljs, N.H.J. (2003). Randomized Study to Compare Balloon Angioplasty and Elective Stent Implantation in Venous Bypass Grafts: The Venestent Study. *Catheter Cardiovasc Interv* 2003, Vol, 60, No. 4, (December 2003), pp. 452-457.

Hassantash, S-A; Bikdeli, B; Kalantarian, S; Sadeghian, M. & Afshar, H. (2008). Pathophysiology of Aortocoronary Saphenous Vein Bypass Graft Disease. *Asian Cardiovasc Thorac Ann* 2008, Vol 16, No. 4, (August 2008) pp. 331-336.

Hillegass, W.B.; Dean, N.A.; Liao, L.; Rhinehart, R.G. & Myers, P. R. (2001) Treatment of no-reflow and impaired flow with the nitric oxide donor nitroprusside following percutaneous coronary interventions: Initial human clinical experience. *J Am Coll Cardiol, Vol. 37, No. 5, (April 2001), pp. 1335-1343.*

Hillegass, W.B. (2011). DES in SVGs: Safe and at least short-term effective. *Catheter Cardiovasc Interv*. Vol 77, No. 3, (February 2011), pp. 356-357.

Hiscock, M.; Oqueli, E. & Dick, R. (2007). Percutaneous Saphenous Vein Graft Intervention – A Review. *Heart Lung and Circulation*, 2007; Vol. 16, Suppl. 3, (2007), pp. S51-S55.

Hong, M.K.; Mehran, R.; Dangas, G.; Mintz, G.S.; Lansky, A.; Kent, K.M.; Pichard, A.D.; Satler, L.F.; Stone, G.W. & Leon. M.B. (2000).Comparison of time course of target lesion revascularization following successful saphenous vein graft angioplasty versus successful native coronary angioplasty. *Am J Cardiol*, Vol. 82, No. 2, (January 2000), pp. 256-258.

Jonas, M.; Stone, G.W.; Mehran, R.; Hermiller, J.; Feldman, R.; Herrmann, H.C.; Cox, D.A.; Kuntz, R.E.; Popma, J.J. & Rogers, C. for the filterWire EX randomized evaluation (FIRE) investigators. (2005). Platelet glycoprotein IIb/IIIa receptor inhibition as adjunctive during saphenous vein graft stenting: differential effects after randomization to occlusion or filter-based embolic protection. *Eur Heart J*, Vol. 27, No. 8, (April 2006), pp. 920-928.

Keeley, E.C.; Velez, C.A.; O'Neill, W.W. & Safian, R. D. (2001). Long-term clinical outcome and predictors of major adverse cardiac events after percutaneous interventions on saphenous vein grafts. *J Am Coll Cardiol*, Vol 38, No. 3, (September 20010), pp. 659-665.

Lansky, A.J.; Yang, Y.M.; Khan, Y.; Costa, R.A.; Pietras, C.; Tsuchiya, Y.; Cristea, E.; Collins, M.; Mehran, R.; Dangas, G. D. ; Mosess, J.W.; Leon, M.B. & Stone, G.W. (2006). Treatment of coronary artery perforations complicating percutaneous coronary intervention with a polytetrafluoroethylene-covered stent graft. *Am J Cardiol*, Vol. 98, No. 3, (August 2006), pp. 370-374.

Leborgne, L.; Cheneau, E.; Pichard, A.; Ajani, A.; Pakala, R.; Yazdi, H.; Satler, L.; Kent, K.; Suddath, W.O.; Pinnow, E.; Canos, D. & Waksman, R. (2003). Effect of direct stenting on clinical outcome in patients treated with percutaneous coronary intervention on saphenous vein graft. *Am Heart J*, Vol. 146, No. 3, (September 2003), pp. 501-506.

Lee, M.; Park, S-J.; Kandzari, D.E.; Kirtane, A.J.; Fearon, W.F.; Brilakis, E.S.; Vermeersch, P.; Kim, Y-H.; Waksman, R.; Mehilli, J.; Mauri, L. & Stone, G.W. (2011). Saphenous vein graft intervention. *J Am Coll Cardiol Interv*, Vol. 4, No. 8, (August, 2011), pp. 831-843.

Lozano, I.; Lopez-Palop, R.; Pinar, E; Saura, D.; Fuertes, J; Rondán, J.; Suárez, E.; Valdéz, M. & Morís, C. (2005). Direct stenting in saphenous vein grafts. Immediate and long-term results. *Rev Esp Cardiol*, Vol. 58, No. 3, (December 2005), pp. 270-277.

Lupi A.; Navarese, E.P.; Lazzero, M.; Sansa, M.; De Servi, S.; Serra, A.; Bongo, A.S. & Buffon, A. (2011) Drug-eluting stents vs. bare metal stents in saphenous vein graft disease. - Insights from a meta-analysis of 7,090 patients. *Circ J*, Vol.75, No. 2, (February 2011), pp. 280-289.

Mauri, L.; Cox, D.; Hermiller, J.; Massaro, J.; Wahr, J.; Tay, S.W.; Jonas, M.; Popma, J.J.; Pavliska, J.; Wahr, D. & Rogers, C.(2007). The PROXIMAL Trial: Proximal Protection During Saphenous Vein Graft Intervention Using the Proxis Embolic Protection System. A Randomized, Prospective, Multicenter Clinical Trial. *J Am Coll Cardiol*, Vol. 50, No. 15, (October 2007), pp.1442–1449.

Mehilli, J.; Richard, G.; Neumann, F.J.; Massberg, S.; Laugwitz, K.L.; Pache, J.; Hausleiter, J.; Ott, I.; Fusaro, M.; Ibrahim, T.; Schömig, A. & Kastrati A. (2011). ISAR-CABG: Randomized, Superiority Trial of Drug-Eluting-Stent and Bare Metal Stent in Safenous Vein Graft Lesions. Paper presented at: American College of Cardiology 2011 Scientific Sessions. New Orleans, LA. April 4, 2011.

McFadden, E.P.; Stabile, E.; Regar, E.; Cheneau, E.; Ong, A.T.L.; Kinnaird, T.; Suddath, W.O.; Weissman, N.J.; Torguson, R.; Kent, K.M.; Pichard, A.D.; Satler, L.F.; Waksman, R. & Serruys, P.W. (2004). Late thrombosis in drug-eluting coronary stents after discontinuation of antiplatelet therapy. *Lancet*, Vol. 364, No. 9444, (October 2004), pp. 1519-1521.

Michishita, I. (2011). The final answer? - For the treatment of saphenous vein graft disease, drug-eluting stents versus bare-metal stents. *Circ J*, Vol. 75, No. 2, (February 2011), pp. 261-262.

Morís, C.; Lozano, I.; Martín, M.; Juán Rondán, J. & Avanzas, P. (2009) Embolic protection devices in saphenous percutaneous intervention. *Eurointervention*, Vol. 5, Supplement D, (May 2009), pp. D45-D50.

Morrison, D.A.; Crowley, S.T.; Veerakul, G.; Barbiere, C.C.; Grover, F. & Sacks J. (1993). Percutaneous Transluminal Angioplasty of Saphenous Vein Grafts for Medically Refractory Unstable Angina. *J Am Coll Cardiol*, Vol 23, No 5, (April 1994), pp. 1066-1070.

Motwani, J.G. & Topol, E.J. (1998). Aortocoronary Saphenous Vein Graft Disease. Pathogenesis, Predisposition, and Prevention. *Circulation*, Vol. 97, No. 9, (March 1998), pp. 916-931.

Murphy, G.J. & Angelini G.D. (2004). Insights into the pathogenesis of vein graft disease: lessons from intravascular ultrasound. *Cardiovascular Ultrasound*, 2:8 (July 2004), Available from: http://www.cardiovascularultrasound.com/content/2/1/8

Nguyen, T.; Pham, L.; Cheem, TH.; Douglas, JS.; Hermiller, J.; & Cindy Grines (2004). Approach to the patient with prior bypass surgery. *J Interven Cardiol* 2004; 17:339-346.

Ong, A.T.L.; McFadden, E.P.; Regar, E.; de Jaegere, P.P.T.; van Domburg, R.T. & Serruys, P.W. (2005). Late Angiographic Stent Thrombosis (LAST) Events With Drug-Eluting Stents. *J Am Coll Cardiol,* Vol. 45, No. 12, (June 2005), pp. 2088-2092.

Pregowsky, J.; Tyczynski, P.; Mintz, GS.; Kim, S-W.; Witkowski, A.; Waksman, R.; Pichard, A.; Satler, L.; Kent, K.; Kruk, M.; Bieganski, S.; Ohlmann, P. & Weissman, NJ. (2005). Incidence and Clinical Correlates of Ruptured Plaques in Saphenous Vein Grafts. An Intravascular Ultrasound Study. *J Am Coll Cardiol,* Vol 45, No. 12, (June 2005), pp.1974-1979.

Roffi, M.; Mukherjee, D.; Chew, D.P.; Bhatt, D.L.; Cho L.; Robbins, M.A.; Ziada, K.M.; Brennan, D.M.; Ellis, S.G. & Topol, E.J. (2002). Lack of benefit from intravenous platelet glycoprotein IIb/IIIa receptor inhibition as adjunctive treatment for percutaneous interventions of aortocoronary bypass grafts. A pooled analysis of five randomized clinical trials. *Circulation,* Vol. 106, No 24, (December 2002), pp. 3063-3067.

Savage, M.P.; Douglas, J.S.; Fischman, D.L.; Pepine, C.J.; King III, S.B.; Werner, J.A.; Bailey, M.D.; Overlie, P.A.; Fenton, S.H.; Brinker, J.A.; Leon, M.B. & Goldberg, S. for the Saphenous Vein De Novo Trial Investigators. (1997). Stent placement compared with balloon angioplasty for obstructed coronary bypass grafts. *N Engl J Med,* Vol 337,No. 11, (September 1997), pp. 740-747.

Schächinger, V.; Hamm, C.W.; Münzel, T.; Haude, M.; Baldus, S.; Grube, E.; Bonzel, T.; Konorza, T.; Köster, R.; Arnold, R.; Haase, J.; Probst, P.; Vom Dahl, J.; Neumann, F-J.; Mudra, H.; Hennen, B.; Thiele, L. & Zeihr, A.M. for the STING (STent IN Grafts) Investigators. (2003). A Randomized Trial of Polytetrafluoroethylene-Membrane-Covered Stents Compared With Conventional Stents in Aortocoronary Saphenous Vein Grafts. *J Am Coll Cardiol,* Vol. 42, No. 8, (Oct 2003), pp. 1360-1369.

Silber, S.; Albertsson, P.; Avilés, F.F; Camici, P.G.; Colombo, A.; Hamm, C.; Jørgensen, E.; Marco, J.; Nordrehaug, J-E.; Ruzyllo, W.; Urban, P.; Stone, G.W. & Wijns, W. (2005). Guidelines for Percutaneous Coronary Interventions: The Task Force for Percutaneous Coronary Interventions of the European Society of Cardiology. *Eur Heart J,* Vol. 26, No. 8, (April 2005), pp. 804-847.

Stankovic, G.; Colombo, A.; Presbitero, P.; van den Branden, F.; Inglese, L.; Cernigliaro, C.; Niccoli, L.; Bartorelli, A.L.; Rubartelli, P.; Reifart, N.; Heyndrickx, G.R.; Saunamäki, K.; Morice, M.C.; Sgura, F.A. & Di Mario, C. (2003). Randomized evaluation of polytetrafluoroethylene-covered stent in saphenous vein grafts: The Randomized Evaluation of polytetrafluoroethylene COVERed stent in Saphenous vein grafts (RECOVERS) Trial. *Circulation,* Vol. 108, No. 1, (July 2003), pp. 37-42.

Stone, G.W.; Rogers, C.; Hermiller, J.; Feldman, R.; Hall, P.; Haber, R.; Masud, A.; Cambier, P.; Caputo, R.P.; Turco, M.; Kovach, R.; Brodie, B.; Hermann, H. C.; Kuntz, R. E; Popma, J.J.; Ramee, S. & Cox, D.A. (2003) for the FilterWire EX Randomized Evaluation (FIRE) Investigators. Randomized comparison of distal protection with a filter-based catheter and balloon occlusion and aspiration system during percutaneous intervention of diseased saphenous vein aorto-coronary bypass grafts. *Circulation,* Vol. 108, No. 5, (August 2003), pp. 548-553.

Stone, G.W.; Goldber, S.; O'Shaughnessy, C.; Midei M.; Siegel, R.M.; Cristea, E.; Dangas, G.; Lansky, A. J. & Mehran, R. (2011). 5-Year Follow-Up of Polytetrafluoroethylene-Covered Stents Compared With Bare-Metal Stents in Aortocoronary Saphenous

Vein Grafts. The Randomized BARRICADE (Barrier Approach to Restenosis: Restrict Intima to Curtail Adverse Events) Trial. *J Am Coll Cardiol Intv*, Vol. 4, No. 3, (March 2011), pp. 300-309.

Turco, M.A.; Buchbinder M.; Popma, J.J.; Wissman, N.J.; Mann, T.; Doucet, S.; Johnson, W.L.; Greenberg, J.D.; Leadley, K. & Russell,M.E. (2006). Pivotal, randomized U.S. study of the Symbiot™ covered stent system in patients with saphenous vein graft disease: eight-month angiographic and clinical results from the Symbiot III Trial. *Catheter Cardiovasc Interv*, Vol 68, No 3, (September 2006), pp. 379-388.

Vermeersch, P.; Agostoni, P.; Verheye, S.; Van der Heuvel, P.; Convens, C.; Bruining, N.; Van den Branden, F. & Van Langenhove, G. (2006). Randomized double-blind comparison of Sirolimus-eluting stent versus bare-metal stent implantation in diseased saphenous vein grafts. Six month angiographic, intravascular ultrasound, and clinical follow-up of the RRISC Trial. *J Am Coll Cardiol*, Vol. 48, No. 12, (December 2006), pp. 2423-2431.

Vermeersch, P.; Agostoni, P.; Verheye, S.; Van der Heuvel, P.; Convens, C.; Bruining, N.; Van den Branden, F. & Van Langenhove, G. for the DELAYED RRISC (Death and Events at Long-term follow-up AnalYsis: Extended Duration of the Reduction of Restenosis In Saphenous vein grafts with Cypher stent) Investigators. (2007). Increased late mortality after Sirolimus-eluting stents versus bare-metal stents in diseased saphenous vein grafts. Results from the randomized DELAYED RRISC Trial. *J Am Coll Cardiol*, Vol. 50, No. 3, (July 2007), pp. 261-267.

Vlodaver, Z . &Edwards, J.E. (1973). Pathologic analysis in fatal cases following saphenous vein coronary arterial bypass. *Chest*, Vol 64, No.5, (November 1973), pp. 555-563.

White, J. (2006). TCT 2005 Late-breaking trials promise to influence practice patterns. *J Interven Cardiol*, Vol 19, No. 1, (February 2006), pp. 113-116.

6

Drug Eluting Balloon

S. Sharma[1], N. Kukreja[2] and D. A. Gorog[2,3]
[1]*Frimley Park Hospital NHS Trust,*
[2]*East and North Hertfordshire NHS Trust,*
[3]*Imperial College, London*
UK

1. Introduction

Since the first percutaneous transluminal coronary angioplasty (PTCA) performed by Andreas Gruntzig in 1977 the technology has evolved significantly. Progress of PTCA has seen the development of many devices, some of which are still in use and many others that have fallen in disuse. The main limitation of the plain old balloon angioplasty (POBA) was the problem of elastic vascular recoil causing abrupt vessel closure and restenosis. The patho-mechanism of restenosis that occurs following balloon angioplasty involves negative vascular remodeling, elastic recoil and thrombosis at the site of injury {Moreno, 1999}. While the thrombus formation can be reduced by use of antiplatelet drugs, the restenosis threat remains. Early restenosis occurred in as many as 30% of angioplasty cases. This led to the development of the metal stent to exert radial force on the vessel wall and thus prevent elastic recoil. Although stents reduced restenosis, their use led to the realisation of a different and new challenge of in stent restenois (ISR). This occurs mainly due to neointima formation {Mach, 2000,Mudra et al, 1997, Hoffman et al, 1996, Kearney et al, 1997} that is principally composed of proliferating smooth muscle cells (SMC) and extra cellular matrix {Geary et al, 2003, Grewe et al, 1999}. By the late 1990s, it was acknowledged that although the incidence of ISR was lower than that of restenosis following balloon angioplasty {Serruys et al, 1991}, it occurred in 15-30% of patients, and possibly more frequently in certain subgroups {Holmes et al, 2002}.

2. Treatment of restenosis

Over the years there have been intensive research efforts to identify possible pharmacotherapeutic regimens to prevent the neointimal restenotic process. Although most experimental studies and some small initial clinical studies showed promise, subsequent large randomized trials have been disappointing {Faxon, 1995, Bertrand et al, 1997, Boccuzzi et al, 1998, Serruys et al, 2000, Faxon, 2002}. Failure to achieve significant reduction in ISR with systemic drug therapy led to the exploration of the concept of local drug delivery. Local drug delivery (LDD), in theory, should achieve greater local drug concentration with lower overall dose compared to systemic therapy, to help achieve maximal tissue effects while minimizing undesired systemic toxicity. It also has the advantage of being able to utilize drugs with low systemic bioavailability or short half-life. Many devices have been developed to administer drugs or genetic material locally to the site of injury {Sharma et al, 2011}. Studies have shown that local administration of pharmacologic agents directly at the site of coronary intervention is an effective means of delivering sufficient amount of drug into the injured arterial tissue site to cause an anti-restenotic therapeutic effect { Schwartz et al, 2004}.

Various approaches for local drug delivery have been tried including nanoparticles, contrast media and drug delivery balloons, such as porous {Herdeg et al, 2000} and double balloons {Oberhoff et al, 2001}. Other options for treating ISR included POBA using either conventional or cutting balloons, implanting a stent inside the stent, rotablation or brachytherapy. However, most of these techniques were not adopted into widespread clinical use due to their various shortcomings and limitations. Until recently, stent-based local drug delivery using drug-eluting stents (DES) is still considered the percutaneous treatment of choice for coronary restenosis. As the process of neo intimal hyperplasia occurs locally due to endothelial injury caused by the metallic stent, it seems logical to use the stent itself to deliver a drug locally in order to overcome this problem.

Thus DES have become the mainstay of intervention for coronary atherosclerotic disease {Kirtane et al, 2009}. However, DES use is limited by small but unpredictable risk of late stent thrombosis due to withdrawal of antiplatelet therapy { McFadden et al, 2004}, delayed mal-apposition {Kozuma et al, 1999}, delayed vascular healing as a result of initial anti-proliferative effect {Jakabcin et al, 2008}, or a hypersensitivity reaction to the drug, polymer coating or both { Finn et al, 2007}.

ISR continues to occur with DES, although at a lower rate compared to BMS. However, the relative massive increase in number of DES implantations in recent years means the problem of ISR although less in relative terms compared to BMS, still causes a problem in absolute terms requiring a significant number of repeat procedures every year globally and remains a treatment challenge {Maisel, 2007}. Treatment of restenosed DES with a second DES is associated with risk of subsequent restenosis of up to 43% {Lemos et al, 2008}. The ideal treatment of a coronary stenosis would eliminate both the stent and the polymer related late problems, while at the same time deliver an antiproliferative agent to reduce the risk of restenosis.

3. Drug eluting balloons

Old-style balloon angioplasty married to the latest in drug-eluting technology, resulting in a drug eluting balloon (DEB), may be an effective alternative to stenting, in particular to overcome the problems of restenosis and ISR. Such a device would potentially overcome the drawbacks of stenting, polymer-related delayed endothelialization, and stent delivery, while at the same time providing homogenous drug delivery to the vessel wall, allowing earlier endothelialization and flexibility of use in complex lesions. However, its limitations include the failure to provide a mechanical scaffold for the prevention of acute recoil and the problem of not being able to treat dissection flaps.

Drug eluting balloons achieve LDD by means of an angioplasty balloon coated with drugs such as paclitaxel, which are well established in DES technology. One of the commercially approved devices, the SeQuent® Please (Braun, Germany) balloon catheter (Fig. 1) has a folded balloon, which is homogenously coated with paclitaxel embedded in contrast medium coating. Paclitaxel (3 µg/ 373mm2 balloon surface) is the pharmacologically active substance whereas the contrast medium has a matrix builder function to facilitate immediate release of drug during balloon inflation {Scheller & Speck, 2009}.

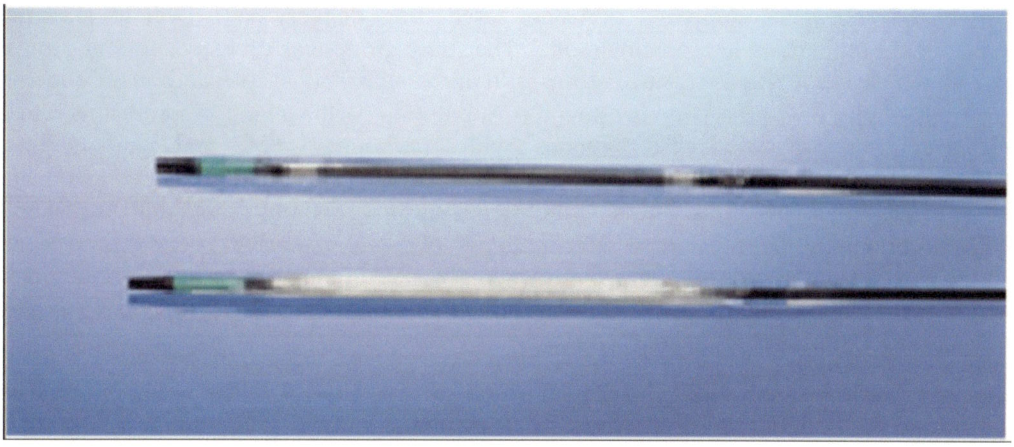

Fig. 1. Photograph of SeQuent (top) and the paclitaxel coated SeQuent® Please balloon catheter (bottom).

The ideal drugs for local delivery should be lipophilic in nature, rapidly adsorbed and have a high retention rate by the vessel intima, in order to exert maximal beneficial effects {Baumbach et al, 1999}. Paclitaxel is a lipophilic drug and bind tightly to various cell constituents {Rowinsky et al, 1995}, resulting in effective local retention at the site of delivery { Creel et al , 2000} and it exerts a long-lasting effect in the cell due to structural alteration of the cytoskeleton. Thus, paclitaxel, with its lipophilic nature, combined with the fact that adding a small amount of hydrophilic contrast medium {Scheller et al, 2003} enhances its solubility, makes it well suited for delivery on a drug-delivery balloon. Various other drugs like, sirolimus, zotarolimus, rapalog and others are being studied currently as a possible alternative to paclitaxel for coating the PTCA balloon {Schnorr et al, 2010}.

3.1 Pre- clinical data

The first preclinical study was conducted by Scheller et al {Scheller et al, 2004}. In this study stainless steel stents (n = 40; diameter: 3.0–3.5 mm; length: 18 mm) were implanted in the left anterior descending and circumflex coronary arteries of pigs. Both conventional uncoated and three different types of paclitaxel-coated coronary angioplasty balloons were used, and contact with vessel wall was maintained for 1 min. The results were assessed by quantitative angiography and histomorphometric studies of the stented arteries. There was a marked reduction (up to 63%) of parameters characterizing ISR in the paclitaxel-coated balloon group, without evidence of increased inflammation in proximity to the stent struts or any effect on re-endothelialisation of the struts. They also showed that paclitaxel-coated balloons lose only 6% of the drug when introduced into the coronary circulation and retracted without inflation. Approximately 80% of the drug is released during inflation, suggesting rapid transfer of the drug from the balloon to the vessel wall without much loss. In this study, the percentage of drug recovered from the vessel wall was at a maximum (17.3%) when a premounted stent on a coated balloon was used, compared with postdilatation using a coated balloon (15.6%) or the coated balloon on its own (8.7%).

Speck and colleagues compared non-stent-based drug delivery with DES in reducing neointimal proliferation in a porcine model. The study group was divided into four groups as follows; Group A was the control group with uncoated balloons, BMS and 'plain' contrast medium. Group B was the same treatment as A, but with paclitaxel in the contrast medium. Group C was paclitaxel-coated balloons, with pre-mounted BMS and plain contrast medium. Finally, group D was sirolimus-eluting stents, non-coated balloons, and plain contrast medium. At 4 weeks, assessment of stenosis was carried out using angiography and histomorphometry. The most impressive inhibition of neointimal proliferation was achieved in the coated balloon group - the neointimal area was 2.4 mm2 ± 0.3 ($p < 0.01$ vs. all other groups), compared with 5.2 mm2 ± 0.3 in group A, 4.3 mm2 ± 0.3 in group B, and 3.8 mm2 ± 0.3 in group D {Speck et al, 2006}.

Cremers and colleagues studied the relationship between the inflation time and dose of placlitaxel on the DEB, on effectiveness in reducing neo-intimal proliferation in a porcine model {Cremers et al, 2009 a}. DEB technology was shown to be effective in reducing neointimal proliferation regardless of the balloon inflation time (10 s, 60 s and two 60 s inflations) and dose (up to a total amount of 10 µg paclitaxel/mm^2 balloon surface). This study showed that drug transfer occurs very early after balloon inflation and also demonstrated the safety profile of applying several balloon inflations within the same vessel either using the same or additional balloons.

In a comparative study of two different types of DEB (Original Paccocath-coating, similar to SeQuent®Please, B. Braun, Germany and DIOR®, Eurocor, Germany) on a porcine coronary overstretch model it was demonstrated that much better results were obtained with the matrix-coated Paccocath DEB compared with the roughened surface DIOR balloon, suggesting that inhibition of neointimal proliferation is dependent on the coating method used {Cremers et al, 2009 b}. In a comparative DEB performance study by Joner et al, in a porcine model of advanced coronary restenosis, significant heterogeneity of neointimal suppression was seen between the devices tested {Joner et al, 2011}

3.2 Use of DEB in the human coronary

The first reports of DEB use in humans were the Paccocath ISR I and ISR II studies in 2006. These were randomized, double-blind German multicenter clinical trials to assess the efficacy and tolerability of a paclitaxel-coated balloon catheter in the treatment of coronary ISR {Scheller et al, 2006, 2008}. Scheller and colleagues enrolled 108 patients (52 and 56 patients in each study) with a single ISR lesion to undergo balloon angioplasty either using a 3mcg/mm2 iopromide-paclitaxel coated balloon (PACCOCATH, Bayer Schering Pharma) or a standard uncoated balloon of the same type. The primary end point of angiographic in-segment late lumen loss was markedly different in the two groups. They reported that at 6-month follow-up, in-segment late lumen loss was 0.81 ± 0.79 mm in the uncoated balloon group, versus 0.11 ± 0.45 mm ($p < 0.001$) in the drug-coated balloon group. By 12 months, only two patients in the coated balloon group required target vessel re-vascularization (p =

0.001), compared with 20 in the control group. A sustained clinical effect of the DEB was noted at 24 months with no subacute thrombosis or other safety concerns.

The Paclitaxel-Eluting PTCA-balloon catheter in Coronary Artery Disease (PEPCAD I-SVD) was a Phase II nonrandomized, open label, uncontrolled, efficacy study evaluating the use of a DEB catheter (SeQuent Please, B. Braun, Germany) for the treatment of small vessel coronary artery disease in 118 patients (reference diameter of 2.25–2.8 mm and lesion length ≤ 22 mm). If the angiographic result was not satisfactory at the end of the procedure, the subjects could be treated with any device, but a bare metal stent was recommended. After 6 months, de novo lesions treated solely with DEB or in combination with BMS (28% of patients) showed a 17.3% binary restenosis rate, and at 1 year 11.7% target lesion revascularization (TLR) and 15% major adverse cardiovascular event rate {Scheller, 2008}. However, in the patients who received DEB alone ($n = 82$) without additional stent insertion, the binary restenosis rate was only 5.5%. The somewhat higher restenosis rate in the total population may have been attributable to 'geographic mismatch' between the DEB-treated area and the subsequently stented surface area.

The PEPCAD II-ISR trial was a prospective, randomized study directly comparing the paclitaxel-eluting balloon catheter (SeQuent Please, B. Braun, Germany) to the paclitaxel-eluting stent (Taxus®, Boston Scientific, MA, USA) in 131 patients with ISR, followed up for 6 months. The main inclusion criteria encompassed diameter stenosis of ≥70% and ≤22 mm in length, with a vessel diameter of 2.5 to 3.5 mm. In 6.2% of the Taxus stent group, the stent was undeliverable and a balloon catheter had to be used instead. Clopidogrel was given for 3 months post treatment to the balloon group and 6 months to the stent group. Patients treated with the drug-eluting balloon experienced a 7.0% ISR compared with 20.3% in the group. Adverse cardiac events occurred in 22% of the stent group and in 9% of the coated balloon group ($p = 0.08$), driven predominantly by reduced need for target lesion revascularisation (TLR), which was 6.3 and 15.4% in the balloon and stent groups, respectively {Unverdorben et al, 2009}. These findings suggested that DEB is at least as efficacious and as well tolerated as DES in treating ISR.

PEPCAD III {Hamm, 2009} was a prospective, randomised, multi-centre, Phase II pilot study which compared the combination of paclitaxel-coated DEB plus BMS (Coroflex® DEBlue, B. Braun) with the sirolimus eluting CYPHER® stent in the treatment of de novo native coronary stenoses with stent diameters between 2.5 and 3.5 mm and less than 24 mm in length. The primary end point was late lumen loss in treated segment at 9 months assessed angiographically. The 637 patients with stable or unstable angina or documented ischemia (ST-elevation myocardial infarction and non-ST-elevation myocardial infarction excluded) were randomized to undergo PCI with either the paclitaxel DEB plus BMS ($n = 312$) or the sirolimus DES ($n = 325$). The in-stent late lumen loss was 0.41 ± 0.51 mm in the DEB + BMS group compared with 0.16 ± 0.39 mm in the DES group ($p < 0.001$). In segment late lumen loss in the two groups were 0.20 ± 0.52 mm and 0.11 ± 0.40 mm ($p = 0.06$), respectively. Target-vessel revascularization (13.8 vs. 6.9%, $p < 0.01$) and TLR (10.5 vs. 4.7%, $p < 0.01$) rates were also significantly higher in the DEB + BMS subgroup at 9 months. Of the safety end points, the rate of myocardial infarction at 9 months was 4.6 and 0.3% ($p < 0.001$) in the DEB plus BMS and DES groups, respectively. In addition, stent thrombosis by Academic Research Consortium criteria was 2.0 and 0.3%, respectively ($p < 0.05$). These results show that the drug-eluting balloon-stent system did not meet the non-inferiority criteria versus the CYPHER stent and the safety aspects need further investigation

In a study of 20 patients, in the Drug-Eluting Balloon In Bifurcation Utrecht [DEBIUT] registry {Fanggiday et al, 2008}, Fanggiday assessed the efficacy and safety of different type of DEB in treating bifurcation lesions. The bifurcation lesions (main and side branch) were treated with the paclitaxel-coated DIOR balloon followed by BMS implantation only in the main branch. At 4-months follow-up, no major acute coronary events and no subacute vessel closure were reported. There was no angiographic follow-up performed in this study, making it difficult to assess the results, although the fact that major adverse cardiovascular event rates were not elevated after 4 months indicates that the coating of this balloon is well tolerated, but the small number of cases makes this woefully underpowered.

Recently, The PICCOLETO Trial {Cortese et al, 2010} failed to show the 'non-inferiority' of a paclitaxel-eluting balloon (DIOR, Eurocor, Germany) compared with a paclitaxel eluting stent (Taxus Liberte, Boston Scientific, MA, USA) in terms of restenosis for the treatment of small coronary arteries (≤2.75 mm). This was a small, single-centre, randomized controlled study that intended to randomize eighty patients with stable or unstable angina undergoing PCI in small vessels (≤2.75 mm) to receive either a DES (Taxus Liberte) or a DEB (DIOR). The enrolment into this study was halted after two thirds of the originally intended number of patients because of a marked outcome difference in the two groups. The 6-month angiographic follow-up of the 57 patients revealed that the primary end point was not met, because the DEB group showed higher per cent diameter stenosis (43.6% vs. 24.3%, p=0.029); angiographic restenosis was higher as well (32.1 vs. 10.3%, p=0.043), whereas MACE was 35.7% in the PCB group and 13.8% in the DES group (p=0.054).

The results of the PEPCAD V were presented at the Transcatheter Therapeutics 2009 {Mathey, 2009}. This was a small feasibility and safety trial using DEBs (SeQuent Please, B. Braun) for the treatment of coronary bifurcation disease, specifically by using DEB in main and side branches, a BMS in the main branch, and a provisional BMS strategy in the side branch. Twenty-eight patients were treated in 2 German centres. Achievement of the primary end point (<30% stenosis in the main branch, <50% stenosis in the side branch) at 9 months follow up occurred in 97% and 89% of vessels, respectively. Although there were no deaths during the follow-up, 2 late stent thromboses occurred in the main branch where DEB was used with BMS. Thus this small study indicated evidence of efficacy but the observed late stent thrombosis raised the issue of safety of DEBs used in combination with BMS.

There are several other studies ongoing, evaluating the role of DEB in treatment of coronary artery disease in various clinical settings. Some of them are listed in the table 1.

4. Limitations of DEB

Apart from the uncertainty about the choice of drug and the method used to coat the balloon there are still many more unanswered questions regarding the use of DEB. There have not been many studies to compare the efficacy and safety of different coating methods used. There is a potential risk of systemic toxicity with the loss of drug. As the device is meant for single use it may not be very cost-effective in long lesions or other situations requiring multiple inflations and with each application the systemic toxicity is potentially higher. It definitely lacks the scaffold effect of a stent that is highly desirable in many clinical situations such as the treatment of acute vessel dissection and acute vessel recoil. With ongoing studies hopefully the device should improve and perhaps overcome some of these limitations.

Study Name	Brief Description of study	Estimated completion
DEB-AMI	Use of DEB in STEMI	2013
PEPCAD DES	DEB use in DES ISR	May 2011
KISSING DEBBIE	Use of kissing DEB in Bifurcation lesion	2011
PEPCAD-BIF	DEB in bifurcation lesions	November 2012
ISAR DESIRE 3	Treatment of ISR with DEB vs. DES vs. POBA	July 2014
SEDUCE	OCT analysis of DEB vs. DES treatment of restenosis	December 2015
PEPCAD IV	DEB in native coronary stenosis of Diabetic patients	September 2011
PEPCAD CTO	DEB in treatment of chronic total occlusion	September 2014
INDICOR	BMS +DEB post dilatation vs DEB predilation + BMS implantation	April 2012
PEPCAD DEB	DEB vs. DES in De-novo coronary stenosis	March 2015
WinDEB Study	Pressure wire guided DEB vs. DES use in SVD	Not Recruiting yet
VIBER	IVUS assisted DEB use	Recruiting

Table 1. Ongoing trials for DEB use in coronary intervention (Source Clinical Trials.gov)

5. Summary

With increasing numbers of coronary revascularisations taking place globally, the challenges and late complications of percutaneous intervention are also growing. The search for an ideal device for PTCA is ongoing. The problem of restenosis is very well described as the 'Achilles heel' of coronary intervention. It not only necessitates repeat procedures but also significant symptoms in patients and the treatment is challenging. After the failure of systemic pharmacotherapy, local drug delivery at the coronary lesion site is the current treatment strategy for restenosis and the stent-based platform is the most extensively used. The limitations of DES {Sharma et al, 2010} and problems of late stent thrombosis have shifted the treatment goal from procedural success to keeping the long-term problems minimal.

The concept of DEB originated more than a decade ago but only has come into clinical use recently. Although it showed some initially promising results in animal study and first in man trials, the subsequent studies have failed to demonstrate their superiority over more traditional approaches. DEB certainly seems to offer promise in the treatment of ISR, and possibly in de novo lesions in small coronary vessels. In such scenarios it has several advantages over DES: it helps to avoid the double/triple metal layer which results in making the coronary vasculature into a metal jacket, thereby distorting the anatomy; it potentially provides homogenous drug distribution in the vessel wall, thus reducing the effects of delayed endothelialization of stent struts; it is free of the polymer matrix used in DES, thus removing the stimulus for late thrombosis; advantages are observed despite a shorter period of dual antiplatelet therapy usage, thus probably reducing costs and problems associated with prolonged dual antiplatelet treatment; and may have a role in small, tortuous, heavily calcified coronaries or bifurcation lesions, where DES continues to underperform.

The 2010 European Society of Cardiology Myocardial revascularisation guidelines suggest considering DEB use in treatment of BMS restenosis and for DEB with proven efficacy/safety profile, according to the respective lesion characteristics of the studies {ESC & EACTS, 2010}. Overall the data available so far does not convince us that DEB will replace all DES. Further studies are required in selective lesion subtypes. It is definitely a promising new treatment strategy on the coronary interventionist's shelf.

6. References

Baumbach A et al. (1999). Baumbach A, Herdeg C, Kluge M, Oberhoff M, Lerch M, Haase KK, Wolter C, Schröder S & Karsch KR. Local drug delivery: impact of pressure, substance characteristics, and stenting on drug transfer into the arterial wall. *Catheter. Cardiovasc. Interv.* 47(1), May 1999, 102–106

Bertrand M et al. (1997). Bertrand ME, McFadden EP, Fruchart JC, Van Belle E, Commeau P, Grollier G, Bassand JP, Machecourt J, Cassagnes J, Mossard JM, Vacheron A, Castaigne A, Danchin N & Lablanche JM. Effect of pravastatin on angiographic restenosis after coronary balloon angioplasty. The PREDICT Trial Investigators. Prevention of Restenosis by Elisor after Transluminal Coronary Angioplasty.*J Am Coll Cardiol,* 30 (4), Oct 1997, 863-869.

Boccuzzi SJ et al. (1998). Boccuzzi SJ, Weintraub WS, Kosinski AS, Roehm JB & Klein JL. Aggressive lipid lowering in post coronary angioplasty patients with elevated cholesterol (the Lovastatin Restenosis Trial). *Am J Cardiol,* 81(5), Mar 1998, 632-636

Cortese et al. (2010). Cortese B, Micheli A, Picchi A, Coppolaro A, Bandinelli L, Severi S & Limbruno U. Paclitaxel-coated balloon versus drug-eluting stent during PCI of small coronary vessels, a prospective randomised clinical trial. The PICCOLETO study. *Heart.* 96(16), Aug 2010, 1291-6

Creel CJ et al. (2000). Creel CJ, Lovich MA & Edelman ER. Arterial paclitaxel distribution and deposition. *Circ. Res.*, 86(8), Apr 2000, 879–884

Cremers B et al. (2009 a). Cremers B, Speck U, Kaufels N, Mahnkopf D, Kühler M, Böhm M & Scheller B. Drug-eluting balloon: very short-term exposure and overlapping. *Thromb. Haemost.* 101(1), Jan 2009, 201–206.

Cremers B et al. (2009 b). Cremers B, Biedermann M, Mahnkopf D, Böhm M & Scheller B. Comparison of two different paclitael coated balloon catheters in the porcine coronary restenosis model. *Clin. Res. Cardiol.* 98(5): May 2009, 325–330

ESC & EACTS, (2010). The Task Force on Myocardial Revascularization of the European Society of Cardiology (ESC) and the European Association for Cardio-Thoracic Surgery (EACTS), Guidelines on myocardial revascularization. *Eur Heart J*, 31(20), Oct 2010, 2501-2555

Fanggiday JC et al. (2008). Fanggiday JC, Stella PR, Guyomi SH & Doevendans PA. Safety and efficacy of drug-eluting balloons in percutaneous treatment of bifurcation lesions the DEBIUT (drug-eluting balloon in bifurcaton utrecht) registry *Catheter.Cardiovasc. Interv.* 71(5), Apr 2008, 629–635.

Faxon DP, (2002). Faxon DP. Systemic drug therapy for restenosis: "Déjà vu all over again". *Circulation*, 106(18), Oct 2002, 2296-2298.

Faxon DP, (1995). Faxon DP. Effect of high dose angiotensin-converting enzyme inhibition on restenosis: Final results of the MARCATOR Study. *J Am Coll Cardiol*, 25(2), Feb1995, 362-369

Finn et al. (2007). Finn AV, Nakazawa G, Joner M, Kolodgie FD, Mont EK, Gold HK & Virmani R. Vascular responses to drug eluting stents: importance of delayed healing. *Arterioscler Thromb Vasc Biol.* 27(7), Jul 2007, 1500-10

Geary et al. (2003). Geary RL, Williams JK, Golden D, Brown DG, Benjamin ME & Adams MR. Time course of cellular proliferation, intimal hyperplasia, and remodeling following angioplasty in monkeys with established atherosclerosis. A nonhuman primate model of restenosis. *Arterioscler Thromb Vasc Biol.* 16(1), Jan 2003, 34-43

Grewe et al. (1999). Grewe PH, Deneke T, Machraoui A, Barmeyer J & Müller KM. Acute and chronic tissue response to coronary stent implantation: pathologic findings in human specimen. *J. Am. Coll. Cardiol.* 35(1), Jan 1999, 157–163.

Hamm, (2009). Hamm CW. PEPCAD III. Presented at: American Heart Association, 14 November 2009.

Herdeg et al. (2000). Herdeg C, Oberhoff M, Baumbach A, Blattner A, Axel DI, Schröder S, Heinle H & Karsch KR. Local paclitaxel delivery for the prevention of restenosis: biological effects and efficacy in vivo (Double Balloon). *J. Am. Coll. Cardiol.*; 35(7), Jun 2000, 1969–1976.

Hoffman et al (1996). Hoffmann R, Mintz GS, Dussaillant GR, Popma JJ, Pichard AD, Satler LF, Kent KM, Griffin J & Leon MB. Patterns and mechanisms of in-stent restenosis: a serial intravascular ultrasound study. *Circulation*; 94(6), Sep 1996, 1247–1254.

Holmes et al. (2002). Holmes DR Jr, Savage M, LaBlanche JM, Grip L, Serruys PW, Fitzgerald P, Fischman D, Goldberg S, Brinker JA, Zeiher AM, Shapiro LM, Willerson J, Davis BR, Ferguson JJ, Popma J, King SB 3rd, Lincoff AM, Tcheng JE, Chan R, Granett JR & Poland M.Results of prevention of restenosis with tranilast and its outcomes (PRESTO) trial. *Circulation;* 106(10). Sep 2002, 1243–1250

Jakabcin et al. (2008). Jakabcin J, Bystron M, Spacek R, Veselka J, Kvasnak M, Kala P, Malý J & Cervinka P.The lack of endothelization after drug-eluting stent implantation as a cause of fatal late stent thrombosis. *J Thromb Thrombolysis.* 26(2), Oct 2008, 154–8.

Joner M et al. (2011). Joner M, Byrne RA, Lapointe JM, Radke PW, Bayer G, Steigerwald K & Wittchow E. Comparative assessment of drug-eluting balloons in an advanced porcine model of coronary restenosis. *Thromb Haemost.* 105(5), May 2011, 864-72.

Kearney M et al. (1997). Kearney M, Pieczek A, Haley L, Losordo DW, Andres V, Schainfeld R, Rosenfield K & Isner JM. Histopathology of in-stent restenosis in patients with peripheral artery disease. *Circulation;* 95(8), Apr 1997, 1998–1200.

Kirtane AJ et al. (2009). Kirtane AJ, Gupta A, Iyengar S, Moses JW, Leon MB, Applegate R, Brodie B, Hannan E, Harjai K, Jensen LO, Park SJ, Perry R, Racz M, Saia F, Tu JV, Waksman R, Lansky AJ, Mehran R & Stone GW. Safety and efficacy of drug-eluting and bare metal stents: comprehensive meta-analysis of randomized trials and observational studies. *Circulation;* 119(25), Jun 2009, 3198-206

Kozuma K et al. (1999). Kozuma K, Costa MA, Sabaté M, Serrano P, van der Giessen WJ, Ligthart JM, Coen VL, Levendag PC & Serruys PW. Late stent malapposition occurring after intracoronary beta-irradiation detected by intravascular ultrasound. *J Invasive Cardiol.* 11(10), Oct 1999, 651–5.

Lemos PA et al. (2008). Lemos PA, Hoye A, Goedhart D, Arampatzis CA, Saia F, van der Giessen WJ, McFadden E, Sianos G, Smits PC, Hofma SH, de Feyter PJ, van Domburg RT & Serruys PW.Clinical, angiographic, and procedural predictors of angiographic restenosis after sirolimus-eluting stent implantation incomplex patients: an evaluation from the Rapamycin-Eluting Stent Evaluated at Rotterdam Cardiology Hospital (RESEARCH) study: *Circulation;* 109(11): Mar 2008, 1366–1370

Mach, (2000). Mach F. Toward new therapeutic strategies against neointimal formation in restenosis. Atheroscler. *Thromb. Vasc. Biol.* 20(7), Jul 2000, 1699–1700.

Maisel (2007). Maisel WH. Unanswered questions - drug-eluting stents and the risk of late thrombosis. *N. Engl. J. Med.* 356(10), Mar 2007981–984.

Mathey (2009). Mathey DG, PEPCAD V: the bifurcation study. Presened at TCT 2009; San Francisco, California.

McFadden EP et al. (2004). McFadden EP, Stabile E, Regar E, Cheneau E, Ong AT, Kinnaird T, Suddath WO, Weissman NJ, Torguson R, Kent KM, Pichard AD, Satler LF, Waksman R & Serruys PW Late thrombosis in drug-eluting coronary stents after discontinuation of antiplatelet therapy. *Lancet,* 364(9444), Oct 2004, 1519–21

Moreno PR, (1999). Moreno PR, Palacios IF, Leon MN, Rhodes J, Fuster V & Fallon JT.Histopathologic comparison of human coronary in-stent and post-balloon angioplasty restenotic tissue. *Am. J. Cardiol.* 84(4) Aug 1999, 462–466.

Mudra H et al. (1997). Mudra H, Regar E, Klauss V, Werner F, Henneke KH, Sbarouni E & Theisen K. Serial follow-up after optimized ultrasound guided deployment of Palmaz-Schatz stents. *Circulation,* 95(2), Jan 1997, 363–370.

Oberhoff M et al. (2001). Oberhoff M, Kunert W, Herdeg C, Küttner A, Kranzhöfer A, Horch B, Baumbach A & Karsch KR. Inhibition of smooth muscle cell proliferation after local drug delivery of the antimitotic drug paclitaxel using a porus balloon catheter. *Basic Res. Cardiol.* 96(3), May 2001, 275–282.

Rowinsky & Donehower 1995. Rowinsky EK, Donehower RC. Paclitaxel (Taxol). *N. Engl. J. Med.* 35(15), Apr 1995, 1004–1014

Scheller B, 2008. PEPCAD I & II. Presented at: European Association of Percutaneous Cardiovascular Intervention, 13 May 2008.

Scheller B & Speck U, 2009. Chapter 4. In B. (Ed.), The drug coated balloon—History and clinical applications (pp. 53). Germany: UNI-MED Verlag AG

Scheller B et al. (2003). Scheller B, Speck U, Romeike B, Schmitt A, Sovak M, Böhm M & Stoll HP. Contrast media as carriers for local drug delivery successful inhibition of neointimal proliferation in the porcine coronary stent model. *Eur. Heart J.*;24(15), Aug 2003,1462–1467.

Scheller B et al. (2004). Scheller B, Speck U, Abramjuk C, Bernhardt U, Böhm M & Nickenig G. Paclitaxel balloon coating, a novel method for prevention and therapy of restenosis. *Circulation,* 110(7), Aug 2004, 810–814.

Scheller B et al. (2006). Scheller B, Hehrlein C, Bocksch W, Rutsch W, Haghi D, Dietz U, Böhm M & Speck U. Treatment of coronary in-stent restenosis with a paclitaxel-coated balloon catheter. *N. Engl. J. Med.* 355(20), Nov 2006, 2113–2124.

Scheller B et al. 2008. Two year follow-up after treatment of coronary in-stent restenosis with a paclitaxel-coated balloon catheter. *Clin. Res. Cardiol.* 97(10), Oct 2008, 773–781.

Schnorr B et al. (2010). Schnorr B, Kelsch B, Cremers B, Clever YP, Speck U & Scheller B. Paclitaxel-coated balloons-Survey of preclinical data. *Minerva Cardioangiol.* 58(5), Oct 2010, 567-82.

Schwartz RS et al. (2004). Schwartz RS, Chronos NA & Virmani R. Preclinical restenosis models and drug-eluting stents: Still important, still much to learn. *J Am Coll Cardiol.* 44(7), Oct 2004, 1373-1385

Serruys PW et al. (1991). Serruys PW, Strauss BH, Beatt KJ, Bertrand ME, Puel J, Rickards AF, Meier B, Goy JJ, Vogt P, Kappenberger L, Angiographic follow-up after placement of a self-expanding coronary-artery stent. *N. Engl. J. Med.* 324(1): Jan1991, 13–17

Serruys PW et al. (2000). Serruys PW, Foley DP, Höfling B, Puel J, Glogar HD, Seabra-Gomes R, Goicolea J, Coste P, Rutsch W, Katus H, Bonnier H, Wijns W, Betriu A, Hauf-Zachariou U, van Swijndregt EM, Melkert R & Simon R. Carvedilol for prevention of restenosis after directional coronary atherectomy: Final results of the European carvedilol atherectomy restenosis (EUROCARE) trial. *Circulation.* 101(13): Jan 2000, 1512-1518.

Speck U et al. (2006). Speck U, Scheller B, Abramjuk C, Breitwieser C, Dobberstein J, Boehm M & Hamm B. Neointima inhibition: comparison of effectiveness of non-stent based local drug delivery and a drug eluting stent in porcine coronary arteries. *Radiology,* 240(2), Aug 2006, 411–418

Sharma S et al. (2010). Sharma S, Kukreja N, Christopoulos C & Gorog DA. Drug-eluting balloon: new tool in the box. *Expert Rev Med Devices,* 7(3), May2010, 381-8.

Sharma S et al. (2011). Sharma S, Christopoulos C, Kukreja N & Gorog DA. Local drug delivery for percutaneous coronary intervention. *Pharmacol Ther.* 129(3), Mar 2011, 260-6

Unverdorben M et al. (2009). Unverdorben M, Vallbracht C, Cremers B, Heuer H, Hengstenberg C, Maikowski C, Werner GS, Antoni D, Kleber FX, Bocksch W, Leschke M, Ackermann H, Boxberger M, Speck U, Degenhardt R & Scheller B. Paclitaxel-coated balloon catheter versus paclitaxel-coated stent for the treatment of coronary in-stent restenosis. *Circulation,* 119(23), Jun 2009, 2986–2994.

7

Cardiac Postconditioning: An Additional Therapy to Limit Cell Death Following Myocardial Infarction

Sandrine Lecour, Lionel Opie and Sarin J. Somers
Hatter Cardiovascular Research Institute, University of Cape Town
South Africa

1. Introduction

1.1 The concept of lethal reperfusion injury

Following acute myocardial infarction (AMI), early reperfusion therapy with thrombolytic therapy or primary percutaneous coronary intervention therapy (PCI) is the best way to salvage the heart by limiting the infarct size and preserving the left ventricular function. The early survival benefits of reperfusion are probably sustained lifelong and after 20 years, the survival rate of 27% in patients treated with conventional therapy is increased to 37% in patients treated with reperfusion therapy (thrombolytics and/or PCI) (van Domburg *et al.* 2005).

However, the benefits of reperfusion come at a price as restoration of the blood flow in the coronary arteries can paradoxically cause myocardial injury. Lethal reperfusion injury manifests itself clinically as stunned myocardium, arrhythmias and endothelial damage (Yellon and Hausenloy 2007). Although still unclear, the mechanisms behind reperfusion injury involve multiple processes including an increase in oxidative stress (Bolli *et al.* 1989), inflammatory damage (Vinten-Johansen 2004), a change in myocyte osmolarity (Garcia-Dorado and Oliveras 1993), calcium loading (Dong *et al.* 2006, Murphy *et al.* 1987) and a change in pH (figure 1) (Inserte *et al.* 2011).

The rapid return of blood in the ischemic myocardium generates an oxidative stress which itself can mediate myocardial injury (Zweier 1988). The release of reactive oxygen species consecutive to the oxidative stress may generate a degree of myocardial injury superior to ischemia alone, partly due to the reduced bioavailability of the potent vasodilator nitric oxide in the vasculature (Zweier and Talukder 2006). The oxidative stress also contributes to the excessive increase of intracellular calcium inducing cardiomyocyte death by hypercontracture and inadequate opening of the mitochondrial permeability transition pore (mPTP) opening (Piper *et al.* 1998). The opening of this pore leads to uncoupled oxidative phosphorylation , depletion of adenosine triphosphate (ATP) and death (Hausenloy and Yellon 2003). Myocardial ischemia causes a progressive decrease in intra- and extra-cellular pH (Inserte *et al.* 2011). At the onset of reperfusion, the removal of extracellular protons and the correction of intracellular acidosis exerts an adverse effect due, in part, to the intracellular sodium and calcium overload (Piper *et al.* 1996). An upregulation of cell adhesion molecules during the first hours of reperfusion leads to the accumulation of neutrophils in the infarcted area, causing vascular plugging and the release of more reactive oxygen species (Vinten-Johansen 2004).

According to animal studies, lethal reperfusion injury may represent between 20% and 70% of the total amount of the irreversible myocardial damage, therefore constituting a major therapeutic target. In this regard, the experimental discovery of ischemic pre- and postconditioning (Zhao *et al.* 2003) represents a promising therapy to limit lethal reperfusion injury.

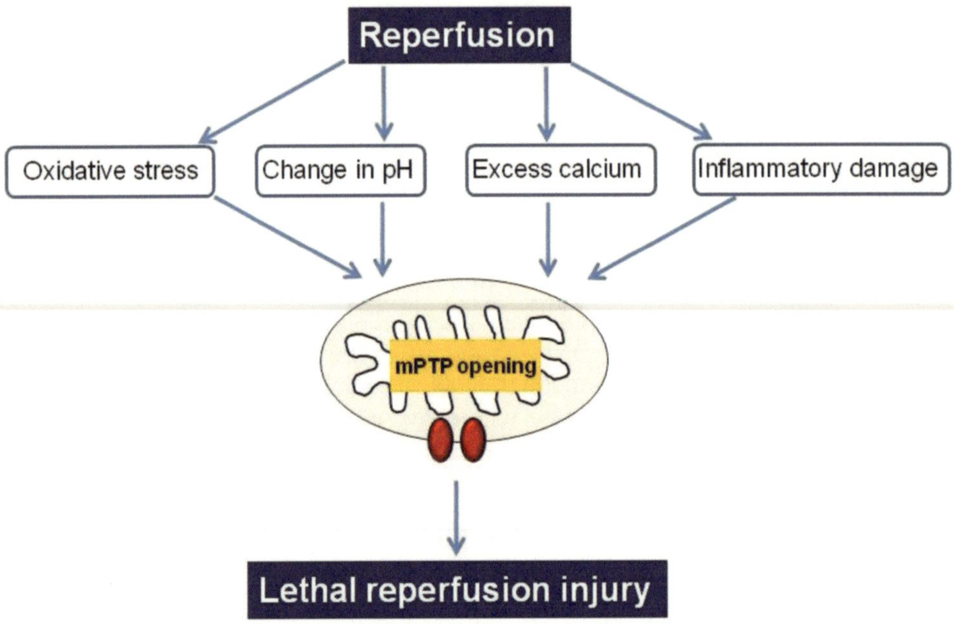

Fig. 1. The concept of lethal reperfusion injury

At the onset of reperfusion, an oxidative stress, a rapid increase in pH, an excess of intra- and extracellular calcium and an inflammatory process facilitate the opening of the mitochondrial permeability transition pore, leading to lethal reperfusion injury.

2. Ischemic preconditioning

2.1 Genesis of an intrinsic cardioprotective solution

In 1986, Murry et al. published a seminal paper describing a phenomenon whereby four cycles of five minutes of coronary artery occlusions with intermittent reperfusion prior to a prolonged 40 minutes occlusion, attenuated infarct size to 25% in the canine myocardium (Reimer *et al.* 1986). Initially, they found that brief periods of ischemia reduced the rate of ATP depletion during subsequent ischemic episodes. Intermittent reperfusion also served to prevent the cumulative effects of ischemic injury by washing out potentially harmful catabolites such as lactate, hydrogen ions (H^+) and ammonia (NH_4). The reduction in ATP depletion was associated with the limitation in infarct size. Given these findings and that the procedure could be reproduced successfully, this cardioprotective phenomenon was termed 'ischemic preconditioning' (IPC) (Murry *et al.* 1986).

This model of cardioprotection is referred to as 'classic' or early preconditioning and is short-lived, with the preconditioned state lasting for only 1-4 hours (figure 2) (Murry *et al.* 1991). However, within 24 hours of the preconditioning stimulus, a late phase of protection, known as delayed preconditioning or the second window of protection, is evident but is less robust and more prolonged, lasting up to 72 hours after the preconditioning stimulus (Baxter *et al.* 1997). Classic IPC exerts its protective effects via the modification of existing proteins. In contrast, delayed preconditioning allows for the *de novo* synthesis of cytoprotective proteins (Bolli *et al.* 2007). Another distinction between the two phases is that although classic IPC limits infarct size, it does not protect against postischemic myocardial contractile dysfunction or stunning. Conversely, late IPC reduces myocardial cell death and preserves left ventricular function (Bolli *et al.* 2007). These disparities suggest that late IPC would provide greater clinical benefits in terms of greater and longer lasting protection.

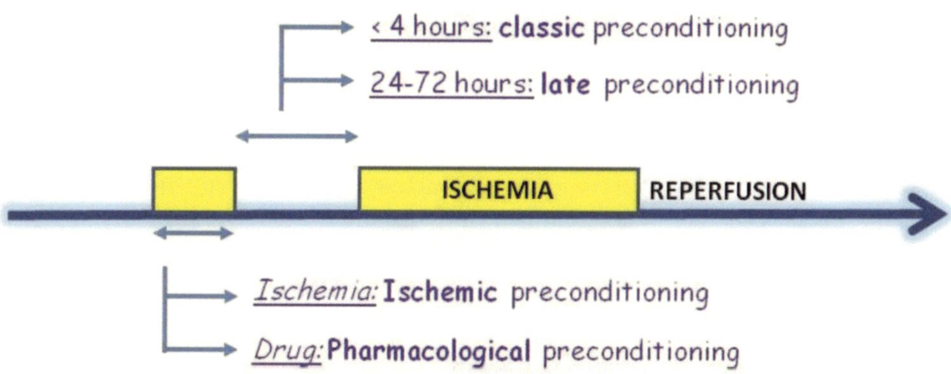

Fig. 2. Schematic representation of classic and delayed postconditioning

2.2 Remote preconditioning

Further research into the development of IPC yielded the discovery that remote ischemia distant to the heart can elicit a similar cardioprotective response as IPC of the local coronary artery. Four brief occlusions of the circumflex branches lasting 5 minutes and interspersed by 5 minutes of reperfusion had a remote infarct reducing effect on the ischemic canine myocardium supplied by the left anterior descending artery (Przyklenk *et al.* 1993). This protective effect was termed remote preconditioning. Subsequent studies have shown that ischemic bursts could be successfully applied to organs such as the intestine (Gho *et al.* 1996), skeletal muscle (Addison *et al.* 2003) and kidney (Pell *et al.* 1998) and as a result, precondition the myocardium.

2.3 Clinical relevance

Although preconditioning is not applicable for patients with AMI, it may serve to alleviate the high risk of myocardial infarction in patients with unstable angina. Furthermore, preconditioning strategies can be applied prior to coronary artery bypass graft (CABG)

surgery to prevent a potentially injurious ischemia insult. A proof-of concept study supporting remote preconditioning of the upper limb in adult patients prior to elective CABG showed significantly reduced serum troponin-T levels (Hausenloy *et al.* 2007). The cardiac remote ischemic preconditioning (CRISP) study implemented remote preconditioning (induced by three 5-minute inflations of a blood pressure to 200 mmHg in the upper arm and followed by three 5-minute reperfusion intervals) before elective PCI in a randomized control trial (Hoole *et al.* 2009). Subject who received the remote IPC had reduced cardiac troponin I release, suffered from less chest pain and ECG ST-segment deviation. In addition, there was a reported improvement in the major adverse cardiac and cerebral event (MACCE) rate. The beneficial use of remote IPC has also been successfully translated to children with congential defects undergoing a cardiopulmonary bypass (Cheung *et al.* 2006).

3. Ischemic postconditioning: A promising therapy to limit reperfusion injury

Discovered in 2003, ischemic postconditioning, achieved by repetitive brief bouts of ischemia at the onset of reperfusion, protects against reperfusion injury and offers a clinical approach in patients with AMI (Zhao *et al.* 2003). Three episodes of 30 secs of reperfusion and 30 secs of ischemia, performed at the onset of reperfusion following a 60 min ischemic insult in dog hearts, protected against reperfusion injury (Zhao *et al.* 2003). Its infarct limiting effect is comparable to ischemic preconditioning and can reduce the infarct size by up to 80% (figure 3) (Zhao *et al.* 2003). Postconditioning has been successful in multiple animal species such as canines, rats, mice and rabbits (Zhao and Vinten-Johansen 2006). Ischemic pre- and postconditioning, used in combination, did not produce any significant benefit over the strategies used separately, which may suggest the activation of similar protective mechanisms by both phenomena (Halkos *et al.* 2004).

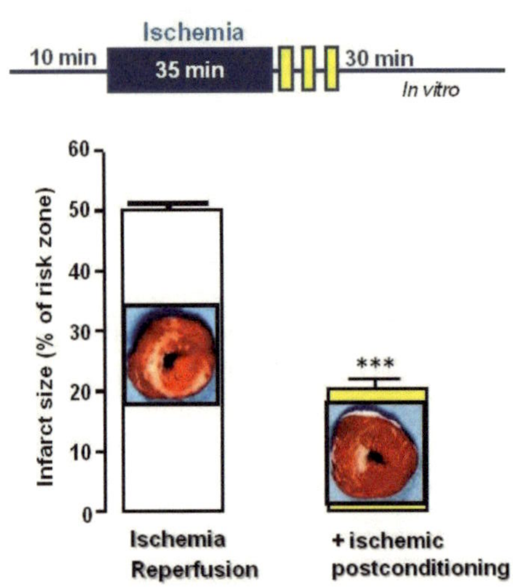

Fig. 3. Ischemic postconditioning decrease infarct size

In animal models subjected to an ischemia-reperfusion insult, ischemic postconditioning performed by short cycles of ischemia-reperfusion at the onset of reperfusion, dramatically reduces the infarct size (dead cells in white).

3.1 Ischemic postconditioning: A rapid translation from bench to bedside

Considering that postconditioning was only discovered in 2003, (Zhao *et al.* 2003) it is remarkable how quickly it made the leap to proof-of-concept clinical trials (figure 4). In 2005, Staat et al published a landmark study whereby postconditioning, applied during the first minutes of reperfusion to AMI patients undergoing emergency PCI, reduced myocardial damage measured through creatine kinase release over 72 hours (Staat *et al.* 2005). After reperfusion by direct stenting, postconditioning simply performed within the first minute of reperfusion by 4 cycles of 1 min inflation/deflation of the angioplasty balloon, reduced the infarct size by 36%. Using more specific endpoints, the same group later confirmed that their postconditioning protocol was associated with a reduction of the infarct size (measured by 201thallium single photon emission computed tomography technique after 6 months) and improved myocardial contractile function (measured by echocardiography) after 1 year (Thibault *et al.* 2008). At 1 year, their pilot study, performed on 38 patients only, showed a 7% increase in the left ventricular ejection fraction in the postconditioned patients (Thibault *et al.* 2008). Animal studies have shown that optimizing the postconditioning protocol is an important process for the success of the therapy (van Vuuren and Lochner 2008). Few human studies seem to confirm this statement. Postconditioning the human heart with three cycles of 30 sec inflation and 30 sec deflation of the angioplasty balloon, within the first 3 min of reperfusion, reduced the infarct size by 27% (Yang *et al.* 2007). In a retrospective analysis of patients undergoing primary angioplasty, the release of creatine kinase in patients who received 4 or more balloon inflations was lower than in patients who received between 1 and 3 balloon inflations (Darling *et al.* 2007).

When measuring the area at risk before reperfusion in patients undergoing primary PCI, the benefit of ischemic postconditioning performed with 4 cycles of 60s reperfusion and 60s reocclusion is not observed in the overall population with ST elevation myocardial infarction but seems to be of value for patients with large areas at risk. Hence, the regression analysis in which the final infarct size was related to the myocardial area at risk showed a significant difference between the control and postconditioning groups (Sorensson *et al.*).

With regards to long term benefit of ischemic postconditioning, a study of 43 patients suggested that the protective effect on cardiac function tends to persist beyond 3 years, but larger studies are needed to confirm its long term effect (Garcia *et al.* 2010).

The benefit of postconditioning can be extended to cardiac surgery. In patients undergoing a valve replacement under cold blood cardioplegic arrest, postconditioning (performed by 3 cycles of 30 sec ischemia and 30 sec reperfusion using aortic clamping) reduced the creatine kinase release, transcardiac neutrophil count and the use of inotropic agents during reperfusion (Luo *et al.* 2008).

Remote postconditioning, whereby the postconditioning protocol applied in one part of the body results in protection of a remote region undergoing ischemia-reperfusion, is successful in animal models (Andreka *et al.* 2007) and may represent a more practical way to protect the human heart than ischemic postconditioning. Recently, remote perconditioning was tested in Danish patients on their way to hospital to receive primary PCI (Botker *et al.*). Remote perconditioning was performed by 4 cycles of 5min inflation/deflation of the blood pressure cuff on the arm of 251 patients. 30 days after reperfusion, the myocardial salvage measured by SPECT imaging was increased by remote perconditioning.

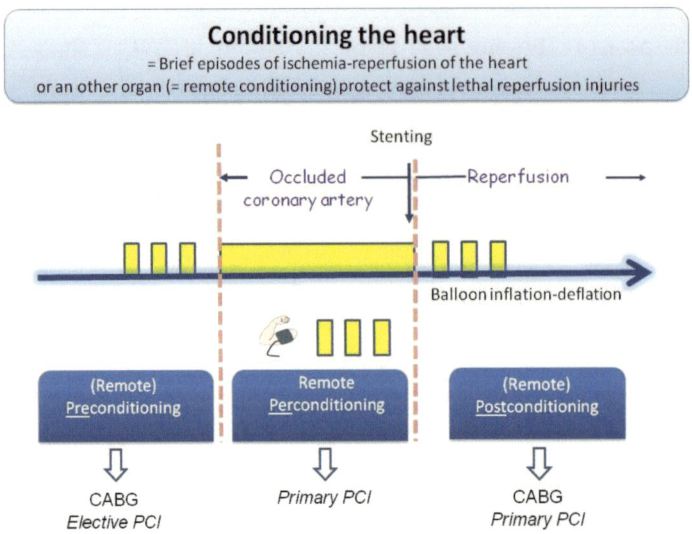

Fig. 4. The concept of conditioning the heart and its clinical applications

3.2 Mechanisms involved in ischemic postconditioning: RISK and SAFE pathways

Following the discovery of ischemic preconditioning in 1986 (Murry *et al.* 1986), intensive research was performed to elucidate the intrinsic prosurvival cascades that can be activated within the heart to limit reperfusion injuries. The delineation of the reperfusion injury salvage kinase (RISK) pathway proved to be a very powerful survival pathway to limit cell death at the onset of reperfusion. More recently, the delineation of another prosurvival signaling cascade termed as the survivor activating factor enhancement (SAFE) pathway and involving the activation of the immune system, offers new potential to limit further reperfusion injury.

3.2.1 RISK pathway

The actual term reperfusion injury salvage kinase (RISK) pathway was first coined in 2002, in a study investigating the signal transduction pathway underlying the infarct-limiting effects of urocortin administered at reperfusion (Schulman *et al.* 2002). Activation of this pathway involves two prosurvival kinases pathways: phosphatidylinositol-3 kinase (PI3K)/Akt and mitogen extraregulated kinase 1/2 (MEK1/2)-extraregulated kinase 1/2 (Erk1/2). Activation of both Erk1/2 and Akt at the onset of reperfusion is generally associated with a reduction of the infarct size and their inhibition with pharmacological agents is often associated with a loss of the infarct sparing effect of many cardioprotective drugs (Hausenloy *et al.* 2011).

In ischemic postconditioning, the RISK pathway is activated at the onset of reperfusion by cell surface receptors including G-protein coupled receptors, cytokine receptors, tyrosine kinase receptors and serine/threonine receptors (Hausenloy and Yellon 2009). Adenosine receptors (Morrison *et al.* 2007) and sphingosine kinase-1 receptors (Jin *et al.* 2008) activate the RISK pathway and it is probable that many other cell-surface implicated as triggers in ischemic postconditoning, such as bradykinin and opioids receptors, also activate the RISK pathway but this remains to be demonstrated directly.

Activation of Akt and Erk1/2 leads to the activation of endothelial nitric oxide synthase (eNOS) and P70S6Kinase (Tsang *et al.* 2004). There are several other protein kinases that have been implicated in ischemic postconditioning signaling which could also be considered as components of the RISK pathway such as protein kinase C (PKC), protein kinase G, p38 mitogen-activated protein kinase (p38MAPK) and Jun N-terminal kinase MAPK.

3.2.2 mPTP and anti-apoptotic signaling pathways activated by the RISK pathway

There are a number of downstream effectors of the RISK pathway which could be responsible for the cardioprotection elicited by ischemic postconditioning. Many of these terminate on the mitochondria an organelle which occupies an essential role in cardiomyocyte survival and death signaling.

The opening of the mitochondrial permeability transition pore (mPTP) at the onset of myocardial reperfusion is a critical determinant of lethal myocardial reperfusion injury, such that pharmacologically inhibiting its opening at this time can reduce myocardial infarct size by 40-50% in both the laboratory (Argaud *et al.* 2005, Hausenloy *et al.* 2002) and clinical setting (Bolli *et al.* 2004). Although the actual identity of the pore-forming units of the mPTP is unknown, several studies have demonstrated mitochondrial cyclophilin-D (CypD) to be a major regulatory component of the mPTP, such that mice lacking CypD appear resistant to mPTP opening and sustain greatly reduced myocardial infarct sizes (Baines *et al.* 2005, Nakagawa *et al.* 2005). The actual mechanism through which the Akt and Erk1/2 components of the RISK pathway mediate mPTP inhibition is unclear, although potential explanations include: (1) the generation of nitric oxide by endothelial nitric oxide synthase (eNOS), a downstream target of the RISK pathway can inhibit mPTP opening (Kim *et al.* 2004); (2) Akt may modulate mitochondrial morphology thereby rendering mitochondria more resistant to mPTP opening (Ong *et al.* 2010); (3) Akt may modulate intracellular calcium handling- by increasing sarcoplasmic reticulum calcium uptake it may prevent mPTP opening (Abdallah *et al.* 2006); (4) Glycogen synthase kinase (GSK3β), a downstream target of both Akt and extracellular regulated kinase (Erk) 1/2 may act as a point of convergence for a variety of pro-survival signaling pathways resulting in mPTP inhibition (Juhaszova *et al.* 2004, Juhaszova *et al.* 2009).

The possibility of recruiting anti-apoptotic signaling pathways had been one of the original reasons for proposing the RISK pathway as a pro-survival signaling pathway, particularly given the close association of apoptotic cell death with the reperfusion phase (Yellon and Baxter 1999). Interestingly, although a large number of potential anti-apoptotic pathways exist downstream of the RISK pathway, relatively few have actually been investigated in the context of cardioprotection, yet alone ischemic postconditioning. These anti-apoptotic mechanisms include: the phosphorylation and inhibition of pro-apoptotic proteins such as BAD (Bcl-2 antagonist of cell death) (Jonassen *et al.* 2001), BAX (Bcl-2-associated X protein) and the activation of anti-apoptotic proteins such as PIM-1 kinase (Hausenloy and Yellon 2009), the effect of which is preservation of mitochondrial integrity and a favorable increase in the anti-apoptotic proteins such as BCL2 (B-cell lymphoma-2) and BCL-XL (B-cell lymphoma-xl).

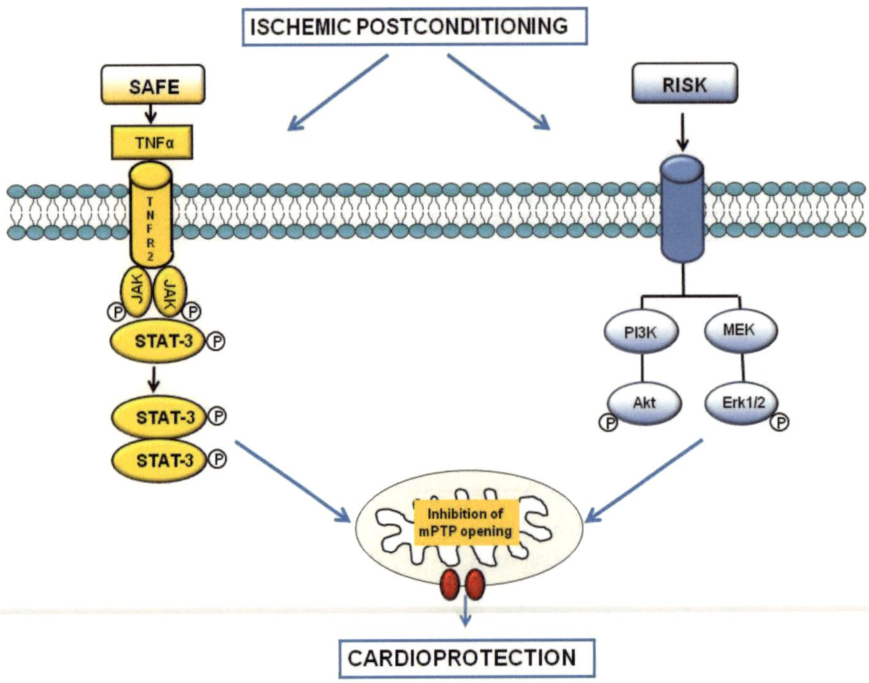

Fig. 5. Prosurvival pathways activated by postconditioning

Ischemic postconditioning activates two powerful prosurvival pathways termed as the SAFE and RISK paths. Both pathways reduce lethal reperfusion injury by limiting the opening of the mitochondrial permeability transition pore (mPTP). SAFE, Survivor Activation Factor Enhancement; TNFα, Tumour Necrosis Factor alpha; JAK, Janus Kinase; STAT-3, Signal Transducer and Activator of Transcription-3, RISK, Reperfusion Injury Salvage Kinase; PI3K, Phosphoinositol 3-Kinase; MEK, Mitogen activated protein kinase Extracellular regulated Kinase; ERK, Extracellular Regulated Kinase.

3.2.3 SAFE pathway

In animal studies, the involvement of the RISK pathway has sparked few inconsistencies, supporting the existence of an alternative prosurvival signal transduction pathway for protecting the ischemic myocardium against lethal reperfusion injury (Lecour 2009b). In this respect, our laboratory has recently described a novel pro-survival pathway, which involves the activation of tumor necrosis factor alpha (TNF) and the transcription factor, signal transducer and activator of transcription 3 (STAT-3), that we have termed as the Survivor Activating Factor Enhancement (SAFE) pathway (figure 5) (Lecour 2009a, b). The SAFE pathway was first discovered in the setting of ischemic preconditioning and its role in ischemic postconditioning has only been recently confirmed.

TNF, a proinflammatory cytokine expressed in all nucleated cell types including cardiomyocytes, exerts its major effects after binding onto its cell surface receptors TNF receptor 1 (TNFR1) and TNF receptor 2 (TNFR2). The two TFNRs differ in their signal pathways with TNFR1 activating both apoptotic and protective signaling whereas TNFR2, although poorly studied, seem to convey prosurvival signaling only (Schulz and Heusch 2009). In a dose and time-dependent manner and function to which type of receptor is activated, TNF can be either protective or deleterious. There are now a large number of experimental data supporting the evidence that ischemic postconditionng requires activation of low concentrations of TNF to confer cardioprotection via TNFR2 (Lecour 2009b). Activation of the receptors phosphorylates the janus kinase (JAK) protein, which in turn, can activate the transcription factor STAT-3. In 2006, the role of STAT-3 in ischemic postconditioning was also suggested in an isolated rat heart model whereby the addition of the JAK/STAT-3 inhibitor AG490 at the onset of reperfusion abolished the cardioprotective effect of ischemic postconditioning (Suleman *et al.* 2006). Both ischemic and pharmacological postconditioning with TNF failed to confer an infarct sparing effect in isolated STAT3-deficient murine hearts subjected to ischemia-reperfusion injury (Boengler *et al.* 2008, Lacerda *et al.* 2009). Furthermore, the absence of protection observed in TNF or TNFR2 knockout mice was associated with the absence of STAT-3 phosphorylation (Lacerda *et al.* 2009). Activation of TNF/TNR2/JAK/STAT-3 may be triggered by various mediators including insulin, angiotensin II, bradykinin, adrenoreceptors, opioids, cannabinoids and sphingosine-1 phosphate (Hausenloy *et al.* 2011).

3.2.4 mPTP and anti-apoptotic signaling pathways activated by the SAFE pathway

TNF-induced protection requires the activation of protein kinase C, the mitochondrial ATP-dependent potassium channel and NFκ-B (Lecour *et al.* 2002, Somers *et al.* 2005). In addition, pharmacological preconditioning with TNF is associated with an increase in mitochondrial free radicals and an addition of free radical scavengers such as mercaptopropionyl glycine abolished its cardioprotective effect (Lacerda *et al.* 2006, Lecour *et al.* 2005a). In contrast, neither p38MAPK, Akt, Erk nor GSK3-β seem to be involved in TNF-induced cardioprotection, therefore suggesting that they do not act as the downstream target of the SAFE pathway (Lacerda *et al.* 2009, Lecour *et al.* 2005b, Tanno *et al.* 2003). STAT3 mediates cardioprotection via the phosphorylation and inactivation of the pro-apoptotic factor Bad (Deuchar *et al.* 2007, Lecour *et al.* 2005b) and Bax (Huffman *et al.* 2008). The mitochondrial permeability transition pore (mPTP) is described as an end-effector of ischemic postconditioning and the RISK pathway and there are now strong evidence that the SAFE pathway may also target the mPTP. Hence, STAT3 expression was demonstrated in mitochondria, playing a role in cell respiration (Wegrzyn *et al.* 2009) and mPTP opening (Boengler *et al.* 2010).

3.3 Targeting the RISK and SAFE paths to limit reperfusion injury

Ischemic postconditioning performed by inflation/deflation of the angioplastic balloon is safe, easy to perform, inexpensive but many patients in remote areas do not have a fast access to a PCI performing facility and ischemic postconditioning has never been tested following thrombolysis. The development of pharmacological drugs which can mimic ischemic postconditioning by activating the prosurvival RISK and SAFE pathways would benefit patients undergoing either PCI or thrombolysis and it would certainly be more practical than ischemic postconditioning.

In this regards, the immunosuppressor drug cyclosporine can bind to the mitochondrial cyclophilin D, thereby inhibiting the opening of the mPTP, a downstream target of both the

RISK and SAFE pathways. In a multicenter single-blinded controlled clinical trial, the effect of cyclosporine A was evaluated in 58 patients with acute ST-elevation myocardial infarction who received an intravenous bolus of 2.5mg/kg of cyclosporine immediately before undergoing PCI, significantly reduced the release of creatine kinase by 40% within the first 72 hours. (Piot *et al.* 2008) Infarct size, assessed on day 5 (by measuring the area of hyperenhancement on magnetic resonance imaging) was significantly reduced. Cyclosporine, routinely used as an immunosuppressive agent, is well known for its toxic side-effects, such as renal and hepatic toxicity and increased susceptibility to infections and cancers. A single bolus injection of cyclosporine did not show any of these side-effects, but larger and longer clinical trials are required to prove the safety and efficacy of cyclosporine as a therapeutic agent following AMI.

Two clinical trials have explored the effect of adenosine in patients with acute myocardial infarction (AMISTAD and AMISTAD II) but the results were mitigated by the haemodynamic effect of the drug. (Mahaffey *et al.* 1999, Ross *et al.* 2005) Although adenosine can successfully reduce the infarct size, it has a vasodilatory and negative chronotropic effect, causing hypotension and bradycardia, thus limiting its clinical application. However, recent experimental studies using polyethylene glycol liposomal adenosine in rats protected against ischemia-reperfusion and reduced the hemodynamic effect of adenosine. (Takahama *et al.* 2009) If this protocol can be applied in a clinical setting, it may limit the side effects of adenosine.

Erythropoietin successfully reduced the infarct size in animal models but its clinical application still needs to be confirmed. (Bullard *et al.* 2005)

3.4 Ischemic postconditioning and comorbidities

At the present, little information is available in humans with regards to the success of ischemic postconditioning with different comorbidities and most of the clinical trials have excluded patients with diabetes/metabolic syndrome. Animal studies have shown that various comorbidities affect the protective effect of postconditioning. Rats with obesity, metabolic syndrome or diabetes become more resistant to the infarct limiting effect of ischemic postconditioning and additional cycles of ischemia-reperfusion are required to achieve a beneficial effect (Hausenloy *et al.* 2011). Similarly, hyperglycemia in rabbits abolishes the cardioprotective effect of ischemic postconditioning (Raphael *et al.*). More recently, depressed rats failed to be protected with ischemic postconditioning (Zhuo *et al.* 2011).

4. Conclusion

Ischemic postconditioning is a safe, simple and inexpensive therapy but several factors need to be taken into consideration for its efficacy. Remote ischemic postconditioning and pharmacological postconditioning present the advantage of being applied in AMI patients with or without PCI. However, the severity and duration of ischemia, the presence of collateral circulation and the algorithm of the postconditioning protocol may all affect the protective effect of ischemic postconditioning against lethal reperfusion injury (Hausenloy *et al.* 2010).

Although small clinical proof-of-concept studies suggest that ischemic postconditioning can protect the human heart against lethal reperfusion injuries, larger clinical trials testing ischemic or pharmacological postconditioning are needed to test the clinical outcome of this phenomenon. In Italy, the POSTAMI trial is currently evaluating the effect of ischemic postconditioning on infarct size (using magnetic resonance imaging) 3 months after ST elevation AMI in 78 patients (Tarantini *et al.* 2010). In Norway, the POSTEMI study is currently evaluating the effect of ischemic postconditioning on infarct size after 4 months by magnetic resonance imaging in 260 patients (Limalanathan *et al.*). Most importantly, the CIRCUS study aims to evaluate whether cyclosporine A, given immediately prior to reperfusion with PCI, can improve clinical outcome in patients with AMI. Conducted in 15 countries and 120 centres, the study will evaluate 1750 patients per group considering cardiac death and hospitalization for in-hospital worsening of heart failure as primary endpoints. The outcome of these larger clinical trials will hopefully conclude that postconditioning should be systematically applied in the management of future patients with AMI.

5. References

Abdallah Y., Gkatzoflia A., Gligorievski D., Kasseckert S., Euler G., Schluter K. D., Schafer M., Piper H. M., Schafer C.: Insulin protects cardiomyocytes against reoxygenation-induced hypercontracture by a survival pathway targeting SR Ca2+ storage 2006 *Cardiovasc Res* Vol.70, No.2, pp.346-53

Addison P. D., Neligan P. C., Ashrafpour H., Khan A., Zhong A., Moses M., Forrest C. R., Pang C. Y.: Noninvasive remote ischemic preconditioning for global protection of skeletal muscle against infarction 2003 *Am J Physiol Heart Circ Physiol* Vol.285, No.4, pp.H1435-43

Andreka G., Vertesaljai M., Szantho G., Font G., Piroth Z., Fontos G., Juhasz E. D., Szekely L., Szelid Z., Turner M. S., Ashrafian H., Frenneaux M. P., Andreka P.: Remote ischaemic postconditioning protects the heart during acute myocardial infarction in pigs 2007 *Heart* Vol.93, No.6, pp.749-52

Argaud L., Gateau-Roesch O., Muntean D., Chalabreysse L., Loufouat J., Robert D., Ovize M.: Specific inhibition of the mitochondrial permeability transition prevents lethal reperfusion injury 2005 *J Mol Cell Cardiol* Vol.38, No.2, pp.367-74

Baines C. P., Kaiser R. A., Purcell N. H., Blair N. S., Osinska H., Hambleton M. A., Brunskill E. W., Sayen M. R., Gottlieb R. A., Dorn G. W., Robbins J., Molkentin J. D.: Loss of cyclophilin D reveals a critical role for mitochondrial permeability transition in cell death 2005 *Nature* Vol.434, No.7033, pp.658-62

Baxter G. F., Goma F. M., Yellon D. M.: Characterisation of the infarct-limiting effect of delayed preconditioning: timecourse and dose-dependency studies in rabbit myocardium 1997 *Basic Res Cardiol* Vol.92, No.3, pp.159-67

Boengler K., Buechert A., Heinen Y., Roeskes C., Hilfiker-Kleiner D., Heusch G., Schulz R.: Cardioprotection by ischemic postconditioning is lost in aged and STAT3-deficient mice 2008 *Circ Res* Vol.102, No.1, pp.131-5

Boengler K., Hilfiker-Kleiner D., Heusch G., Schulz R.: Inhibition of permeability transition pore opening by mitochondrial STAT3 and its role in myocardial ischemia/reperfusion 2010 *Basic Res Cardiol* Vol.105, No.6, pp.771-85

Bolli R., Becker L., Gross G., Mentzer R., Jr., Balshaw D., Lathrop D. A.: Myocardial protection at a crossroads: the need for translation into clinical therapy 2004 *Circ Res* Vol.95, No.2, pp.125-34

Bolli R., Jeroudi M. O., Patel B. S., Dubose C. M., Lai E. K., Roberts R., Mccay P. B.: Direct evidence that oxygen-derived free radicals contribute to postischemic myocardial dysfunction in the intact dog 1989 *Proc Natl Acad Sci U S A* Vol.86, No.12, pp.4695-9

Bolli R., Li Q. H., Tang X. L., Guo Y., Xuan Y. T., Rokosh G., Dawn B.: The late phase of preconditioning and its natural clinical application--gene therapy 2007 *Heart Fail Rev* Vol.12, No.3-4, pp.189-99

Botker H. E., Kharbanda R., Schmidt M. R., Bottcher M., Kaltoft A. K., Terkelsen C. J., Munk K., Andersen N. H., Hansen T. M., Trautner S., Lassen J. F., Christiansen E. H., Krusell L. R., Kristensen S. D., Thuesen L., Nielsen S. S., Rehling M., Sorensen H. T., Redington A. N., Nielsen T. T.: Remote ischaemic conditioning before hospital admission, as a complement to angioplasty, and effect on myocardial salvage in patients with acute myocardial infarction: a randomised trial *Lancet* Vol.375, No.9716, pp.727-34

Bullard A. J., Govewalla P., Yellon D. M.: Erythropoietin protects the myocardium against reperfusion injury in vitro and in vivo 2005 *Basic Res Cardiol* Vol.100, No.5, pp.397-403

Cheung M. M., Kharbanda R. K., Konstantinov I. E., Shimizu M., Frndova H., Li J., Holtby H. M., Cox P. N., Smallhorn J. F., Van Arsdell G. S., Redington A. N.: Randomized controlled trial of the effects of remote ischemic preconditioning on children undergoing cardiac surgery: first clinical application in humans 2006 *J Am Coll Cardiol* Vol.47, No.11, pp.2277-82

Darling C. E., Solari P. B., Smith C. S., Furman M. I., Przyklenk K.: 'Postconditioning' the human heart: multiple balloon inflations during primary angioplasty may confer cardioprotection 2007 *Basic Res Cardiol* Vol.102, No.3, pp.274-8

Deuchar G. A., Opie L. H., Lecour S.: TNFalpha is required to confer protection in an in vivo model of classical ischaemic preconditioning 2007 *Life Sci* Vol.80, No.18, pp.1686-91

Dong Z., Saikumar P., Weinberg J. M., Venkatachalam M. A.: Calcium in cell injury and death 2006 *Annu Rev Pathol* Vol.1, pp.405-34

Garcia-Dorado D., Oliveras J.: Myocardial oedema: a preventable cause of reperfusion injury? 1993 *Cardiovasc Res* Vol.27, No.9, pp.1555-63

Garcia S., Henry T. D., Wang Y. L., Chavez I. J., Pedersen W. R., Lesser J. R., Shroff G. R., Moore L., Traverse J. H.: Long-term follow-up of patients undergoing postconditioning during ST-elevation myocardial infarction 2010 *J Cardiovasc Transl Res* Vol.4, No.1, pp.92-8

Gho B. C., Schoemaker R. G., Van Den Doel M. A., Duncker D. J., Verdouw P. D.: Myocardial protection by brief ischemia in noncardiac tissue 1996 *Circulation* Vol.94, No.9, pp.2193-200

Halkos M. E., Kerendi F., Corvera J. S., Wang N. P., Kin H., Payne C. S., Sun H. Y., Guyton R. A., Vinten-Johansen J., Zhao Z. Q.: Myocardial protection with postconditioning is not enhanced by ischemic preconditioning 2004 *Ann Thorac Surg* Vol.78, No.3, pp.961-9; discussion 969

Hausenloy D. J., Baxter G., Bell R., Botker H. E., Davidson S. M., Downey J., Heusch G., Kitakaze M., Lecour S., Mentzer R., Mocanu M. M., Ovize M., Schulz R., Shannon R., Walker M., Walkinshaw G., Yellon D. M.: Translating novel strategies for cardioprotection: the Hatter Workshop Recommendations 2010 *Basic Res Cardiol* Vol.105, No.6, pp.677-86

Hausenloy D. J., Lecour S., Yellon D. M.: Reperfusion injury salvage kinase and survivor activating factor enhancement prosurvival signaling pathways in ischemic postconditioning: two sides of the same coin 2011 *Antioxid Redox Signal* Vol.14, No.5, pp.893-907

Hausenloy D. J., Maddock H. L., Baxter G. F., Yellon D. M.: Inhibiting mitochondrial permeability transition pore opening: a new paradigm for myocardial preconditioning? 2002 *Cardiovasc Res* Vol.55, No.3, pp.534-43

Hausenloy D. J., Mwamure P. K., Venugopal V., Harris J., Barnard M., Grundy E., Ashley E., Vichare S., Di Salvo C., Kolvekar S., Hayward M., Keogh B., Macallister R. J., Yellon D. M.: Effect of remote ischaemic preconditioning on myocardial injury in patients undergoing coronary artery bypass graft surgery: a randomised controlled trial 2007 *Lancet* Vol.370, No.9587, pp.575-9

Hausenloy D. J., Yellon D. M.: Cardioprotective growth factors 2009 *Cardiovasc Res* Vol.83, No.2, pp.179-94

Hausenloy D. J., Yellon D. M.: The mitochondrial permeability transition pore: its fundamental role in mediating cell death during ischaemia and reperfusion 2003 *J Mol Cell Cardiol* Vol.35, No.4, pp.339-41

Hoole S. P., Heck P. M., Sharples L., Khan S. N., Duehmke R., Densem C. G., Clarke S. C., Shapiro L. M., Schofield P. M., O'sullivan M., Dutka D. P.: Cardiac Remote Ischemic Preconditioning in Coronary Stenting (CRISP Stent) Study: a prospective, randomized control trial 2009 *Circulation* Vol.119, No.6, pp.820-7

Huffman L. C., Koch S. E., Butler K. L.: Coronary effluent from a preconditioned heart activates the JAK-STAT pathway and induces cardioprotection in a donor heart 2008 *Am J Physiol Heart Circ Physiol* Vol.294, No.1, pp.H257-62

Inserte J., Ruiz-Meana M., Rodriguez-Sinovas A., Barba I., Garcia-Dorado D.: Contribution of delayed intracellular pH recovery to ischemic postconditioning protection 2011 *Antioxid Redox Signal* Vol.14, No.5, pp.923-39

Jin Z. Q., Karliner J. S., Vessey D. A.: Ischaemic postconditioning protects isolated mouse hearts against ischaemia/reperfusion injury via sphingosine kinase isoform-1 activation 2008 *Cardiovasc Res* Vol.79, No.1, pp.134-40

Jonassen A. K., Sack M. N., Mjos O. D., Yellon D. M.: Myocardial protection by insulin at reperfusion requires early administration and is mediated via Akt and p70s6 kinase cell-survival signaling 2001 *Circ Res* Vol.89, No.12, pp.1191-8

Juhaszova M., Zorov D. B., Kim S. H., Pepe S., Fu Q., Fishbein K. W., Ziman B. D., Wang S., Ytrehus K., Antos C. L., Olson E. N., Sollott S. J.: Glycogen synthase kinase-3beta mediates convergence of protection signaling to inhibit the mitochondrial permeability transition pore 2004 *J Clin Invest* Vol.113, No.11, pp.1535-49

Juhaszova M., Zorov D. B., Yaniv Y., Nuss H. B., Wang S., Sollott S. J.: Role of glycogen synthase kinase-3beta in cardioprotection 2009 *Circ Res* Vol.104, No.11, pp.1240-52

Kim J. S., Ohshima S., Pediaditakis P., Lemasters J. J.: Nitric oxide: a signaling molecule against mitochondrial permeability transition- and pH-dependent cell death after reperfusion 2004 *Free Radic Biol Med* Vol.37, No.12, pp.1943-50

Lacerda L., Smith R. M., Opie L., Lecour S.: TNFalpha-induced cytoprotection requires the production of free radicals within mitochondria in C(2)C(12) myotubes 2006 *Life Sci*

Lacerda L., Somers S., Opie L. H., Lecour S.: Ischaemic postconditioning protects against reperfusion injury via the SAFE pathway 2009 *Cardiovasc Res* Vol.84, No.2, pp.201-8

Lecour S.: Activation of the protective Survivor Activating Factor Enhancement (SAFE) pathway against reperfusion injury: Does it go beyond the RISK pathway? 2009a *J Mol Cell Cardiol* Vol.47, No.1, pp.32-40

Lecour S.: Multiple protective pathways against reperfusion injury: a SAFE path without Aktion? 2009b *J Mol Cell Cardiol* Vol.46, No.5, pp.607-9

Lecour S., Rochette L., Opie L.: Free radicals trigger TNFalpha-induced cardioprotection 2005a *Cardiovasc Res* Vol.65, No.1, pp.239-43

Lecour S., Smith R. M., Woodward B., Opie L. H., Rochette L., Sack M. N.: Identification of a novel role for sphingolipid signaling in TNF alpha and ischemic preconditioning mediated cardioprotection 2002 *J Mol Cell Cardiol* Vol.34, No.5, pp.509-18

Lecour S., Suleman N., Deuchar G. A., Somers S., Lacerda L., Huisamen B., Opie L. H.: Pharmacological preconditioning with tumor necrosis factor-alpha activates signal transducer and activator of transcription-3 at reperfusion without involving classic prosurvival kinases (Akt and extracellular signal-regulated kinase) 2005b *Circulation* Vol.112, No.25, pp.3911-8

Limalanathan S., Andersen G. O., Hoffmann P., Klow N. E., Abdelnoor M., Eritsland J.: Rationale and design of the POSTEMI (postconditioning in ST-elevation myocardial infarction) study *Cardiology* Vol.116, No.2, pp.103-9

Luo W., Li B., Chen R., Huang R., Lin G.: Effect of ischemic postconditioning in adult valve replacement 2008 *Eur J Cardiothorac Surg* Vol.33, No.2, pp.203-8

Mahaffey K. W., Puma J. A., Barbagelata N. A., Dicarli M. F., Leesar M. A., Browne K. F., Eisenberg P. R., Bolli R., Casas A. C., Molina-Viamonte V., Orlandi C., Blevins R., Gibbons R. J., Califf R. M., Granger C. B.: Adenosine as an adjunct to thrombolytic therapy for acute myocardial infarction: results of a multicenter, randomized, placebo-controlled trial: the Acute Myocardial Infarction STudy of ADenosine (AMISTAD) trial 1999 *J Am Coll Cardiol* Vol.34, No.6, pp.1711-20

Morrison R. R., Tan X. L., Ledent C., Mustafa S. J., Hofmann P. A.: Targeted deletion of A2A adenosine receptors attenuates the protective effects of myocardial postconditioning 2007 *Am J Physiol Heart Circ Physiol* Vol.293, No.4, pp.H2523-9

Murphy J. G., Marsh J. D., Smith T. W.: The role of calcium in ischemic myocardial injury 1987 *Circulation* Vol.75, No.6 Pt 2, pp.V15-24

Murry C. E., Jennings R. B., Reimer K. A.: New insights into potential mechanisms of ischemic preconditioning 1991 *Circulation* Vol.84, No.1, pp.442-5

Murry C. E., Jennings R. B., Reimer K. A.: Preconditioning with ischemia: a delay of lethal cell injury in ischemic myocardium 1986 *Circulation* Vol.74, No.5, pp.1124-36

Nakagawa T., Shimizu S., Watanabe T., Yamaguchi O., Otsu K., Yamagata H., Inohara H., Kubo T., Tsujimoto Y.: Cyclophilin D-dependent mitochondrial permeability transition regulates some necrotic but not apoptotic cell death 2005 *Nature* Vol.434, No.7033, pp.652-8

Ong S. B., Subrayan S., Lim S. Y., Yellon D. M., Davidson S. M., Hausenloy D. J.: Inhibiting mitochondrial fission protects the heart against ischemia/reperfusion injury 2010 *Circulation* Vol.121, No.18, pp.2012-22

Pell T. J., Baxter G. F., Yellon D. M., Drew G. M.: Renal ischemia preconditions myocardium: role of adenosine receptors and ATP-sensitive potassium channels 1998 *Am J Physiol* Vol.275, No.5 Pt 2, pp.H1542-7

Piot C., Croisille P., Staat P., Thibault H., Rioufol G., Mewton N., Elbelghiti R., Cung T. T., Bonnefoy E., Angoulvant D., Macia C., Raczka F., Sportouch C., Gahide G., Finet G., Andre-Fouet X., Revel D., Kirkorian G., Monassier J. P., Derumeaux G., Ovize M.: Effect of cyclosporine on reperfusion injury in acute myocardial infarction 2008 *N Engl J Med* Vol.359, No.5, pp.473-81

Piper H. M., Balser C., Ladilov Y. V., Schafer M., Siegmund B., Ruiz-Meana M., Garcia-Dorado D.: The role of Na+/H+ exchange in ischemia-reperfusion 1996 *Basic Res Cardiol* Vol.91, No.3, pp.191-202

Piper H. M., Garcia-Dorado D., Ovize M.: A fresh look at reperfusion injury 1998 *Cardiovasc Res* Vol.38, No.2, pp.291-300

Przyklenk K., Bauer B., Ovize M., Kloner R. A., Whittaker P.: Regional ischemic 'preconditioning' protects remote virgin myocardium from subsequent sustained coronary occlusion 1993 *Circulation* Vol.87, No.3, pp.893-9

Raphael J., Gozal Y., Navot N., Zuo Z.: Hyperglycemia inhibits anesthetic-induced postconditioning in the rabbit heart via modulation of phosphatidylinositol-3-kinase/Akt and endothelial nitric oxide synthase signaling *J Cardiovasc Pharmacol* Vol.55, No.4, pp.348-57

Reimer K. A., Murry C. E., Yamasawa I., Hill M. L., Jennings R. B.: Four brief periods of myocardial ischemia cause no cumulative ATP loss or necrosis 1986 *Am J Physiol* Vol.251, No.6 Pt 2, pp.H1306-15

Ross A. M., Gibbons R. J., Stone G. W., Kloner R. A., Alexander R. W.: A randomized, double-blinded, placebo-controlled multicenter trial of adenosine as an adjunct to reperfusion in the treatment of acute myocardial infarction (AMISTAD-II) 2005 *J Am Coll Cardiol* Vol.45, No.11, pp.1775-80

Schulman D., Latchman D. S., Yellon D. M.: Urocortin protects the heart from reperfusion injury via upregulation of p42/p44 MAPK signaling pathway 2002 *Am J Physiol Heart Circ Physiol* Vol.283, No.4, pp.H1481-8

Schulz R., Heusch G.: Tumor necrosis factor-alpha and its receptors 1 and 2: Yin and Yang in myocardial infarction? 2009 *Circulation* Vol.119, No.10, pp.1355-7

Somers S., Lacerda L., Opie L., Lecour S.: NFkB triggers TNF induced cardioprotection in C2C12 2005 *J Mol Cell Cardiol* Vol.38, pp.1040-1041

Sorensson P., Saleh N., Bouvier F., Bohm F., Settergren M., Caidahl K., Tornvall P., Arheden H., Ryden L., Pernow J.: Effect of postconditioning on infarct size in patients with ST elevation myocardial infarction *Heart* Vol.96, No.21, pp.1710-5

Staat P., Rioufol G., Piot C., Cottin Y., Cung T. T., L'huillier I., Aupetit J. F., Bonnefoy E., Finet G., Andre-Fouet X., Ovize M.: Postconditioning the human heart 2005 *Circulation* Vol.112, No.14, pp.2143-8

Suleman N., Opie L., Lecour S.: Ischemic postconditioning confers cardioprotection via phosphorylation of STAT-3 2006 *J Mol Cell Cardiol* Vol.40, No.6, pp.977

Takahama H., Minamino T., Asanuma H., Fujita M., Asai T., Wakeno M., Sasaki H., Kikuchi H., Hashimoto K., Oku N., Asakura M., Kim J., Takashima S., Komamura K., Sugimachi M., Mochizuki N., Kitakaze M.: Prolonged targeting of ischemic/reperfused myocardium by liposomal adenosine augments cardioprotection in rats 2009 *J Am Coll Cardiol* Vol.53, No.8, pp.709-17

Tanno M., Gorog D. A., Bellahcene M., Cao X., Quinlan R. A., Marber M. S.: Tumor necrosis factor-induced protection of the murine heart is independent of p38-MAPK activation 2003 *J Mol Cell Cardiol* Vol.35, No.12, pp.1523-7

Tarantini G., Favaretto E., Napodano M., Perazzolo Marra M., Cacciavillani L., Babuin L., Giovagnoni A., Renda P., De Biasio V., Plebani M., Mion M., Zaninotto M., Mistrorigo F., Panfili M., Isabella G., Bilato C., Iliceto S.: Design and methodologies of the POSTconditioning during coronary angioplasty in acute myocardial infarction (POST-AMI) trial 2010 *Cardiology* Vol.116, No.2, pp.110-6

Thibault H., Piot C., Staat P., Bontemps L., Sportouch C., Rioufol G., Cung T. T., Bonnefoy E., Angoulvant D., Aupetit J. F., Finet G., Andre-Fouet X., Macia J. C., Raczka F., Rossi R., Itti R., Kirkorian G., Derumeaux G., Ovize M.: Long-term benefit of postconditioning 2008 *Circulation* Vol.117, No.8, pp.1037-44

Tsang A., Hausenloy D. J., Mocanu M. M., Yellon D. M.: Postconditioning: a form of "modified reperfusion" protects the myocardium by activating the phosphatidylinositol 3-kinase-Akt pathway 2004 *Circ Res* Vol.95, No.3, pp.230-2

Van Domburg R. T., Sonnenschein K., Nieuwlaat R., Kamp O., Storm C. J., Bax J. J., Simoons M. L.: Sustained benefit 20 years after reperfusion therapy in acute myocardial infarction 2005 *J Am Coll Cardiol* Vol.46, No.1, pp.15-20

Van Vuuren D., Lochner A.: Ischaemic postconditioning: from bench to bedside 2008 *Cardiovasc J Afr* Vol.19, No.6, pp.311-20

Vinten-Johansen J.: Involvement of neutrophils in the pathogenesis of lethal myocardial reperfusion injury 2004 *Cardiovasc Res* Vol.61, No.3, pp.481-97

Wegrzyn J., Potla R., Chwae Y. J., Sepuri N. B., Zhang Q., Koeck T., Derecka M., Szczepanek K., Szelag M., Gornicka A., Moh A., Moghaddas S., Chen Q., Bobbili S., Cichy J., Dulak J., Baker D. P., Wolfman A., Stuehr D., Hassan M. O., Fu X. Y., Avadhani N., Drake J. I., Fawcett P., Lesnefsky E. J., Larner A. C.: Function of mitochondrial Stat3 in cellular respiration 2009 *Science* Vol.323, No.5915, pp.793-7

Yang X. C., Liu Y., Wang L. F., Cui L., Wang T., Ge Y. G., Wang H. S., Li W. M., Xu L., Ni Z. H., Liu S. H., Zhang L., Jia H. M., Vinten-Johansen J., Zhao Z. Q.: Reduction in myocardial infarct size by postconditioning in patients after percutaneous coronary intervention 2007 *J Invasive Cardiol* Vol.19, No.10, pp.424-30

Yellon D. M., Baxter G. F.: Reperfusion injury revisited: is there a role for growth factor signaling in limiting lethal reperfusion injury? 1999 *Trends Cardiovasc Med* Vol.9, pp.245-249

Yellon D. M., Hausenloy D. J.: Myocardial reperfusion injury 2007 *N Engl J Med* Vol.357, No.11, pp.1121-35

Zhao Z. Q., Corvera J. S., Halkos M. E., Kerendi F., Wang N. P., Guyton R. A., Vinten-Johansen J.: Inhibition of myocardial injury by ischemic postconditioning during reperfusion: comparison with ischemic preconditioning 2003 *Am J Physiol Heart Circ Physiol* Vol.285, No.2, pp.H579-88

Zhao Z. Q., Vinten-Johansen J.: Postconditioning: reduction of reperfusion-induced injury 2006 *Cardiovasc Res* Vol.70, No.2, pp.200-11

Zhuo C., Wang Y., Wang X., Wang Y., Chen Y.: Cardioprotection by ischemic postconditioning is abolished in depressed rats: role of Akt and signal transducer and activator of transcription-3 2011 *Mol Cell Biochem* Vol.346, No.1-2, pp.39-47

Zweier J. L.: Measurement of superoxide-derived free radicals in the reperfused heart. Evidence for a free radical mechanism of reperfusion injury 1988 *J Biol Chem* Vol.263, No.3, pp.1353-7

Zweier J. L., Talukder M. A.: The role of oxidants and free radicals in reperfusion injury 2006 *Cardiovasc Res* Vol.70, No.2, pp.181-90

8

DES Overview: A Historical and Current Review of Pivotal Clinical Trial Programs

Susan Bezenek, Poornima Sood, Wes Pierson, Chuck Simonton and Krishna Sudhir
Abbott Vascular, Santa Clara, CA
USA

1. Introduction

The focus of this chapter is drug-eluting stents (DES) for the treatment of coronary artery disease (CAD). The clinical trial programs for the main DES approved by the Food and Drug Administration (FDA) for the treatment of CAD are presented. CAD is the leading cause of death in both men and women around the world. In the United States alone, there is a coronary event that occurs every 25 seconds and someone will die from a coronary event every minute (Roger et al., 2011). The current treatment options for ischemic CAD include medications, percutaneous interventions, and surgery to perform coronary artery bypass grafting (CABG). According to the American Heart Association (AHA) 2011 Statistics Update, the total number of percutaneous coronary interventions (PCI) procedures performed in 2007 was 1,178,000 compared to 408,000 CABG operations. With risk factors like obesity and diabetes prevalence increasing globally, the number of CAD interventions will likely continue to rise in the future and require more specialized treatment options for more complex lesions and patient populations.

In past decades, percutaneous angioplasty (PTCA) or plain old balloon angioplasty (POBA) was used to treat obstructive coronary lesions but had frequent incidence of abrupt closure and restenosis. The use of bare metal stents (BMS) helped to address the limitations of PTCA, as evident by reduced angiographic restenosis and target vessel revascularizations (TVR) in earlier clinical trials. The results of these trials led to the first FDA approved balloon-expandable BMS, the Palmaz-Schatz stent (Cordis Corp; a Johnson and Johnson Company) and the Gianturco-Roubin coil stent (Cook Inc, Bloomington, IN) (Fischman et al., 1994; Serruys et al., 1994). Compared to PTCA, the development of BMS reduced the need for urgent CABG associated with abrupt closures and restenosis, but the need for repeat procedures persisted (Doostzadeh et al., 2010). Although BMS provided the structural support to prevent abrupt closures, arterial wall recoil, and negative arterial wall remodeling, the problem of neointimal hyperplasia was not remedied by BMS. Some of the earlier trials evaluating BMS demonstrated that restenosis occurred in about 20% of cases by 6 months (Doostzadeh et al., 2009). The development of DES emerged and intended to deliver localized pharmaceutical agents targeted to reduce restenosis.

In order for DES to optimize therapeutic benefits with minimal risks, several factors must be considered. The stent cell design, strut thickness, polymer technology, mechanism of drug, and pharmacokinetics must all be considered to minimize vessel injury and prevent delayed healing while allowing appropriate endothelialization and avoiding loss of coating integrity, especially during stent delivery and expansion. In order to evaluate the safety and efficacy of DES, the early trials were designed with a BMS comparator arm and used similar endpoints as the previous BMS trials. DES were originally compared to BMS in the RAVEL, TAXUS I, ENDEAVOR I, and SPIRIT FIRST first-in-man clinical trials. These early clinical trials favored the DES arms with reduction in restenosis, major adverse cardiac events (MACE), and revascularizations compared to BMS (Grube et al., 2003; Morice et al., 2002; Moses et al., 2003; Serruys et al., 2002a). DES appeared to address the needs for safe and efficacious PCI for ischemic coronary arterial disease. The underlying metal stent of a DES system provided the structural support to reduce abrupt closure and recoil, while covering the outside of the stent with a platform to deliver pharmaceutical agents that reduced neointimal hyperplasia. As a result, DES replaced BMS as the predominant PCI therapy for suitable patients over the past decade. To date, there are four main commercially available DES manufacturers in the U.S. that will be highlighted in this chapter; Cordis-Johnson and Johnson, Boston Scientific, Medtronic, and Abbott Vascular. Although improved clinical outcomes with these DES have been evident, the risk of stent thrombosis (ST) was previously believed to be one of the potential draw backs of DES compared to BMS. The FDA Circulatory Advisory Panel released a statement following an extensive panel review of trial results and noted that there was no subsequent increase in deaths or MIs from ST in patients treated with DES per the on-label, approved indication (FDA, 2006). The use of dual antiplatelet therapy (DAPT) has been recommended up to 12 months following the procedure in patients that are not at high risk for bleeding per the ACCF/AHA/SCAI 2007 guidelines (King, 2007). The ideal duration of DAPT continues to be explored as DES is now utilized in more high risk patients and in real-world settings. The current improvements for DES focus on drug delivery platforms and bioresorbable stents that may remove potential contributing factors of the stent that cause stent thrombosis. Therefore, this chapter will conclude with an overview of new stent technology currently being evaluated in clinical trials.

2. CYPHER® and NEVO™

The first DES to be approved in the U.S by the FDA in 2003 was CYPHER, manufactured by Cordis Corp; a Johnson and Johnson Company. The CYPHER stent is the Bx Velocity bare metal stent comprised of 316L stainless steel and has three non-eroding polymer coatings with the active drug, sirolimus loaded throughout the coating, but outside of the stent. The basecoat of the stent contains a combination of two non-erodible polymers; n-butyl methylacrylate (PBMA) and polyethylene co-vinyl acetate (PEVA). The two polymers are mixed in a combination with the sirolimus and applied to a parylene C treated stent, which is covered lastly by a drug-free polymer coating of PBMA (accessed online at http://www.cordislabeling.com). The polymer coating thickness is 13.7 μm and as an early stent design, the strut thickness is subsequently one of thickest (140 μm). The CYPHER stent sizes available range from 8 mm - 33 mm long and diameter sizes of 2.25 mm - 3.50 mm with a maximum sirolimus dose of 314 μg. Sirolimus (rapamycin) has lipophilic properties that favor the diffusion across cell membranes of the smooth muscle cells. It is not well understood, but thought that once in the cell, sirolimus binds to the FKBP12 cytoplasmic intracellular protein, which subsequently inhibits the mammalian target of rapamycin (mTOR) regulatory enzyme. The inhibition of mTOR interrupts the cell cycle at the G1 phase and will subsequently inhibit proliferation of smooth muscle cells (Sousa et al., 2001).

The CYPHER stent was approved for commercialization in the U.S. based on the results from the RAVEL and SIRIUS trials. The CYPHER stent received a clinical indication to improve coronary artery lumen diameter in patients with ischemic de novo coronary lesions measuring ≤ 30 mm long in native coronary arteries measuring ≥ 2.25 mm and ≤ 3.5 mm in diameter (accessed online at http://www.cordislabeling.com). The RAVEL study was a randomized, multicenter, double-blind trial that evaluated the CYPHER sirolimus-eluting stent system (SES) compared to the Bx Velocity BMS in single *de novo* coronary lesion treatable by a single 18 mm length stent. The trial enrolled 120 patients in the CYPHER arm and 118 patients in the control (BMS) arm. As reported by Morice et al. and Serruys et al. (2002) (Morice et al., 2002; Serruys et al., 2002b), the primary endpoint of in-stent late loss (LL) favored the CYPHER arm and the angiographic binary restenosis (ABR) rate was 0% in the CYPHER arm compared to 26.6% in the BMS arm at 6 months. The CYPHER arm also favored in clinical endpoint results, as no events of target lesion revascularization (TLR) or target vessel revascularization (TVR) occurred at one year, compared to the BMS arm rates of 23.7% and 26.0%, respectively (Morice et al., 2002; Serruys et al., 2002b). With the promising results demonstrated in the RAVEL trial, the CYPHER stent was evaluated in longer lesions between 15 and 33 mm in length in the SIRIUS trial. There were 533 patients enrolled in the CYPHER arm and 525 patients in the Bx Velocity arm. The SIRIUS trial was a randomized 1:1 multicenter trial and was the pivotal trial that led to FDA approval in the U.S. Compared to the RAVEL trial, the SIRIUS trial enrolled patients with more complex characteristics, such as diabetes, overlapping stent usage, and longer lesions. The mean lesion length in the CYPHER sirolimus-eluting stent system (SES) arm in the RAVEL trial was 9.56 mm compared to 14.4 mm in the SIRIUS trial (Htay and Liu, 2005). The primary endpoint was target vessel failure (TVF; defined as target vessel revascularization, cardiac death or Q-wave and non-Q-wave MI not clearly attributed to a vessel other than the target vessel) and showed statistical significance in favor of the SES arm compared to the Bx Velocity BMS arm, respectively (8.8% versus 21.0%, $p < 0.001$) and also demonstrated significant reductions in TLR rates for the SES arm compared to the BMS arm at 1 year, respectively (4.1% versus 16.6%, $p < 0.001$) (Holmes, 2003).

Trials conducted in Europe and Canada that evaluated CYPHER compared to the Bx Velocity, the E-SIRIUS and C-SIRIUS trials showed consistent results that favored the SES arms compared to the BMS arms. The TLR rates remained numerically lower in the SES arm (4.0%) compared to the BMS arm (20.9%) in the E-SIRIUS trial and also the C-SIRIUS trial (4.0% versus 18.0%, respectively) (Schampaert et al., 2004; Schofer et al., 2003). Following FDA approval in 2003, post-marketing surveillance was initiated in the CYPHER Stent Post-Market Registry in 2003 and the e-SELECT post-market Registry in 2006. The post-market trials were designed as open-label, single-arm, multicenter trials that enrolled real-world treated patients. The CYPHER Stent Post-market registry enrolled up to 15,000 patients and the e-SELECT trial enrolled up to 2070 patients to continue monitoring safety and surveillance required by the FDA. Since the initial approval, multiple registries out of the U.S (OUS) have been initiated as well, such as in Israel, China, and India. The SIRIUS 2.25 mm pivotal trial was conducted to evaluate the safety and efficacy of the SES 2.25mm stent for the reduction of angiographic binary restenosis at 6 months in patients with reference vessel diameters between 2.0 and 2.5 mm and lesion lengths ≤ 20 mm. The trial was a non-randomized, multicenter, prospective trial that compared propensity scores matched results from plain old balloon angioplasty (POBA), Palmaz Schatz, and Bx VELOCITY to the SES 2.25mm treated patients. The outcomes were favorable for the SES 2.25 mm stent arm and were consistent with previous CYPHER trials. Table 1 below highlights the first-in-man (FIM), pivotal, and post-marketing trials conducted for the CYPHER DES.

Trial	Design	Sample size	Primary endpoint	SES treatment arm	BMS treatment arm	P value
RAVEL	Randomized, multi-center	238	In-stent late loss at 6 months	0.01±0.33 mm	0.80±0.53 mm	P < 0.001
SIRIUS	Randomized multicenter	1,058	Target vessel failure (TVF)* at 9 months	8.6%	21.0%	P < 0.001
CYPHER Post-Marketing Surveillance Registry (2003)	Open label, single arm, multicenter	2067	Major adverse cardiac event (MACE)▲ and TLR at 1 year	MACE 7.3% TLR 4.6%	Not applicable (NA)	Not applicable (NA)
e-SELECT Registry (2006)	Open label, single arm, multicenter	15,000	Composite of stent thrombosis (ST) per ARC-definite/ probable at 3 years	1.0% (1 yr) (3 yr data not available to date)	Not applicable (NA)	Not applicable (NA)

*TVF = target vessel revascularization, cardiac death, or Q-wave and non-Q-wave MI not clearly attributed to a vessel other than the target vessel. ▲MACE = death, Q-wave and non-Q-wave MI, and emergent coronary artery bypass graft (CABG), target lesion revascularization (TLR).

Table 1. Clinical trials evaluating the CYPHER SES

One of the challenges faced with these earlier pivotal trials (SIRIUS and RAVEL) was the small sample sizes that were underpowered to discern differences in stent thrombosis (ST) rates between the DES and the BMS arms (Morice et al., 2007; Weisz et al., 2006). As registries collected data on larger populations, a potential increased safety risk of stent thrombosis was questioned with DES use compared to BMS (Lagerqvist et al., 2007; Moreno et al., 2005). During the 2006 FDA Circulatory Advisory Panel, it was concluded that expanded use of DES beyond the approved indication in more complex patients may contribute to the incidence of ST in DES (FDA, 2006). The antiplatelet medication recommendations were also modified to extend clopidogrel usage for up to 12 months for those patients treated with DES that are not at high risk for bleeding in order to potentially reduce ST events (King et al., 2007). As more long term data has become available over the past decade, the concern for increased ST in DES has diminished while strategic new stent technology has been evolving into next generation stent designs.

The next generation of DES under development by Cordis is the NEVO™ sirolimus-eluting stent system (NEVO SES) that has a cobalt chromium alloy platform with reservoirs loaded with a bioabsorbable polymer, polyglycolic lactic acid (PGLA), combined with sirolimus. The strut thickness (100 µm) is thinner than the original CYPHER SES platform and there is an open-cell design that may aid in conformability and flexibility. One of the potential benefits of the reservoir technique for localized drug delivery on a stent, is that the surface area of polymer exposure to the vessel is reduced, which may help to reduce sensitivity or inflammatory responses to polymer that result in events. Furthermore, the NEVO SES elutes sirolimus within 90 days from implant while the PGLA degrades, leaving only a bare metal scaffold in place which may help reduce ST attributed to permanent polymer coatings (Otake et al., 2011a).

The NEVO ResElution-1 trial was a randomized, multicenter, prospective trial that was designed to demonstrate the non-inferiority of NEVO SES compared to a second generation paclitaxel-eluting stent (PES), the TAXUS® Liberté® PES (see 3.0 below) in terms of in-stent late loss at 6 months. The trial enrolled 394 patients and met the primary endpoint; NEVO SES was non-inferior to TAXUS Liberté for in-stent late loss, respectively (0.13 ± 0.31 and 0.36± 48, p <0.001) and demonstrated more uniform suppression of neointimal hyperplasia (Spaulding, 2011). Numerically lower rates of MACE, death, MI, and revascularization have also been demonstrated in favor of the NEVO SES arm compared to the TAXUS Liberté arm through 24 months, as well as no events of ST in the NEVO SES arm (Spaulding, 2011). The NEVO ResElution-1 IVUS sub-study was also conducted and enrolled 100 patients and had 3D intravascular ultrasound (IVUS) studies available on 64 patients at 6 months, which showed that a significant reduction in neointimal obstruction occurred in the NEVO SES arm (5.5 ± 11.0%) compared to the TAXUS Liberté arm (11.5 ± 9.7%), p = 0.02 (Otake et al., 2011a). There was no event of ST in the NEVO SES arm at 6 months compared to 1 event in the TAXUS Liberté arm, and clinical outcomes were overall comparable for death, MI, and TLR (Otake et al., 2011a). Long-term follow-up will continue in the NEVO-SES trial through 5 years. On June 15th, 2011 however, it was announced that CYPHER and NEVO clinical trial programs would be ending due to production cost and declining market share, thus ending future CYPHER-biodegradable new stent technologies for the treatment of CAD.

3. TAXUS® and PLATINUM™

The TAXUS Express2™ paclitaxel eluting stent system (PES) was initially approved by the FDA in 2004, becoming the second DES to be commercially available in the U.S. The TAXUS Express2 PES utilizes paclitaxel as the active drug agent, which is a plant based alkaloid that disrupts the cellular microtubules by binding to tubulin and subsequently arrests the cell cycle at the M phase (Rowinsky and Donehower, 1995). The earliest TAXUS DES implanted in humans was the NIR™ stainless steel closed cell design. The uncoated NIR BMS was used as the scaffold in the TAXUS I, II, and III trials and it is coated with a paclitaxel dose of 1 µg/mm² (Halkin and Stone, 2004). The biphasic polymer-controlled drug release of this stent design elutes paclitaxel in two phases; an initial burst release phase within the first 48 hours followed by a slower release phase over the next 10 days (Halkin and Stone, 2004). The TAXUS Express[1] and TAXUS Express[2] were later utilized in the pivotal trials (TAXUS IV and TAXUS V) and also had a stainless steel platform with tandem cell architecture and strut thickness of 132 µm and a non-degradable TRANSLUTE™ polymer-coating containing paclitaxel. The TRANSLUTE polymer coating thickness is approximately 16 µm and consists of polylactide-co-caprolactone, which provides a uniform and controlled release of paclitaxel with a drug density of 1 µg/mm^2 (Hellige and Windecker, 2009). There are three profiles that were developed and the paclitaxel to polymer ratios for fast, moderate, and slow release profiles are 35:65, 25:75, and 8.8:91.2, respectively, with varying degrees of drug release over time (Acharya and Park, 2006). The long-term retention of paclitaxel within the stent has raised concerns over delayed healing or hypersensitivities that may contribute to the development of very late stent thrombosis (Joner et al., 2006).

The first-in-man trial evaluating a PES was the TAXUS I trial that compared TAXUS NIR PES to the bare-metal stent (BMS) counterpart. TAXUS I was designed as a multicenter RCT that enrolled approximately 61 patients and had a primary endpoint of major adverse cardiac events (MACE) at 30 days follow-up. Patients were randomized 1:1 to receive a single 12 mm long TAXUS-SR PES or BMS in de novo coronary vessels measuring 3.0-3.5 mm diameter (Halkin and Stone, 2004). Although the study was designed primarily to evaluate safety, the low late loss and neointimal hyperplasia in the TAXUS arm suggested benefits of this DES when compared to the BMS counterpart similarly observed in the RAVEL and SIRIUS trials. At 30 days, there was no difference observed in MACE rates, as both the TAXUS and the BMS arms had no events and numerically low rates persisted at one year in favor of the TAXUS NIR arm respectively, 3.0% versus 10.0% (Colombo et al., 2003; Grube et al., 2003). At six months, the in-stent LL in the TAXUS NIR arm was 0.36 ± 48 mm compared to 0.71 ± 0.47 mm in the BMS arm (p value = 0.008) and the neointimal hyperplasia volume was 14.8 ± 10.8 compared to 21.6 ± 10.7 mm^3 (p value = 0.028), respectively (Halkin and Stone, 2004). The TAXUS II trial was also designed as a multicenter RCT but expanded enrollment to approximately 536 patients that were randomized to either TAXUS SR (n = 131), TAXUS MR (135), or the NIR BMS (n = 134) counterpart. The primary endpoint was % in-stent volume obstruction at 6 months and was statistically significant in favor of the TAXUS SR and TAXUS MR patients compared to the BMS treated patients ($p < 0.001$) (Colombo et al., 2003). The in-stent LL and TLR rates continued to favor the TAXUS SR and MR treated patients through long-term follow-up as well with no late thrombosis events occurring between two and three year follow-up in the DES treated patients.

The feasibility to treat patients with in-stent restenosis was explored in TAXUS III which was designed as an uncontrolled, single-arm, multicenter pilot study. The trial enrolled 28 patients treated with TAXUS PES for in-stent restenosis following previous BMS treatment and was further explored in the TAXUS V-ISR trial, which enrolled 396 patients and compared TAXUS PES (195 patients) to balloon angioplasty followed by vascular brachytherapy (201 patients) (Stone et al., 2006; Tanabe et al., 2003). The results supported the safety and efficacy of TAXUS PES compared to vascular brachytherapy, with numerically lower rates of stent thrombosis, MACE, MI, and TLRs compared to the BMS arm (Lasala et al., 2006).

TAXUS IV was designed as randomized, controlled, multicenter trial that enrolled approximately 1,314 patients in the U.S for the treatment of single vessel disease with de novo coronary lesions. The primary endpoint was TVR at 9 months and compared the TAXUS Express PES to BMS in patients with reference vessel diameter (RVD) of 2.5 -3.75 mm and de novo lesions measuring 10-28 mm in length to be coverable by a single stent (Halkin and Stone, 2004). The baseline characteristics were notably well matched between the DES and the BMS arm, as the mean RVD and lesion lengths were the same in both arms, respectively 2.75 mm and 13.4 mm. At 9 months, statistically significant differences were noted between the TAXUS DES and BMS in the primary endpoint, as well as for MACE and TLR. The primary endpoint results for TVR at 9 months was 8.5% in the TAXUS DES arm compared to 15.0% in the BMS arm ($p = 0.0002$), as well as showing significance in TLR at 9 months (Halkin and Stone, 2004). The TLR rates were statistically significant at 9 months in favor of the TAXUS DES arm in patients with orally medicated treated diabetes ($p < 0.0001$) and non-diabetes ($p < 0.0001$), with the exception of patients with insulin treated diabetes ($p = 0.32$) (Halkin and Stone, 2004). For the safety endpoints of death, MI, and stent thrombosis (ST) were non-significant at 9 months in the overall population and suggested that clinical safety was not compromised in exchange for more efficacy with the use of DES.

To further evaluate the TAXUS Express PES in more complex patient populations, the TAXUS V and TAXUS VI clinical trials aimed to evaluate results when compared to BMS. The TAXUS V clinical trial was a randomized, multicenter trial that enrolled 1156 patients with de novo lesions measuring 10-46 mm in length in reference vessel diameters between 2.25 - 4.0 mm; a minimum of 200 patients each with a 2.25 mm diameter or a 4.0 mm diameter were enrolled, as well as a minimum of 300 patients with overlapping stents (Halkin and Stone, 2004). The rates of the primary endpoint of TVR at 9 months were higher in the DES arm than previously observed in the earlier trials, yet still demonstrated a statistically significant difference compared to the BMS arm at 9 months ($p = 0.0184$) (Stone et al., 2005). TAXUS VI trial was designed to evaluate the performance of TAXUS Express compared to BMS and was a multicenter, randomized controlled trial with a primary endpoint of TVR at 9 months and enrolled 446 patients. The results of the primary endpoint revealed that TAXUS Express TVR rates at 9 months were numerically lower than the TAXUS Express rates from the TAXUS V trial, but both continued to outperform the BMS counterpart in reducing revascularization events (Dawkins et al., 2005). Following approval of the TAXUS Express, the ARRIVE I and II post-market surveillance registries were initiated to continue to monitor safety in 'real-world' setting patients that receive treatment with the TAXUS Express. Patients enrolled in the post-market registries or all-comer trials may not have been eligible in the previous RCTs that have specific inclusion and exclusion criteria, and thus may give a broader perspective of how the stent performs in real clinical practice with more complex patient and lesion subsets. The ARRIVE-1 was the first post-market registry for TAXUS and enrolled over 2000 patients and the ARRIVE-II registry enrolled over 4,000 patients (Dobies, 2007; Lasala et al., 2006). Boston Scientific pooled the data from these registries and was able to show that TAXUS was used in patient populations more complex than previously evaluated in the RCTs, such as bifurcation lesions, acute myocardial infarction, and ostial lesions (Lasala et al., 2006).

Trial	Design	Sample size	Primary endpoint	PES treatment arm	BMS treatment arm	P value
TAXUS I	Randomized multicenter	61	MACE at 30 days	0.0%	0.0%	Not significant (under powered)
TAXUS II	Randomized, multicenter	536	% in-stent volume obstruction at 6 months	SR 7.9% MR 7.8%	23.2% 20.5%	P < 0.001 P < 0.001
TAXUS IV	Randomized multicenter	1,314	TVR at 9 months	4.7%	11.3%	P < 0.001
TAXUS V	Randomized multicenter	1,156	TVR at 9 months	12.1%	17.3%	P = 0.0184
TAXUS VI	Randomized, multicenter	446	TVR at 9 months	9.1%	19.4%	P = 0.0027
ARRIVE I & II Pooled post-marketing surveillance	Open label, single arm, multicenter	7,492	TAXUS stent related cardiac events at 1 year	9.5%	Not applicable	Not applicable

Table 2. Clinical trials evaluating TAXUS paclitaxel-eluting stents

The next generation of TAXUS stent was the TAXUS Liberté PES evaluated in the ATLAS program and was conducted similarly to the TAXUS Express program, with an ATLAS de novo, ATLAS expansion, and OLYMPIA registry. These trials evaluated unmet needs in DES and aimed to expand the indications for use in these more complex lesion and patients. The TAXUS Liberté stent was approved for commercialization in the U.S by the FDA on April 12, 2005 and uses the same open-cell design, Translute polymer, and paclitaxel drug as the TAXUS Express system yet has thinner polymer (17 μm) and thinner struts (97 μm). The ATLAS trial was a single-arm, multicenter trial that used a historical control group with matched lesions from the TAXUS IV and V clinical trials. The primary endpoint was non-inferiority compared to the historic control group in terms of TVR at 9 months. The TAXUS Liberté stent demonstrated non-inferiority compared to the historic control, despite having more complex patients evaluated in the TAXUS Liberté arm (Turco, 2008). The ATLAS program expanded to evaluate small vessel and long lesion treatment with the TAXUS Liberté stent in the ATLAS Small Vessel 2.25 mm and ATLAS Long Lesion clinical trials (Table 3).

Trial	Design	Sample size	Primary endpoint	PES treatment arm	Comparator arm	P value
TAXUS ATLAS (TAXUS Liberté)	Single arm compared to historical TAXUS IV and V PES control group, multicenter	871	TVR at 9 months	7.95%	7.01%	P non-inferiority = 0.0487
TAXUS Liberté ATOM - ATLAS Small Vessel (Expansion)	Single arm compared to DES and BMS, multicenter	261	% Diameter stenosis at 9 months	32.2%	PES 39.6% BMS 40.1%	$p < 0.0001$
TAXUS ATLAS Long Lesion	Single arm compared to historical TAXUS IV and V PES control group, multicenter	150	% Diameter stenosis at 9 months	31.4%	35.5%	$p < 0.0001$
ION - PERSEUS	Randomized, multicenter compared to TAXUS Express	1264	TLF at 12 months	5.6%	6.1%	$p = 0.003$
ION - Small Vessel	Open label, single arm, compared to BMS	224	In-stent late loss at 9 months	0.38 ± 0.51	0.80 ± 0.53	$p < 0.0001$

Accessed at http://www.bostonscientific.com/templatedata/imports/collateral/eDFU/

Table 3. Clinical trials evaluating TAXUS Liberté and ION Element stents

The most recent generation of DES developed by Boston Scientific, the Platinum Element ION PES (ION), has additional design changes from the TAXUS Liberté that aim to further improve patient outcomes. Studies have suggested that various alloys provide different strength and allow for thinner struts that subsequently enhance healing and may reduce revascularizations (Ako et al., 2007; Joner et al., 2008; Kastrati et al., 2001). The Platinum ION PES system was approved by the FDA on April 22, 2011 as the latest generation of DES and utilizes a platinum chromium alloy stent but uses the same polymer and drug as the TAXUS Express with the same concentration (1 μg/mm^2). The improved design offers thinner struts (81 μm) and thin polymer layer (14.9 μm). The ION stent system has been evaluated in the PERSEUS clinical trial for the treatment of *de novo* coronary lesions of ≤ 28 mm length in vessels measuring between 2.75 - 4.0 mm. The PERSEUS clinical trial is a randomized controlled trial comparing the ION stent system to the TAXUS Express stent and has a primary endpoint of target lesion failure (TLF) at 12 months. The primary endpoint was met and the ION stent demonstrated non-inferiority compared to the well established TAXUS Express stent in terms of TLF at 12 months. The ION stent has also been evaluated in vessel sizes ≥ 2.25 and < 2.75 mm diameter and lesion lengths ≤ 20 mm in the ION Small Vessel trial versus the performance of BMS from TAXUS IV and V historical comparator arms (Table 3). The primary endpoint was in-stent late loss at 9 months and superiority ($p < 0.0001$) was met compared to the BMS control arm and furthermore, ION has also demonstrated comparable results to the TAXUS Liberté stent (Meredith, 2011). From the first generation TAXUS NIR to the Platinum ION systems, the PES clinical trial program established safety and efficacy for the treatment of coronary artery lesions. Boston Scientific has also developed a drug-eluting stent with a biodegradable polymer, the JACTAX™ PES further discussed in section 8. In addition, the XIENCE V stent is also distributed as the PROMUS everolimus-eluting stent (EES) by Boston Scientific noted in Section 5.

4. ENDEAVOR® and RESOLUTE™

The Endeavor zotarolimus-eluting stent system (ZES) is the first DES manufactured by Medtronic, Inc., Santa Rosa, CA. The stent received FDA approval for commercialization in the U.S in February, 2008. The Endeavor DES utilizes the Driver BMS cobalt alloy stent and a phosphorylcholine lipophilic (PC) polymer coating outside of the stent for delivery of zotarolimus, which is an anti-proliferative drug eluted within 14 days and faster than the first generation DES. Another DES that utilizes zotarolimus was the ZoMaxx stent system manufactured by Abbott Vascular and became commercially available outside of the U.S. Zotarolimus is a highly lipophilic anti-proliferative drug that rapidly is dissolved and has been found to inhibit neointimal hyperplasia (Garcia-Touchard et al., 2006). The thin strut design (91μm) with the added benefit of rapid drug elution allows for rapid endothelialization, reduced inflammation and the promotion of healing.

The Endeavor ZES was first studied in the Endeavor I single-arm, multicenter clinical trial and enrolled 100 patients with de novo coronary lesions measuring ≤ 15 mm in length in vessels with diameter sizes between 3.0-3.5 mm. The primary efficacy endpoint was in-stent late loss at 4 months and was 0.33 ± 0.36 mm and the primary safety endpoint was MACE at 30 days and was 1.0% for the Endeavor ZES (Meredith et al., 2005). The Endeavor II clinical trial enrolled 1,197 patients and was a randomized multicenter trial comparing Endeavor ZES to the Driver BMS for treatment of single *de novo* lesion measuring > 14 mm and ≤ 27 mm in vessel diameters between 2.25 – 3.5 mm. The primary endpoint was TVF at 9 months and the Endeavor arm (7.9%) demonstrated non-inferiority to the Driver BMS arm (15.1%) at 9 months ($p = 0.0001$) (Fajadet et al., 2006). The Endeavor II clinical trial was extended as a continued access trial (Endeavor II CA) and enrolled 296 additional patients in a single arm allowing single lesion treatment < 20 mm in vessel sizes 2.25 - 3.5 mm.

The Endeavor III randomized multi-center trial enrolled 436 patients (3:1) comparing the Endeavor ZES to Cypher SES for single *de novo* lesion treatment measuring > 14 mm and ≤ 27 mm in vessel diameters between 2.25 - 3.5 mm. The primary endpoint was in-segment late loss at 8 months and the Endeavor arm demonstrated numerically higher late loss (0.34 ± 0.44 mm) compared to the Cypher SES arm (0.13 ± 0.32) (Kandzari et al., 2006). Endeavor IV was the pivotal randomized clinical trial that enrolled 1,548 patients with a single de novo lesion measuring ≤ 27 mm in vessels measuring 2.5 mm-3.5 mm, thus restricting the small vessel sizes that had previously been evaluated in Endeavor I, II, and III. The trial had a clinical composite endpoint of target vessel failure (TVF; defined as cardiovascular death, MI, and target vessel revascularization) at 9 months and also included angiographic and IVUS endpoints. The primary endpoint was met and the Endeavor stent demonstrated non-inferiority compared to the TAXUS Express PES at 9 months respectively, (6.6% versus 7.1%, $p < 0.001$), (Leon et al., 2010). Based on the results from the Endeavor II, III, and IV, it was evident that the Endeavor stent outperformed the Driver BMS in terms of reducing TLR, but the same outcome was not observed when compared to the current gold standard first generation stents (CYPHER and TAXUS). In the Endeavor III trial, the Endeavor arm had numerically higher late loss and TLR rates compared to the CYPHER arm, respectively (6.3% versus 3.5%) (Maeng et al., 2010). In the Endeavor IV trial, the Endeavor arm also had numerically higher TLR rates compared to the TAXUS arm through the 3 year follow-up, respectively (6.5% versus 6.0%) not showing improved efficacy over the first generation DES, which was expected with a next generation DES (Leon et al., 2009). Subsequently, a new DES, known as the RESOLUTE™ ZES was developed by Medtronic to improve upon the Endeavor stent (Maeng et al., 2010).

The RESOLUTE ZES is the newest generation of DES developed by Medtronic currently under evaluation in randomized and all-comer trials that will be seeking FDA approval for commercialization in the U.S. in April, 2011 and has already received C.E. Mark status for outside of the U.S. in 2007. The RESOLUTE ZES utilizes the same stent as in DRIVER and ENDEAVOR and zotarolimus, but uses the BioLinx polymer outside coating for extended release of zotarolimus (Leon, 2011). The RESOLUTE first-in-man trial was a single-arm multicenter trial that enrolled 139 patients and evaluated in-stent late loss compared to the ENDEAVOR ZES matched cohort from Endeavor II. The late loss was reduced by 0.39 mm ($p < 0.001$) with the RESOLUTE stent and the TLR rate was 1.0% at 1 year, suggesting that delayed elution through the RESOLUTE stent design may translate to improved safety and efficacy (Meredith et al., 2009).

The RESOLUTE All-Comers (RAC) trial was the first trial to compare RESOLUTE ZES to the next generation XIENCE V everolimus-eluting stent (EES) manufactured by Abbott Vascular (refer to section 5). The RAC trial is a randomized, open-label, multicenter investigation comparing 2,292 patients randomized 1:1 to RESOLUTE ZES or XIENCE V EES with a primary endpoint of target lesions failure (TLF; defined as cardiac death, target vessel MI, and target lesion revascularization) at 1 year. The RESOLUTE ZES was found to be non-inferior to the XIENCE V EES at 1 year. The RESOLUTE ZES arm TLF rate at 1 year was 8.2% and the XIENCE V EES rate was 8.3% (p = non-inferiority) (Meredith, 2011). The trial evaluated notably more complex patient and lesion types than in the previous ENDEAVOR or RESOLUTE trials where inclusion and exclusion criteria restricted more challenging cases. Clinical outcomes remained comparable overall through two years between treatment arms for death, MI, TLR, and ST events (Meredith, 2011).

Trial	Design	Sample size	Primary endpoint	ZES treatment arm	Comparator arm	P value
Endeavor I	Single-arm, multicenter	100	MACE at 30 days; in-stent LL at 120 days	MACE 1%; in-stent LL 0.33 ± 0.36 mm	Not applicable	Not applicable
Endeavor II	Randomized, multicenter	1,197	TVF at 9 months	7.9%	Driver 15.1%	P = 0.0001
Endeavor III	Randomized, multicenter	436	In-segment late loss at 8 months	0.34 ± 0.44 mm	CYPHER 0.13 ± 0.32 mm	P < 0.001
Endeavor IV	Randomized, multicenter	1,548	TVF at 9 months	6.6%	TAXUS 7.1%	P < 0.001
RESOLUTE	Single-arm, multicenter, feasibility	139	In-stent late loss at 9 months	0.22 ± 0.27 mm	ENDEAVOR II (matched cohort) 0.62 ± 0.46 mm	P < 0.001
RESOLUTE All-Comers (RAC)	Randomized, multicenter	2,292	TLF at 1 year	8.2%	XIENCE V 8.3%	P < 0.001
RESOLUTE U.S.	Single-arm, multicenter	1,402	TLF at 1 year	3.7%	ENDEAVOR (historical) 6.5%	P sup = 0.002

Table 4. Clinical trials evaluating the ENDEAVOR and RESOLUTE zotarolimus eluting stents

A RESOLUTE U.S. trial is being conducted with 1402 patients in the RESOLUTE stent arm and is a single-arm, multicenter trial using Endeavor historical data as a comparator arm to evaluate the primary endpoint of target lesion failure (TLF; defined as cardiac death, target vessel MI, and target lesions revascularization) at 1 year. The RESOLUTE U.S. trial design allowed for 2.25 – 4.2 mm vessel diameter and lesion length ≤ 27 mm (Yeung et al., 2011). The trial evaluated for non-inferiority and superiority using a performance goal from the Endeavor program and was able to demonstrate both non-inferiority and superiority at 1 year in terms of TLF. At 1 year, the RESOLUTE arm main cohort showed a 3.7% rate of TLF compared to 6.5% from the Endeavor historical control arm (p non-infer. < 0.001 and p sup = 0.002) (Leon, 2011). The numerically lower rates of TLF observed in the RESOLUTE arm compared to the historical Endeavor arm may be attributed to change in polymer (BioLinx) with subsequent extended release of zotarolimus. The RESOLUTE clinical trial program continues to follow patient outcomes for long-term follow-up and has also multiple trials currently underway OUS, such as the RESOLUTE International, the RESOLUTE Japan, RESOLUTE ASIA, and RESOLUTE CHINA.

5. XIENCE V® and XIENCE PRIME™

The XIENCE V everolimus-eluting stent (EES) was approved by the FDA on July 2, 2008 and is manufactured by Abbott Vascular. The XIENCE V stent/scaffold is the MULTILINK VISION bare metal stent and it is the thinnest strut platform of the DES approved for commercialization in the US to date. Compared to CYPHER (140 μm), TAXUS EXPRESS (132 μm), TAXUS Liberté (97 μm), and ENDEAVOR (91 μm), the XIENCE V (81 μm) strut remains the thinnest for first and second generation DES in the USA and is comparable to the Platinum Chromium Element stent (81 μm) (Smits, TCT 2009). XIENCE V uses an acrylic polymer primer coating outside of the stent, referred to as PBMA [poly (n-butylmethacrylate)], covered by a fluorinated copolymer coating made of two monomeric compounds (vinylidene fluoride and hexafluoropropylene). XIENCE V was engineered to elute everolimus from a thin (7.8 micron), non adhesive, durable, biocompatible, and fluorinated copolymer (Bezenek et al., 2011). Everolimus is an anti-proliferative drug with anti-inflammatory properties that arrests the cell in the G1 phase. The XIENCE V EES clinical trial program has established a robust body of data. The SPIRIT FIRST study was a first-in-man, multi-center, randomized, controlled trial conducted in Europe to assess the feasibility and performance of the XIENCE V in the treatment of subjects with a single de novo native coronary artery lesion compared to the metallic, uncoated MULTI LINK VISION RX Coronary Stent System (VISION RX CSS). SPIRIT FIRST enrolled approximately 60 patients with reference vessel size of 3 mm and a single lesion length ≤ 12 mm. The primary endpoint was in-stent late loss at 6 months and XIENCE V demonstrated superiority to the MULTI-LINK VISION BMS arm by meeting the primary endpoint with 0.10 ± 0.23 mm late loss compared to the BMS arm late loss of 0.85 ± 0.36 mm (superiority *P* value < 0.0001). The trial was designed with a major secondary endpoint of % volume obstruction (%VO) and the XIENCE V arm demonstrated a 72% reduction in %VO compared to the BMS arm, respectively (8.0% versus 21.0%, p < 0.001). The trial has completed 5 year follow-up and notably, there was no stent thrombosis event reported in either arm in the SPIRIT FIRST study. Safety and efficacy results evident in the SPIRIT FIRST trial led to the SPIRIT II trial.

The SPIRIT II trial was a multi-center randomized trial (3:1) designed to continue assessing the safety and performance of the XIENCE V in the treatment of patients with a maximum of two de novo native coronary artery lesions each in a different epicardial vessel, compared to TAXUS. The SPIRIT II clinical study arm allowed the treatment of de novo lesions ≤ 28 mm in length in coronary arteries with a reference vessel diameter (RVD) ≥ 2.5 mm to ≤ 4.25 mm. Three hundred (300) patients were enrolled in the study; 223 patients were treated with XIENCE V, 59 patients were treated with TAXUS EXPRESS, and 17 patients received TAXUS Liberté. The primary endpoint was in-stent late loss at 6 months and was designed with angiographic and IVUS endpoints. The trial was powered for a major secondary endpoint of in-segment late loss as well. XIENCE V® demonstrated non-inferiority to the TAXUS® arm in terms of the primary endpoint of in-stent late loss. The XIENCE V arm was 0.11 ± 0.27 mm compared to 0.36 ± 0.39 mm in the TAXUS arm ($p < 0.0001$). The primary endpoint demonstrated that XIENCE V® was statistically superior to the TAXUS® (superiority P value < 0.0001). The in-segment late loss results favored the XIENCE V arm compared to the TAXUS arm with a 53% reduction observed at 6 months. The clinical follow-up through 5 years supported the safety and efficacy of the XIENCE V EES and no late catch-up was observed.

The SPIRIT III pivotal clinical trial was designed to demonstrate the non-inferiority of XIENCE V to TAXUS. Conducted in the United States (US) and Japan, the SPIRIT III clinical trial was composed of a randomized clinical trial in the US (RCT) and a non-randomized arm (4.0 mm arm) and one non-randomized arm in Japan. The SPIRIT III RCT was designed as a randomized (2:1), multi-center non-inferiority evaluation of the XIENCE V stent compared to the TAXUS stent and enrolled a total of 1002 patients (669 patients in XIENCE V arm and 333 patients in the TAXUS arm). Treatment of up to two de novo lesions ≤ 28 mm in length in native coronary arteries with RVD ≥ 2.5 mm to ≤ 3.75 mm was permitted. The trial design had a primary efficacy endpoint of in-segment late loss at 8 months and also a co-primary endpoint of TVF at 9 months. In the SPIRIT III RCT arm, XIENCE V was found to be statistically non-inferior to TAXUS (Stone, 2010). The primary endpoint of in-segment LL at 8 months results for the XIENCE V arm was 0.14 ± 41 mm and for the TAXUS arm was 0.28 mm ± 48 mm (p non-inferior < 0.0001). Additionally, since non-inferiority was demonstrated, a superiority analysis of the primary endpoint was performed using a two-sided t-test with alpha = 0.05. The analysis showed the superiority of XIENCE V to the TAXUS arm in terms of the primary endpoint of in-segment LL at 8 months (p superior = 0.0037). The major secondary endpoint of TVF was also met with the XIENCE V arm demonstrating numerically lower rates (7.6%) compared to the TAXUS arm (9.7%) at 9 months (p non-inferior < 0.0001).

As part of the SPIRIT III clinical trial design, the non-randomized 4.0 mm arm was compared to the TAXUS patients of the RCT arm. The SPIRIT III 4.0 mm arm trial demonstrated consistent results with the SPIRIT III RCT arm. The SPIRIT III 4.0 mm non-randomized arm demonstrated non-inferiority of XIENCE V 4.0 mm arm compared to the TAXUS RCT arm in terms of the primary endpoint of in-segment LL at 8 months (p non-inferior < 0.0001). In-segment LL at 8 months was 0.17 ± 0.38 mm for the XIENCE V 4.0 mm arm and 0.28 ± 0.48 mm for the TAXUS RCT arm. The third cohort of the SPIRIT III trial that actively enrolled patients was the SPIRIT III Japan single-arm trial. In the SPIRIT III Japan arm, the XIENCE V arm was also found to be statistically non-inferior to TAXUS RCT arm. The primary endpoint of the trial was met with in-segment LL results of 0.15 ± 0.34 mm for the XIENCE V Japan arm and 0.28 ± 0.48 mm for the TAXUS RCT arm at 8 months. The XIENCE V Japan arm also demonstrated non-inferiority to the TAXUS RCT arm for in-segment LL at 8 months (p non-inferior < 0.0001). No stent thrombosis occurred through two-year follow-up in the XIENCE V Japan arm. Clinical results of treatment with XIENCE V in the SPIRIT III trial supported the safety and efficacy of XIENCE V and since approval in the U.S., has demonstrated long-term follow-up with 5 year results available this year at TCT 2011. In order to expand XIENCE V use to more complex patients, the SPIRIT IV clinical trial was designed to allow for multiple lesions to be treated beyond what was previously evaluated in earlier randomized trials for comparing DES.

The SPIRIT IV clinical trial was a randomized (2:1) multi-center evaluation of the XIENCE V EES compared to the TAXUS PES in the treatment of up to three de novo lesions ≤ 28 mm in length in native coronary arteries with RVD ≥ 2.5 mm to ≤ 3.75 mm. There were 3,687 patients enrolled and they were stratified based on diabetes mellitus status (diabetic vs. non-diabetic) and lesion characteristics (complex vs. non-complex). Complex lesion characteristics included triple vessel treatment, or dual lesions per vessel treatment, or lesions involving RCA-aorto-ostial locations, or bifurcations lesions. The primary endpoint was TLF at 1 year and two major secondary endpoints were also evaluated; TLR and the composite of target vessel MI and cardiac death at 1 year. In the SPIRIT IV clinical trial, XIENCE V demonstrated non-inferiority to TAXUS in terms of the primary endpoint of TLF respectively, (4.2% compared to 6.8%, p non-inferior < 0.0001). Since non-inferiority was demonstrated, the pre-specified superiority test of the primary endpoint was performed. Superiority of XIENCE V over TAXUS for the primary endpoint (p superior = 0.0012) was also met at 1 year.

Additional pre-specified hypothesis tests for non-inferiority and superiority were performed for the major secondary endpoints of TLR and cardiac death or target vessel MI at 1 year. The XIENCE V arm demonstrated non-inferiority to the TAXUS arm in terms of TLR rates at 1 year, respectively (2.5% and 4.6%, p non-inferior < 0.0001). For cardiac death or target vessel MI, the XIENCE V arm also demonstrated non-inferiority to the TAXUS arm respectively, (2.2% compared to 3.2%, p non-inferior < 0.0001). Moreover, the XIENCE V arm also demonstrated superiority (p superior = 0.0012) over the TAXUS arm for TLR, but did not meet superiority (p superior = 0.0899) for cardiac death or target vessel MI at 1 year. The SPIRIT IV trial showed numerically low ARC (definite/probable) ST rates through the two-year follow-up in the XIENCE V arm (0.42%) compared to the TAXUS arm (1.23%), consistent with earlier SPIRIT trials, but in a more complex patient population. A similar finding was observed in the all-comers, single arm post-marketing trial, the XIENCE V USA trial discussed here below.

The XIENCE V USA post-marketing safety and surveillance trial was designed as a single-arm, multicenter, open-label trial that enrolled 5,054 patients in the U.S following FDA approval of the XIENCE V EES in 2008. As part of the requirements for FDA approval, the XIENCE V USA evaluated the real-world usage of the XIENCE V EES in clinical practice and monitor safety outcomes. The primary endpoint is the composite of definite/probable ST rates as defined by the Academic Research Consortium (ARC) definitions and also has a co-primary endpoint of cardiac death and MI at 1 year and will follow patients through 5 year follow-up. As the trial is a post-approval study, the restrictions of inclusion and exclusion criteria do not limit the enrollment and thus provide a perspective of outcomes in patients that have not been evaluated in pivotal RCTs, such as AMI, in-stent restenosis, or chronic total occlusions. Despite having more complex subgroups, the XIENCE V patients have demonstrated consistent results at 1 year with ST rates comparable to the SPIRIT III pivotal trial, which only allowed for a single lesion per vessel treatment of less than 28 mm. At 1 year, the XIENCE V USA ST rate was 0.8% and the cardiac death and MI rate was 6.3% (Hermiller, 2010).

More recently, the XIENCE V nano EES was approved by the FDA in May 2011 for the treatment of small vessels. The XIENCE V nano EES was approved as a line extension to the existing XIENCE V EES based on the results of the SPIRIT Small Vessel (SV) single-arm, multicenter clinical trial. The purpose of the SPIRIT SV trial was to evaluate the safety and efficacy of the 2.25 mm XIENCE V EES in improving coronary luminal diameter in subjects with symptomatic heart disease due to a maximum of two de novo native coronary artery lesions measuring ≤ 28 mm in small vessels (≥ 2.25 mm to < 2.50 mm), each in a different epicardial vessel. The study was designed to enroll up to 150 patients with the first 60 patients enrolled in the angiographic cohort requiring angiographic follow-up at 8 months. The primary endpoint was TLF at 1 year and was required to meet a pre-specified performance goal of 20.4% at 1 year. The study was designed to enroll up to 150 patients with the first 60 patients enrolled in an angiographic cohort requiring angiographic follow-up at 8 months. The 1-year TLF rate was 8.1%and therefore met the performance goal of 20.4% and met the primary endpoint ($p<0.0001$). The mean in-segment late loss at 8 months was 0.16 ± 0.41 mm and the mean in-stent late loss was 0.20 ± 0.40 mm, both slightly higher compared to the in-segment (0.14 ± 0.41 mm) and in-stent late loss (0.16 ± 0.41 mm) reported in the XIENCE V arm of SPIRIT III RCT, yet lower than the in-segment and in-stent late loss for SPIRIT III RCT TAXUS arm, respectively (0.28 ± 0.48 mm and 0.30 ± 0.53 mm).

5.1 XIENCE PRIME™

As observed in the XIENCE V USA post-marketing single-arm trial, the complexity of patients and lesions being treated with DES is requiring more specialized treatments and challenging cases in the catheterization lab. In order to address this market need, the XIENCE PRIME and XIENCE PRIME Long Lesion (LL) EES were developed from the framework of the XIENCE V EES with modifications to further enhance deliverability, flexibility, and stent retention. The XIENCE PRIME utilizes an improved cobalt chromium alloy stent, but the same polymer composition of the poly n-butyl methacrylate (PBMA) primer coating, drug reservoir layer of poly vinylidene fluoride co-hexafluoropropylene (PVDF-HFP), and the same everolimus/polymer weight to weight combination ratio and thickness. XIENCE PRIME also uses the same anti-proliferative drug (everolimus) and has the same drug density ($100 \mu g/cm^2$) as the original XIENCE V EES design. The strut thickness remains one of the thinnest available to date at 81μm. Both the XIENCE V and the XEINCE PRIME were built upon the MULTI-LINK BMS design, but the XIENCE PRIME has the added features of the MULTI-LINK 8™ BMS design, where a link has been made taller and the cell has been lengthened. The delivery system also underwent important modifications that include a smooth rounded tip, designed to enhance tracking, and deliverability, while the shorter balloon taper aims to reduce stent injury.

The objective of the SPIRIT PRIME clinical trial is to evaluate the safety and effectiveness of the XIENCE PRIME™ and XIENCE PRIME LL™ EES in improving coronary luminal diameter in subjects with symptomatic heart disease. The XIENCE PRIME and XIENCE PRIME LL EES enrolled patients with symptomatic heart disease due to de novo native coronary artery lesions (lesion length ≤ 32 mm) with vessel diameters measuring ≥ 2.25 mm and ≤ 4.25 mm. The study was designed as a single-arm, open-label, multi-center non-randomized clinical trial using the core size XIENCE PRIME and XIENCE PRIME LL. Approximately 500 subjects were enrolled; 400 in the Core Size Registry (CSR) and 100 in the Long Lesion Registry (LLR), which included stent lengths of 33 and 38 mm. The primary endpoint of TLF at one year was required to meet pre-specified (per protocol) performance goals (PG); the CSR PG was 9.2% and the PG for the LLR was 19.2%. The XIENCE PRIME met the primary endpoint for both the CSR and the LLR in terms of TLF rates at 1 year with 6.5% for the CSR ($p = 0.0038$) and 12.5% for the LLR ($p = 12.5\%$) as per ARC MI definition.

Thus meeting the primary endpoint, the XIENCE PRIME Pre-Market Approval (PMA) packet has been submitted for FDA approval in April, 2011 by Abbott Vascular and is pending approval for commercialization in the U.S. XIENCE PRIME has already received C.E. Mark for commercialization in Europe since June, 2009. Long-term follow-up continues for XIENCE PRIME, Small Vessel, SPIRIT IV, and XIENCE V USA to further support the robust data supporting the safety and efficacy profile.

Trial	Design	Sample size	Primary endpoint	EES treatment arm	Comparator arm	P value
SPIRIT FIRST	Randomized, multicenter	60	In-stent late-loss at 6 months	0.10 ± 0.23 mm	BMS 0.85 ±0.36 mm	P < 0.001
SPIRIT II	Randomized, multicenter	300	In-stent late-loss at 6 months	0.11 ± 0.27 mm	TAXUS 0.36 ± 0.39 mm	P < 0.0001
SPIRIT III	Randomized, multicenter	1,002	In-segment late loss at 8 months	0.14 ± 0.41 mm	TAXUS 0.28 ± 0.48 mm	$P_{superiority}$ = 0.004
SPIRIT IV	Randomized, multicenter	3,687	TLF at 1 year	4.2%	TAXUS 6.8%	$P_{superiority}$ = 0.001
XIENCE V USA	Single-arm, multicenter, open label	5,054	Composite of Stent Thrombosis	0.8%	Not applicable	Not applicable
SPIRIT Small Vessel (SV)	Single-arm, multicenter, open label	144	TLF at 1 year	8.1%	PG* 20.4%	P < 0.0001
SPIRIT PRIME	Single-arm, multicenter, open label	419 CSR◊ arm 110 LLR▲ arm	TLF at 1 year	CSR 6.5% LLR 12.5%	PG 9.2% PG19.2%	P = 0.034 P = 0.048

Of note, the XIENCE V stent is also distributed as the PROMUS EES by Boston Scientific.
* PG = performance goal; ◊CSR = Core Sample Registry; ▲LLR = Long Lesion Registry

Table 5. Clinical Trials evaluating the XIENCE V and the XIENCE PRIME everolimus-eluting stents

6. Longterm trial results

Key trials discussed above have already completed or are reaching the final year of follow-up. The question of improved clinical outcomes with DES over BMS has been established with long-term safety profiles available from all of the leading manufacturers. The question of which DES has sustained the most improved clinical outcomes remains debatable depending on the patient needs and ability to adhere to the indicated dual antiplatelet therapy recommended of aspirin and clopidogrel, as per the DES PCI recommendations (King et al., 2007). The long-term follow-up available from key DES trials is presented in Table 6.

Trial	Treatment Arms	Follow-up Year	Cardiac death %	MI %	TLR %	TVR %	Stent Thrombosis (ARC def/prob %)
RAVEL (Morice et al., 2007)	CYPHER SES	5	12.1	8.9	10.3	2.7	3.3
	BMS		7.1 (all death)	6.9	26.0 P<0.001	2.6	6.8 (all ARC)
SIRIUS	CYPHER SES	5	4.1	6.2	9.4	16.5	1.2
	BMS		3.6	6.5	24.2 P<0.001	30.5 P<0.001	1.8
TAXUS IV (Ellis et al., 2009a)	TAXUS Express PES	5	4.4	7.2	9.1	16.9	2.2
	BMS		4.5	7.4	20.5 P<0.0001	27.4 P<0.0001	2.1
TAXUS V (Ellis et al., 2009b)	TAXUS Express PES	5	3.8	8.4	16.3	Not available	1.9
	BMS		1.6 P=0.04	5.4	22.3 P=0.005		0.7
ENDEAVOR III (Kandzari et al., 2011)	ENDEAVOR ZES	5	0.3%	1.0%	8.1%	16.9%	0.7%
	CYPHER SES		2.8%	4.6% P=0.03	6.5%	13.0%	0.9%
ENDEAVOR IV (Leon et al., 2010)	ENDEAVOR ZES	3	1.7	2.1	6.5	9.9	1.1
	TAXUS Express PES		2.4	4.9 P=0.005	6.1	10.9	1.7
SPIRIT III (Stone, 2010b)	XIENCE V	4	2.6	4.4	7.6	13.4	1.4
	TAXUS Express		2.6	6.6	10.3	16.1	1.6
SPIRIT IV (Stone, 2010a)	XIENCE V	2	0.9%	2.5%	4.5%	3.9%	0.42%
	TAXUS Express		1.3%	3.9% (P=0.02)	6.9% (P=0.004)	4.3%	1.23% (P=0.008)

(Available significant P values (≤ 0.05) are included above).

Table 6. Long-term Clinical Outcomes Currently Available

7. Current challenges

A challenge that remains when comparing DES head to head across trials is the inconsistency between definitions. In order to address this challenge, the Academic Research Consortium (ARC) developed standardized definitions for clinical trial endpoints (Cutlip et al., 2007). The ARC definitions have now become the gold standard for clinical trial endpoints and definitions of clinical events, such as cardiac deaths, MI, and ST. In addition, clinical events may be retrospectively adjudicated by Clinical Events Committees (CEC) using the ARC definitions for post ad-hoc analysis of events not initially evaluated using the ARC definitions. The ARC definitions particularly met the need of unifying the ST definition that differed across stent manufacturers and clinical trials. One of the main concerns with using DES initially was the additional risk of ST possibly due to delayed healing, inflammation or incompatibility between polymer and the vessel (Lagerqvist et al., 2007; Moreno et al., 2005). First generation DES have observed higher rates of very late ST compared to BMS (Camenzind et al., 2007; Daemen et al., 2007; Farb and Boam, 2007; Pfisterer et al., 2006). Several DES specific characteristics may contribute to the development of ST, such as choice of drug, polymer, and strut thickness. Other patient specific characteristics may contribute, such as patient co-morbidities (diabetes, renal failure and acute MI) and lesion characteristics. Compliance to DAPT and platelet responsiveness also plays a role in ST rates observed in DES (Bezenek et al., 2011). Procedural factors related to smaller luminal dimensions, such as stent under-expansion or malapposition are risk factors for ST, in addition to stent length, multi-stenting, persistent slow flow, positive remodeling, dissections, geographic miss, residual stenosis, and late stent malapposition which have all been related to ST (Bezenek et al., 2011). Furthermore, well established criteria for the duration and dose with existing antiplatelet medication, as well as the role of newly emerging antiplatelet medications does not exist currently. Although the ARC definitions did provide a common reference for ST definitions concerning timing and severity, the appropriate standardized dose of DAPT remains in question with DES use. Despite these challenges however, few DES have emerged as demonstrating a consistent numerically low rate of ST across clinical trials. The XIENCE V and XIENCE PRIME DES remain two of the DES with the lowest ST event profile across RCT, single-arm, and all-comer trials, despite reduced DAPT compliance observed at 2 years in the COMPARE all-comers trial; the combination of stent design, thin struts, bio-compatible polymer coating technologies, and drug may contribute to numerically low ST rates consistently observed (Bezenek et al., 2011).

8. Additional stent technology

In order to address the concern for potential increased risk of late/very late ST with DES, several manufacturers developed biodegradable polymers and bioabsorbable scaffolds that degrade over time. Durable polymers may be associated with increased complications and clinical events and new developments in DES are integrating dissolvable polymers and scaffolds to eliminate this potential problem. Abbott Vascular currently has the ABSORB™ clinical trial program that is evaluating the everolimus-eluting bioresorbable vascular scaffold (BVS) in global clinical trials. The ABSORB BVS clinical trial program is evaluating the safety and efficacy of fully bioabsorbable scaffold that is comprised of a poly-L-lactic acid backbone and has a poly-D, L-lactic acid coating that modulates the release of everolimus. The ABSORB international clinical trials that have enrolled patients thus far include ABSORB Cohorts A and Cohort B and ABSORB EXTEND. The ABSORB Cohort A trial enrolled 30 patients and was designed to evaluate the safety and performance of ABSORB BVS in single de novo lesions. The 4-year clinical event rates remain numerically low with no events of scaffold thrombosis occurring (Chevalier, 2011). The ABSORB Cohort B trial enrolled 101 patients and allowed up to two de novo lesions to be treated. Current 12-month results for Cohort B were presented at the American College of Cardiology (ACC) and reported that no scaffold thrombosis have occurred either by ARC or per protocol definitions as well (Serruys, 2011). The ABSORB EXTEND trial plans to enroll up to 1000 patients at up to 100 international sites and will continue to assess the safety and performance of ABSORB BVS in up to two de novo lesions, allowing for the evaluation of longer lesions and overlapping scaffolds.

As mentioned earlier, the NEVO stent was a new technology in development by Cordis Corporation, Johnson and Johnson, and used polylactic-co-glycolic acid (PGLA) loaded in reservoirs drilled through the struts of a cobalt chromium stent and has subsequently been removed from further development (Belardi, 2011; Otake et al., 2011b). The JACTAX™ biodegradable stent system is developed by Boston Scientific and uses D-lactic polylactic acid (DLPLA) mounted on the TAXUS Liberté stent whose outside coating elutes paclitaxel (Grube et al., 2010; Shand, 2010) . The Biolimus-A9 TM eluting BioMatrix™ stent system (Biosensors Interventional Technologies Pte Ltd, Singapore) incorporates a biodegradable polylactic acid (PLA) coated on the outside of the S-Stent stainless steel stent that scaffolds the artery (Abizaid et al., 2011; Shand, 2010). The Leaders trial was designed to compare the BioMatrix stent to the CYPHR stent and enrolled 1707 patients (randomized 1:1) with a composite clinical primary endpoint of cardiac death, MI, and clinically-indicated target vessel revascularization (Windecker et al., 2008). The primary endpoint was met and BioMatrix demonstrated non-inferiority compared to CYPHER (9.2% versus 10.5%; P=0.003) and has sustained numerically low rats of very-late ARC-defined definite stent thrombosis through 3 years, respectively (0.2% versus 0.9%), (Windecker, 2011; Windecker et al., 2008).

The CardioMind Sparrow is developed by CardioMind, Inc. and is a self-expandable nitinol stent with a PLA/PLGA copolymer biodegradable outside coating (Abizaid et al., 2011). The ELIXER-DES™ is under development by the Elixer Medical Group and has a cobalt-chromium stent as the scaffold and uses polyester or polylactide based biodegradable polymer coating over the outside of the stent. Other technologies are moving toward polymer-free DES as well, such as the BioFreedom™ (Biosensors Inc.), the VESTAsync™ (MIV Therapeutics), and the Optima™ (CID S.r.I) with further specialized designs using biolimus A9, sirolimus, and tacrolimus, respectively (Abizaid et al., 2011). Lastly, endothelium progenitor cell (EPC) capture stents were developed (Genous™ manufactured by OrbusNeich, Florida, USA) coated with CD34 antibodies that were to bind to circulating EPCs. The EPC capture stents have yet to show clinical trials demonstrating safety and efficacy superior to DES and have not become mainstream treatment options to date (Garg et al., 2010).

9. Conclusion

In conclusion, DES has emerged as a treatment of choice for patients that are suitable candidates with no restrictions to physician recommended DAPT medication. The first and next generation DES evaluated in the CYPHER, TAXUS, ENDEAVOR, and XIENCE V clinical programs significantly reduced restenosis compared to BMS and have demonstrated comparable safety outcomes. In order to address potential polymer induced inflammation or delayed healing related safety events in current FDA approved DES, new technologies using biodegradable polymers, polymer-free DES, and bioresorbable stent scaffolds have emerged to further enhance PCI options. Long-term clinical results have clearly supported the safety and efficacy of DES and more specialized DES designs and trials for specific patient and lesion unmet needs continue to be pursued.

10. References

Abizaid A., Costa J.R., Jr., Feres F. (2011) First nine-month complete invasive assessment (angiography, IVUS, and OCT) of the novel NEVO sirolimus-eluting stent with biodegradable polymer. Catheterization and Cardiovascular Interventions 77:49-51. DOI: 10.1002/ccd.22558.

Acharya G., Park K. (2006) Mechanisms of controlled drug release from drug-eluting stents. Adv Drug Deliv Rev 58:387-401.

Ako J., Bonneau H.N., Honda Y., Fitzgerald P.J. (2007) Design criteria for the ideal drug-eluting stent. American Journal of Cardiology 100:3M-9M.

Belardi J.A. (2011) Nevo stent: a successful stent makeover. Catheter Cardiovasc Interv 77:52-3. DOI: 10.1002/ccd.22921.

Bezenek S., Hermiller J., Lansky A., Yaqub M., Hattori K., Cao S., Sood P., Sudhir K. (2011) Low stent thrombosis risk with the XIENCE V(R) everolimus-eluting coronary stent: Evidence from randomized and single-arm clinical trials. Journal of Interventional Cardiology:DOI: 10.1111/j.1540-8183.2011.00628.x. DOI: 10.1111/j.1540-8183.2011.00628.x.

Camenzind E., Steg P.G., Wijns W. (2007) Stent thrombosis late after implantation of first-generation drug-eluting stents: a cause for concern. Circulation 115:1440-1455.

Chevalier B. (2011) ABSORB Cohort B Trial - Evaluation of the ABSORB Bioresorbable Everolimus-Eluting Vascular Scaffold in the Treatment of Patients with de novo Native Coroanry Artery Lesions, Amercian College of Cardiology, netherlands.

Colombo A., Drzewiecki J., Banning A., Grube E., Hauptmann K., Silber S., Dudek D., Fort S., Schiele F., Zmudka K., Guagliumi G., Russell M.E. (2003) Randomized study to assess the effectiveness of slow- and moderate-release polymer-based paclitaxel-eluting stents for coronary artery lesions. Circulation 108:788-794.

Cutlip D.E., Windecker S., Mehran R., Boam A., Cohen D.J., van Es G.A., Steg P.G., Morel M.A., Mauri L., Vranckx P., McFadden E., Lansky A., Hamon M., Krucoff M.W., Serruys P.W. (2007) Clinical end points in coronary stent trials: a case for standardized definitions. Circulation 115:2344-2351.

Daemen J., Wenaweser P., Tsuchida K., Abrecht L., Vaina S., Morger C., Kukreja N., Juni P., Sianos G., Hellige G., van Domburg R.T., Hess O.M., Boersma E., Meier B., Windecker S., Serruys P.W. (2007) Early and late coronary stent thrombosis of sirolimus-eluting and paclitaxel-eluting stents in routine clinical practice: data from a large two-institutional cohort study. Lancet 369:667-678.

Dawkins K.D., Grube E., Guagliumi G., Banning A.P., Zmudka K., Colombo A., Thuesen L., Hauptman K., Marco J., Wijns W., Popma J.J., Koglin J., Russell M.E. (2005) Clinical efficacy of polymer-based paclitaxel-eluting stents in the treatment of complex, long coronary artery lesions from a multicenter, randomized trial: support for the use of drug-eluting stents in contemporary clinical practice. Circulation 112:3306-3313. 10.1161/CIRCULATIONAHA.105.552190.

Dobies D. (2007) ARRIVE I at 2 years, EuroPCR, Barcelona, Spain.

Doostzadeh J., Bezenek S., Cheong W.-F., Sood P., Schwartz L.B., Sudhir K. (2009) Clinical trials in interventional cardiology: focus on the XIENCE drug-eluting stent, in: S. C. Gad (Ed.), Clinical Trials Handbook, Wiley, Hoboken. pp. 397-435.

Doostzadeh J., Clark L.N., Bezenek S., Pierson W., Sood P.R., Sudhir K. (2010) Recent progress in percutaneous coronary intervention: evolution of the drug-eluting stents, focus on the XIENCE V drug-eluting stent. Coronary Artery Disease 21:46-56. DOI: 10.1097/MCA.0b013e328333f550.

Fajadet J., Wijns W., Laarman G.J., Kuck K.H., Ormiston J., Munzel T., Popma J.J., Fitzgerald P.J., Bonan R., Kuntz R.E. (2006) Randomized, double-blind, multicenter study of the Endeavor zotarolimus-eluting phosphorylcholine-encapsulated stent for treatment of native coronary artery lesions: clinical and angiographic results of the ENDEAVOR II trial. Circulation 114:798-806.

Farb A., Boam A.B. (2007) Stent thrombosis redux--the FDA perspective. New England Journal of Medicine 356:984-987.

FDA. (2006) Circulatory System Devices Advisory Panel.

Fischman D.L., Leon M.B., Baim D.S., Schatz R.A., Savage M.P., Penn I., Detre K., Veltri L., Ricci D., Nobuyoshi M., et al. (1994) A randomized comparison of coronary-stent placement and balloon angioplasty in the treatment of coronary artery disease. New England Journal of Medicine 331:496-501. DOI: 10.1056/NEJM199408253310802.

Garcia-Touchard A., Burke S.E., Toner J.L., Cromack K., Schwartz R.S. (2006) Zotarolimus-eluting stents reduce experimental coronary artery neointimal hyperplasia after 4 weeks. European Heart Journal 27:988-993.

Grube E., Silber S., Hauptmann K.E., Mueller R., Buellesfeld L., Gerckens U., Russell M.E. (2003) TAXUS I: six- and twelve-month results from a randomized, double-blind trial on a slow-release paclitaxel-eluting stent for de novo coronary lesions. Circulation 107:38-42.

Grube E., Schofer J., Hauptmann K.E., Nickenig G., Curzen N., Allocco D.J., Dawkins K.D. (2010) A novel paclitaxel-eluting stent with an ultrathin abluminal biodegradable polymer 9-month outcomes with the JACTAX HD stent. JACC Cardiovasc Interv 3:431-8.

Halkin A., Stone G.W. (2004) Polymer-based paclitaxel-eluting stents in percutaneous coronary intervention: a review of the TAXUS trials. Journal of Intervational Cardiology 17:271-182.

Hellige G., Windecker S. (2009) Head-to-head and extrapolated comparisons of different drug-eluting stents: differences in late loss, restenosis, and clinical outcomes. Journal of Interventional Cardiology 22:S48-S63.

Hermiller J. (2010) Early and late stent thrombosis rates in 5,054 real-world patients from XIENCE V USA with and without dual antiplatelet therapy interruptions, EuroPCR, Paris.

Holmes D.R. (2003) 12-month clinical follow-up from SIRIUS, ACC Chicago, USA.

Htay T., Liu M.W. (2005) Drug-eluting stent: a review and update. Vascular Health Risk Management 1:263-276.

Joner M., Finn A.V., Farb A., Mont E.K., Kolodgie F.D., Ladich E., Kutys R., Skorija K., Gold H.K., Virmani R. (2006) Pathology of drug-eluting stents in humans: delayed healing and late thrombotic risk. J Am Coll Cardiol 48:193-202.

Joner M., Nakazawa G., Finn A.V., Quee S.C., Coleman L., Acampado E., Wilson P.S., Skorija K., Cheng Q., Xu X., Gold H.K., Kolodgie F.D., Virmani R. (2008) Endothelial cell recovery between comparator polymer-based drug-eluting stents. Journal of the American College of Cardiology 52:333-42.

Kandzari D.E., Leon M.B., Popma J.J., Fitzgerald P.J., O'Shaughnessy C., Ball M.W., Turco M., Applegate R.J., Gurbel P.A., Midei M.G., Badre S.S., Mauri L., Thompson K.P., LeNarz L.A., Kuntz R.E. (2006) Comparison of zotarolimus-eluting and sirolimus-eluting stents in patients with native coronary artery disease: a randomized controlled trial. Journal of the American College of Cardiology 48:2440-2447.

Kastrati A., Mehilli J., Dirschinger J., Dotzer F., Schuhlen H., Neumann F.J., Fleckenstein M., Pfafferott C., Seyfarth M., Schomig A. (2001) Intracoronary stenting and angiographic results: strut thickness effect on restenosis outcome (ISAR-STEREO) trial. Circulation 103:2816-2821.

King S.B. (2007) Applying drug-eluting stents in clinical practice. American Journal of Cardiology 100:25K-31K.

King S.B., 3rd, Aversano T., Ballard W.L., Beekman R.H., 3rd, Cowley M.J., Ellis S.G., Faxon D.P., Hannan E.L., Hirshfeld J.W., Jr., Jacobs A.K., Kellett M.A., Jr., Kimmel S.E., Landzberg J.S., McKeever L.S., Moscucci M., Pomerantz R.M., Smith K.M., Vetrovec G.W., Creager M.A., Holmes D.R., Jr., Newby L.K., Weitz H.H., Merli G., Pina I., Rodgers G.P., Tracy C.M. (2007) ACCF/AHA/SCAI 2007 update of the Clinical Competence Statement on Cardiac Interventional Procedures: a report of the American College of Cardiology Foundation/American Heart Association/American College of Physicians Task Force on Clinical Competence and Training (Writing Committee to Update the 1998 Clinical Competence Statement on Recommendations for the Assessment and Maintenance of Proficiency in Coronary Interventional Procedures). Circulation 116:98-124.

Lagerqvist B., James S.K., Stenestrand U., Lindback J., Nilsson T., Wallentin L. (2007) Long-term outcomes with drug-eluting stents versus bare-metal stents in Sweden. New England Journal of Medicine 356:1009-1019.

Lasala J.M., Stone G.W., Dawkins K.D., Serruys P.W., Colombo A., Grube E., Koglin J., Ellis S. (2006) An overview of the TAXUS Express, paclitaxel-eluting stent clinical trial program. Journal of Interventional Cardiology 19:422-31.

Leon M.B. (2011) Clinical evaluation of the RESOLUTE zotarolimus-eluting coronary stent system in the treatment of de novo lesions in native coronary arteries (the RESOLUTE US clinical trial), ACC, New Orleans, USA.

Leon M.B., Nikolsky E., Cutlip D.E., Mauri L., Liberman H., Wilson H., Patterson J., Moses J., Kandzari D.E. (2010) Improved late clinical safety with zotarolimus-eluting stents compared with paclitaxel-eluting stents in patients with de novo coronary lesions: 3-year follow-up from the ENDEAVOR IV (Randomized Comparison of Zotarolimus- and Paclitaxel-Eluting Stents in Patients With Coronary Artery Disease) trial. JACC Cardiovasc Interv 3:1043-50.

Leon M.B., Kandzari D.E., Eisenstein E.L., Anstrom K.J., Mauri L., Cutlip D.E., Nikolsky E., O'Shaughnessy C., Overlie P.A., Kirtane A.J., McLaurin B.T., Solomon S.L., Douglas

J.S., Jr., Popma J.J. (2009) Late safety, efficacy, and cost-effectiveness of a zotarolimus-eluting stent compared with a paclitaxel-eluting stent in patients with de novo coronary lesions: 2-year follow-up from the ENDEAVOR IV trial (Randomized, Controlled Trial of the Medtronic Endeavor Drug [ABT-578] Eluting Coronary Stent System Versus the Taxus Paclitaxel-Eluting Coronary Stent System in De Novo Native Coronary Artery Lesions). Journal of the American College of Cardiology: Cardiovascular Interventions 2:1208-1218.

Maeng M., Holm N.R., Kaltoft A., Jensen L.O., Tilsted H.H., Thuesen L., Lassen J.F. (2010) Zotarolimus-eluting versus sirolimus-eluting coronary stent implantation. Interventional Cardiology 2:807-812.

Meredith I.T. (2011) Platinum small vessel 12-month outcomes, EuroPCR, Paris, France.

Meredith I.T., Ormiston J., Whitbourn R., Kay I.P., Muller D., Bonan R., Popma J.J., Cutlip D.E., Fitzgerald P., Prpic R., Kuntz R.E. (2005) First-in-human study of the Endeavor ABT-578-eluting phosphorylcholine-encapsulated stent system in de novo native coronary artery lesions: Endeavor I Trial. EuroIntervention 1:157-164. DOI: EIJV1I2A26 [pii].

Meredith I.T., Worthley S., Whitbourn R., Walters D.L., McClean D., Horrigan M., Popma J.J., Cutlip D.E., DePaoli A., Negoita M., Fitzgerald P.J. (2009) Clinical and angiographic results with the next-generation resolute stent system: a prospective, multicenter, first-in-human trial. Journal of the American College of Cardiology: Cardiovascular Interventions 2:977-985.

Moreno R., Fernandez C., Hernandez R., Alfonso F., Angiolillo D.J., Sabate M., Escaned J., Banuelos C., Fernandez-Ortiz A., Macaya C. (2005) Drug-eluting stent thrombosis: results from a pooled analysis including 10 randomized studies. Journal of the American College of Cardiology 45:954-959.

Morice M.C., Serruys P.W., Barragan P., Bode C., Van Es G.A., Stoll H.P., Snead D., Mauri L., Cutlip D.E., Sousa E. (2007) Long-term clinical outcomes with sirolimus-eluting coronary stents: five-year results of the RAVEL trial. Journal of the American College of Cardiology 50:1299-1304.

Morice M.C., Serruys P.W., Sousa J.E., Fajadet J., Ban Hayashi E., Perin M., Colombo A., Schuler G., Barragan P., Guagliumi G., Molnar F., Falotico R. (2002) A randomized comparison of a sirolimus-eluting stent with a standard stent for coronary revascularization. New England Journal of Medicine 346:1773-1780.

Moses J.W., Leon M.B., Popma J.J., Fitzgerald P.J., Holmes D.R., O'Shaughnessy C., Caputo R.P., Kereiakes D.J., Williams D.O., Teirstein P.S., Jaeger J.L., Kuntz R.E. (2003) Sirolimus-eluting stents versus standard stents in patients with stenosis in a native coronary artery. New England Journal of Medicine 349:1315-1323.

Otake H., Honda Y., Courtney B.K., Shimohama T., Ako J., Waseda K., Macours N., Rogers C., Popma J.J., Abizaid A., Ormiston J.A., Spaulding C., Cohen S.A., Fitzgerald P.J. (2011a) Intravascular ultrasound results from the NEVO ResElution-I trial: a randomized, blinded comparison of sirolimus-eluting NEVO stents with paclitaxel-eluting TAXUS Liberte stents in de novo native coronary artery lesions. Circulation: Cardiovascular Interventions 4:146-154.

Otake H., Honda Y., Courtney B.K., Shimohama T., Ako J., Waseda K., Macours N., Rogers C., Popma J.J., Abizaid A., Ormiston J.A., Spaulding C., Cohen S.A., Fitzgerald P.J. (2011b) Intravascular ultrasound results from the NEVO ResElution-I trial: a randomized, blinded comparison of sirolimus-eluting NEVO stents with paclitaxel-eluting TAXUS Liberte stents in de novo native coronary artery lesions. Circ Cardiovasc Interv 4:146-54.

Pfisterer M., Brunner-La Rocca H.P., Buser P.T., Rickenbacher P., Hunziker P., Mueller C., Jeger R., Bader F., Osswald S., Kaiser C. (2006) Late clinical events after clopidogrel discontinuation may limit the benefit of drug-eluting stents: an observational study of drug-eluting versus bare-metal stents. Journal of the American College of Cardiology 48:2584-2591.

Roger V.L., Go A.S., Lloyd-Jones D.M., Adams R.J., Berry J.D., Brown T.M., Carnethon M.R., Dai S., de Simone G., Ford E.S., Fox C.S., Fullerton H.J., Gillespie C., Greenlund K.J., Hailpern S.M., Heit J.A., Ho P.M., Howard V.J., Kissela B.M., Kittner S.J., Lackland D.T., Lichtman J.H., Lisabeth L.D., Makuc D.M., Marcus G.M., Marelli A., Matchar D.B., McDermott M.M., Meigs J.B., Moy C.S., Mozaffarian D., Mussolino M.E., Nichol G., Paynter N.P., Rosamond W.D., Sorlie P.D., Stafford R.S., Turan T.N., Turner M.B., Wong N.D., Wylie-Rosett J. (2011) Heart disease and stroke statistics--2011 update: a report from the American Heart Association. Circulation 123:e18-e209.

Rowinsky E.K., Donehower R.C. (1995) Paclitaxel (taxol). New England Journal of Medicine 332:1004-1014. DOI: 10.1056/NEJM199504133321507.

Schampaert E., Cohen E.A., Schluter M., Reeves F., Traboulsi M., Title L.M., Kuntz R.E., Popma J.J. (2004) The Canadian study of the sirolimus-eluting stent in the treatment of patients with long de novo lesions in small native coronary arteries (C-SIRIUS). Journal of the American College of Cardiology 43:1110-1115.

Schofer J., Schluter M., Gershlick A.H., Wijns W., Garcia E., Schampaert E., Breithardt G. (2003) Sirolimus-eluting stents for treatment of patients with long atherosclerotic lesions in small coronary arteries: double-blind, randomised controlled trial (E-SIRIUS). Lancet 362:1093-1099.

Serruys P.W. (2011) ABSORB: Evaluation of the Bioresorbable Everolimus-Eluting Vascular Scaffold (BVS) in the Treatment of Patients with De Novo Native Coronary Artery Lesions: 1 Year Angiographic, IVUS, IVUS-VH and OCT results of Cohort B., American College of Cardiology, Netherlands.

Serruys P.W., Regar E., Carter A.J. (2002a) Rapamycin eluting stent: the onset of a new era in interventional cardiology. Heart 87:305-307.

Serruys P.W., de Jaegere P., Kiemeneij F., Macaya C., Rutsch W., Heyndrickx G., Emanuelsson H., Marco J., Legrand V., Materne P., et al. (1994) A comparison of balloon-expandable-stent implantation with balloon angioplasty in patients with coronary artery disease. New England Journal of Medicine 331:489-495. DOI: 10.1056/NEJM199408253310801.

Serruys P.W., Degertekin M., Tanabe K., Abizaid A., Sousa J.E., Colombo A., Guagliumi G., Wijns W., Lindeboom W.K., Ligthart J., de Feyter P.J., Morice M.C. (2002b) Intravascular ultrasound findings in the multicenter, randomized, double-blind RAVEL (RAndomized study with the sirolimus-eluting VElocity balloon-expandable stent in the treatment of patients with de novo native coronary artery Lesions) trial. Circulation 106:798-803.

Shand J. (2010) Drug-eluting stents: the next generation. Interv. Cardiol. 2:341-350.

Sousa J.E., Costa M.A., Abizaid A., Abizaid A.S., Feres F., Pinto I.M., Seixas A.C., Staico R., Mattos L.A., Sousa A.G., Falotico R., Jaeger J., Popma J.J., Serruys P.W. (2001) Lack of neointimal proliferation after implantation of sirolimus-coated stents in human coronary arteries: a quantitative coronary angiography and three-dimensional intravascular ultrasound study. Circulation 103:192-195.

Spaulding C. (2011) The NEVO RES-1 study: a randomized, multi-center comparison of the NEVO reservoir-based sirolimus-eluting stent with the TAXUS Liberte paclitaxel-eluting stent: 2-year outcomes, EuroPCR, Paris, France.

Stone G.W. (2010) Comparison of everolimus-eluting and paclitaxel-eluting stents: First report of the four-year clinical outcomes from the SPIRIT III trial, TCT, Washington D.C., USA.

Stone G.W., Ellis S.G., O'Shaughnessy C.D., Martin S.L., Satler L., McGarry T., Turco M.A., Kereiakes D.J., Kelley L., Popma J.J., Russell M.E. (2006) Paclitaxel-eluting stents vs vascular brachytherapy for in-stent restenosis within bare-metal stents: the TAXUS V ISR randomized trial. Journal of the American Medical Association 295:1253-1263.

Stone G.W., Ellis S.G., Cannon L., Mann J.T., Greenberg J.D., Spriggs D., O'Shaughnessy C.D., DeMaio S., Hall P., Popma J.J., Koglin J., Russell M.E. (2005) Comparison of a polymer-based paclitaxel-eluting stent with a bare metal stent in patients with complex coronary artery disease: a randomized controlled trial. Journal of the American Medical Association 294:1215-1223.

Tanabe K., Serruys P.W., Grube E., Smits P.C., Selbach G., van der Giessen W.J., Staberock M., de Feyter P., Muller R., Regar E., Degertekin M., Ligthart J.M., Disco C., Backx B., Russell M.E. (2003) TAXUS III Trial: in-stent restenosis treated with stent-based delivery of paclitaxel incorporated in a slow-release polymer formulation. Circulation 107:559-564.

Turco M. (2008) TAXUS ATLAS 3-Year Clinical Results, TCT, Washington, D.C, USA.

Weisz G., Leon M.B., Holmes D.R., Jr., Kereiakes D.J., Clark M.R., Cohen B.M., Ellis S.G., Coleman P., Hill C., Shi C., Cutlip D.E., Kuntz R.E., Moses J.W. (2006) Two-year outcomes after sirolimus-eluting stent implantation: results from the Sirolimus-Eluting Stent in de Novo Native Coronary Lesions (SIRIUS) trial. Journal of the American College of Cardiology 47:1350-1355.

Windecker S. (2011) BioMatrix Flx - New Generation DES, Euro-PCR, Europe.

Windecker S., Serruys P.W., Wandel S., Buszman P., Trznadel S., Linke A., Lenk K., Ischinger T., Klauss V., Eberli F., Corti R., Wijns W., Morice M.C., di Mario C., Davies S., van Geuns R.J., Eerdmans P., van Es G.A., Meier B., Juni P. (2008) Biolimus-eluting stent with biodegradable polymer versus sirolimus-eluting stent with durable polymer for coronary revascularisation (LEADERS): a randomised non-inferiority trial. Lancet 372:1163-73.

Yeung A.C., Leon M.B., Jain A., Tolleson T.R., Spriggs D.J., Mc Laurin B.T., Popma J.J., Fitzgerald P.J., Cutlip D.E., Massaro J.M., Mauri L. (2011) Clinical evaluation of the RESOLUTE zotarolimus-eluting coronary stent system in the treatment of de novo lesions in native coronary arteries: the RESOLUTE US clinical trial. Journal of the American College of Cardiology 57:1778-1783.

9

Rotablation in the Drug Eluting Stent Era

Petros S. Dardas
St Luke's Hospital, Thessaloniki
Greece

1. Introduction

In the field of interventional cardiology, heavily calcified coronary lesions (HCCL) pose great technical challenges and are associated with a high frequency of restenosis and target lesion revascularization (TLR) (Moses et al, 2004). The prevalence of severe calcium, defined as superficial (calcium at the intimal-lumen interface or closer to the lumen than to the adventitia) with greater than 180° arc, is estimated to present itself in 12% of cases using angiographic imaging. When IVUS guidance is used, it is seen in approximately 26% of cases (Figure 1) (Mintz et al, 2005).

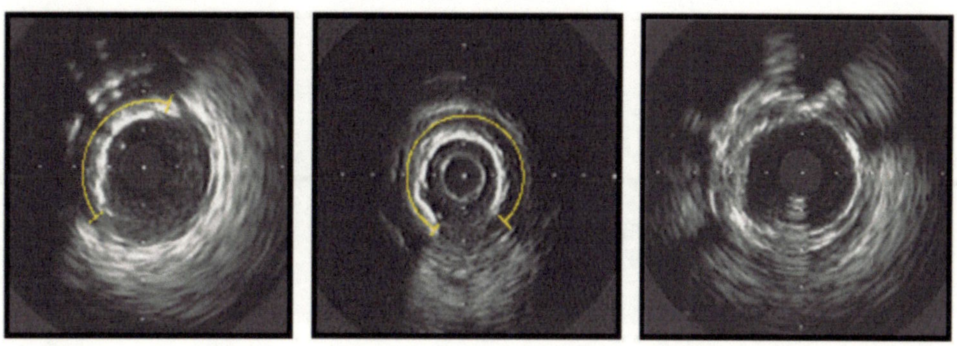

Fig. 1. Calcium distribution: Left: 180^0, in the center: 270^0, Right: superficial and deep

Occasionally, the degree of calcification and/or the geometry of the plaque prevent the crossing of the lesion with balloon or stent. Adequate lesion preparation before stent implantation remains an essential component of contemporary practice of coronary stent implantation in patients with complex lesions to improve both immediate and long-term outcomes. In heavily calcified lesions preparation with high-pressure balloon inflation may occasionally succeed but is often inadequate, or may create vessel wall rupture (undilatable lesion, figure 2) (Hoffmann et al, 1998).

In an attempt to overcome challenges posed by calcification, a number of devices and techniques have been developed. One such advance is rotational atherectomy, in which a rotating brass burr (figure 3) mounted on a flexible drive shaft and coated with diamond chips pulverizes a portion of the fibrous, calcified, inelastic plaque, modifies the plaque compliance, and leaves a smooth, nonendothelialized surface with intact media (figure 4).

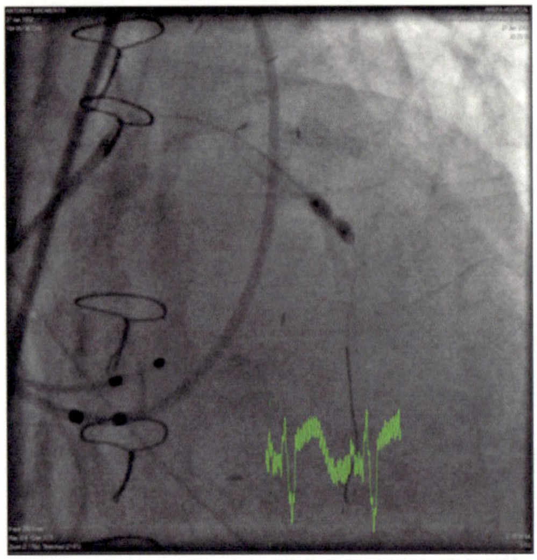

Fig. 2. Undilatable lesion
An undilatable lesion revealed by balloon inflation.

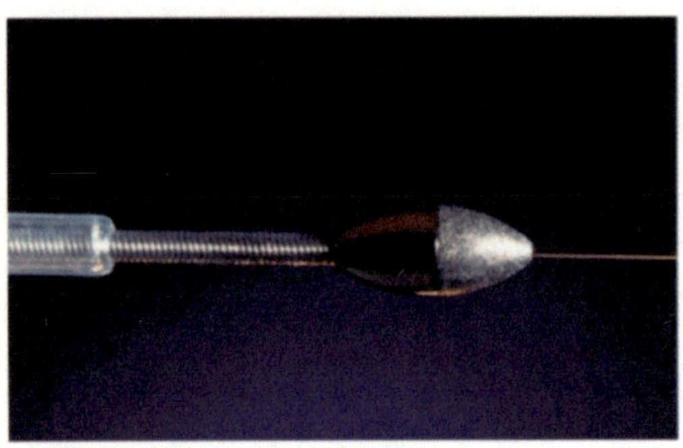

Fig. 3. Rotablator
The rotablator uses a rotating brass burr coated with diamond chips, mounted on to a flexible drive shaft.

Rotational atherectomy overcomes this obstacle through plaque modification of the calcified lesion; however, without adjunctive stenting, restenosis rates remain high (Warth, et al, 1994). Bare metal stents reduce restenosis rates in both calcified and noncalcified coronary lesions with and without atherectomy; however, restenosis and subsequent TLR rates continue to exceed 10-20% (Serruys et al, 1994; Fischman et al, 1994; Rankin et al, 1999; Cutlip et al, 2002). Drug eluting stents (DES) further reduce restenosis and TLR in both calcified and noncalcified lesions (Moses et al, 2003; Stone et al, 2004). Despite this benefit, the delivery of DES remains challenging in complex coronary anatomy, including eccentric, extensively calcified lesions. In order to obtain the desired long-term effectiveness of DES, successful initial implantation must be accomplished; therefore, aggressive lesion preparation becomes essential for these patient subsets.

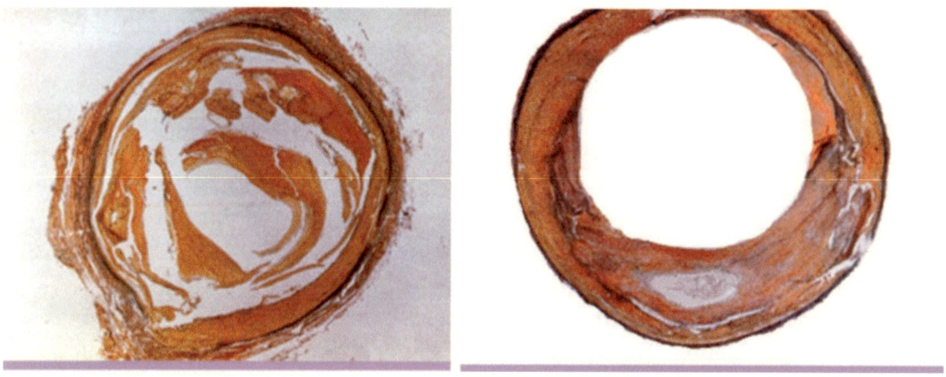

Fig. 4. Histology
Histology cross-sections post balloon (left) and post Rota (right).

Whether the benefit of DES persists after the vessel injury caused by rotational atherectomy is unknown. Rotablation followed by DES implantation (Rota-DES) for complex severely calcified lesions is a rational combination that has not been thoroughly evaluated. The limited studies with rotablation and DES showed promising results with no long term safety concerns. In these studies, a subtle observation was made suggesting that rotablation prior to DES implantation in such lesions may have an add-on effect on long term outcome compared to DES alone (Clavijo et al, 2006; Rao et al, 2006; Khattab et al, 2007). Therefore, the goal of this chapter is to investigate the immediate and long term outcomes of patients who are treated with rotational atherectomy to facilitate the delivery of DES in heavily calcified lesions. In addition, a full overview of the technique, the pros and cons, the advantages and complications and its applications in various lesion subsets will be provided.

2. RotA- general concepts

The technique of RotA was invented at the start of the 1980s by David Auth and has been used during angioplasty for more than 20 years (Reisman et al, 1996). The method is most effective in the modification of calcified plaques, facilitating stent placement during angioplasty. The treatment of HCCL (as opposed to non-calcified lesions) with angioplasty has been associated with a lower success rate and a higher incidence of complications (Wilensky et al, 2002). The geometry and inflexibility of HCCL often does not permit successful approach and correct stent deployment (Hoffmann et al, 1998). In addition, balloon dilatation and stent deployment in HCCL carry a higher risk of dissection and rupture. RotA devices use a rotating brass burr that pulverizes a portion of the fibrous, calcified, inelastic plaque, modifies the plaque compliance, and leaves a smooth, nonendothelialized surface with intact media (Mintz et al, 1992; Kovach et al, 1993). RotA is based on the principle of differential atherectomy, namely selective atherectomy of the fibrous and calcified plaque (Reisman, 1996). (Figure 5) Successful RotA results in the creation of a smooth vessel lumen, suitable for the successful performance of balloon angioplasty and stenting at the site of the lesion (Ellis et al, 1994).

The findings of the various studies have created some general guiding rules for the optimized use of RotA (Brown et al, 1997; Reifart et al, 1997; Whitlow et al, 2001; Dill et al, 2000; Buchbinder et al, 2001; vom Dahl J et al, 2002; Goldberg et al, 2000):

1. It is essential to use specific guiding catheters with sufficient support and coaxial fitting.
2. The atherectomy speed must be approximately 140000 rpm, although there is no clear cut-off and some operators use 150,000 rpm.
3. The intermittent application of RotA within lesion is preferred; usually "pecking" technique is used, where the burr is moved forward and backward the lesion, without pushing the rotablator into the lesion
4. Starting with smaller burrs reduces the plaque burden to the distal bed and a patent lumen is achieved in a shorter period of time
5. A RotA technique with 2 burrs may be chosen in order to reduce the incidence of the no-reflow phenomenon. The smaller burr (usually 1.25 mm) is used first, followed by a larger burr based on the size of the vessel, aiming at a burr/vessel ratio that does not exceed 0.6-0.7. However sometimes a single small burr is sufficient
6. Bigger burrs may debulk more of the lesion but they also may damage/activate more blood cells
7. In cases of extensive rotablation and large amount of debulking, glycoprotein IIb/IIIa inhibitors is recommended.
8. The duration of RotA application should not exceed 15-20 sec, with immediate cessation if the revolutions drop by >5000 rpm
9. During RotA, 500 ml of heparinised (5000 units) normal saline solution with 5 mg verapamil and 1000 µg nitroglycerine is administered locally, with a view to preventing thrombus formation and vascular spasm, and avoiding the no-reflow phenomenon.

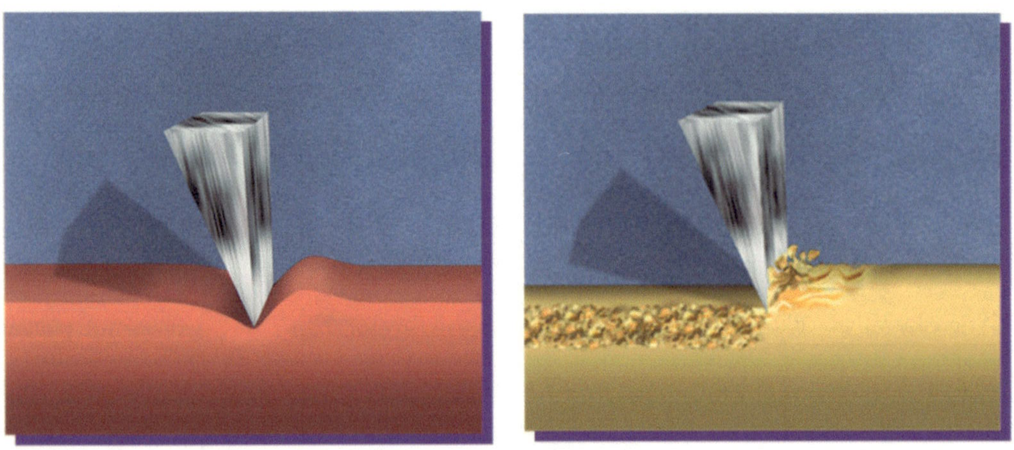

Fig. 5. Differential atherectomy
The concept of differential atherectomy: the rotablation preferentially ablates inelastic, calcified, atherosclerotic tissue.

3. RotA Indications and technique according to lesion specification

The absolute indication for RotA is the heavily calcified lesions (HCCL), localized or extended, and mainly the presence of a circumferential calcium ring where the lesion is undilatable by balloon angioplasty (Figures 6 and 7).

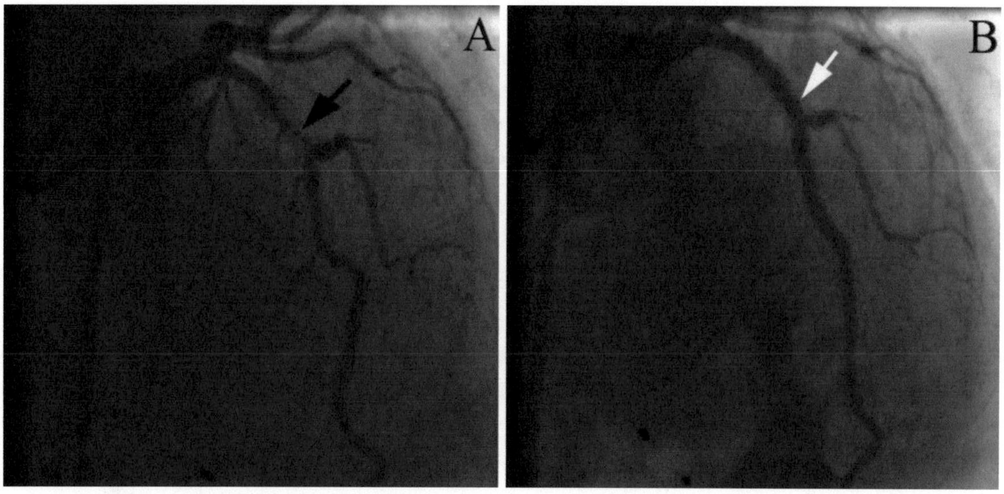

Fig. 6. Longitudinal calcified LAD lesion
A. Localised calcified longitudinal lesion of the left anterior descending artery before the origin of the first diagonal branch (black arrow).
B. Restoration of vessel patency with the combination of rotational atherectomy and drug-eluting stent (white arrow).

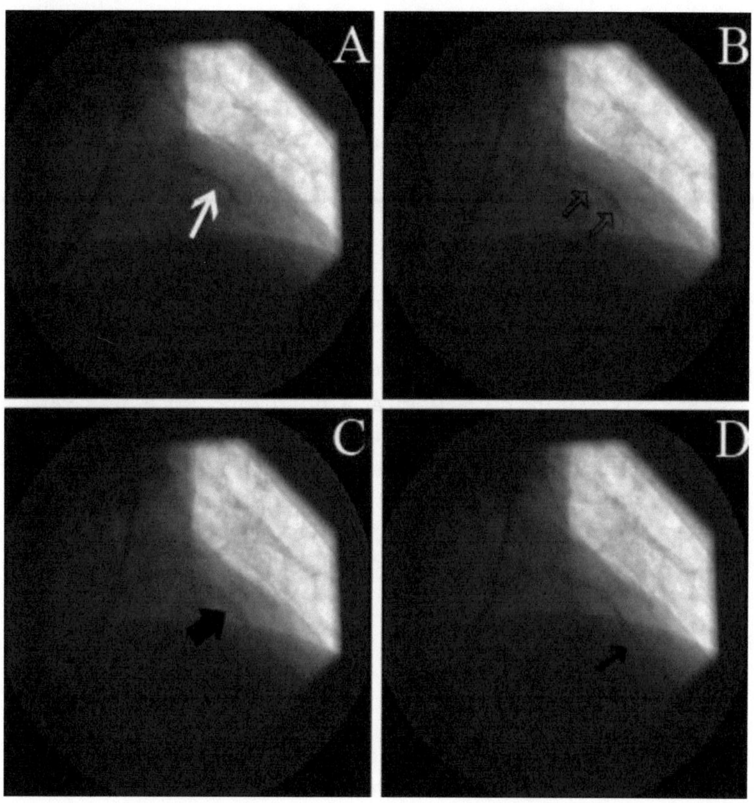

Fig. 7. Unsucessful treatment of calcified LAD lesion with POBA

The lesion in Figure 6 had previously been treated unsuccessfully using direct balloon dilatation without rotational atherectomy of the calcified plaque. A. Attempt to deploy the balloon (white arrow). B. Incomplete deployment of proximal end of the balloon (open arrows). C. Rupture of the angioplasty balloon (thick black arrow). D. The result of the rupture is the characteristic escape of contrast medium distal to the balloon (thin black arrow).

Other indications are ostial lesions with severe fibrosis with or without calcification, and balloon-inaccessible lesions, provided that the Rotawire can cross the lesion.

- In cases with multiple HCCL in the same vessel (tandem lesions) (Figure 8), segmental RotA is preferred. Because of the potential for a large quantity of plaque debris, a stepped burr approach is recommended. Interpolated low pressure balloon angioplasty may be helpful in improving flow, can also localize the areas of resistance and improve vasospasm.
- In ostial lesions (specifically in RCA) (figure 9) the frequent fibrocalcific characteristics of these lesions make them well suited for rotablation treatment. Coaxial placement of the guiding catheter is mandatory (assess in two projections-best RAO). Straight alignment of the guide catheter is essential in order to center the guidewire (extra support). The lie of the guidewire is essential and keeping the tip just beyond the lesion may improve the centering.
- In bifurcation lesions the mainstay of treatment is branch preservation and adequate lumen in both limbs. Rotablation should be started at the most difficult to wire branch first. Use low burr-artery ratios (<0.5) especially when there is angulation present.
- In coronary arteries with severe tortuosity the main issue is to avoid perforation. Keeping the tip of the guidewire just beyond the lesion is essential in order to reduce sidewall tension. A stepped-burr approach and the use of undersized burrs are recommended. The activated burr should be advanced at low speed ensuring that there is no wire tension. Ablation of normal tissue can occur if the tension on the wall exceeds the elasticity of the vessel (wire bias) (Figure 10).
- Failed PCI is either due to inability to cross the lesion or dilate. These lesions are frequently calcified. The decision to use rotablation should be made early, before large dissections appear.
- The inability to cross a CTO with a balloon catheter occurs in approximately 7% of all CTOs that are successfully crossed with a guidewire. RotA is a safe and effective technique to overcome this frustrating situation (Figure 11). Chronic total occlusions are well suited for rotational atherectomy and treatment is only limited by the ability to cross the lesion with the guidewire. Conventional guidewires should be used and exchange for the rota-wire with a OTW catheter. These lesions are frequently fibrocalcific. Initiating treatment with the smallest burrs (1.25 mm) is the safest approach.

4. RotA complications

Possible but rare complications include myocardial infarction, emergency CABG, coronary artery dissection, no reflow phenomenon, due to peripheral embolization, perforation or severe coronary artery spasm (Cavusoglu et al, 2004). The strict application of the general rules for the optimal use of RotA mentioned above, eliminates the possibility of any complication.

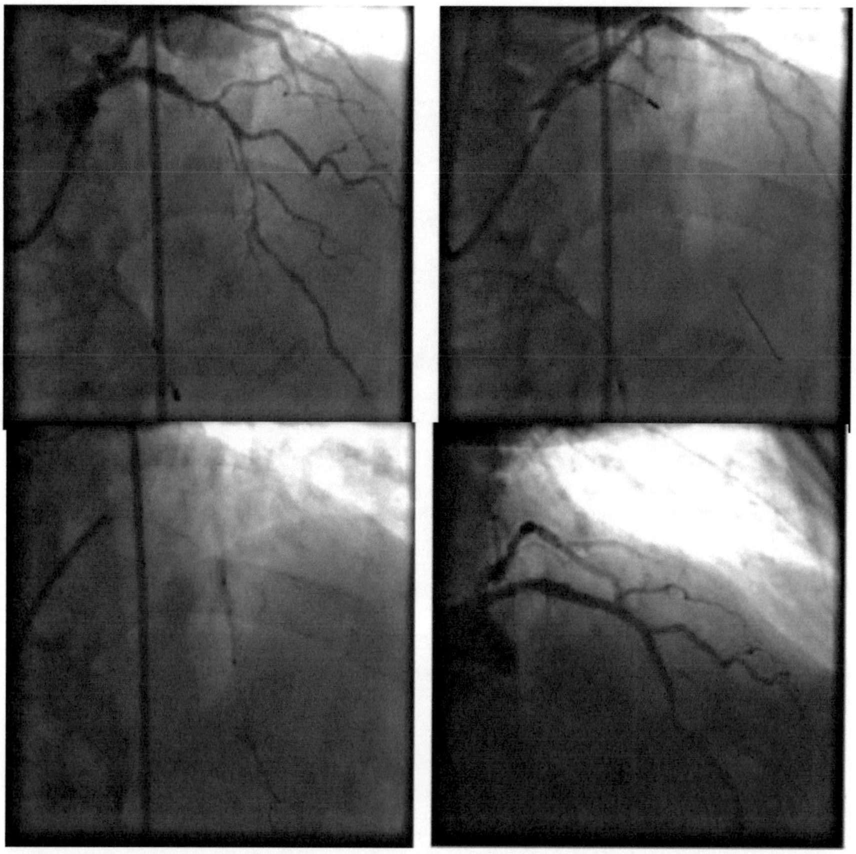

Fig. 8. Tandem calcified LAD lesion
Tandem LAD lesions before, after Rota (segmental approach) and final result after DES.

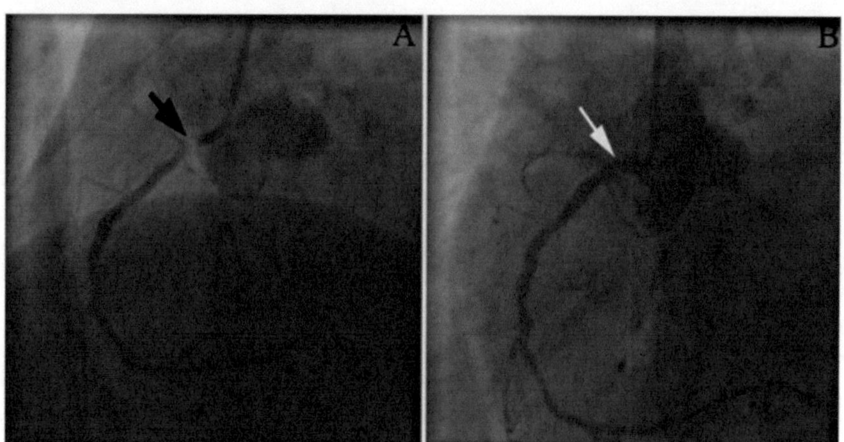

Fig. 9. Calcified ostial RCA lesion
A. Calcified ostial lesion in the right coronary artery (black arrow). B. Restoration of vessel patency with the combination of rotational atherectomy and drug-eluting stent (white arrow).

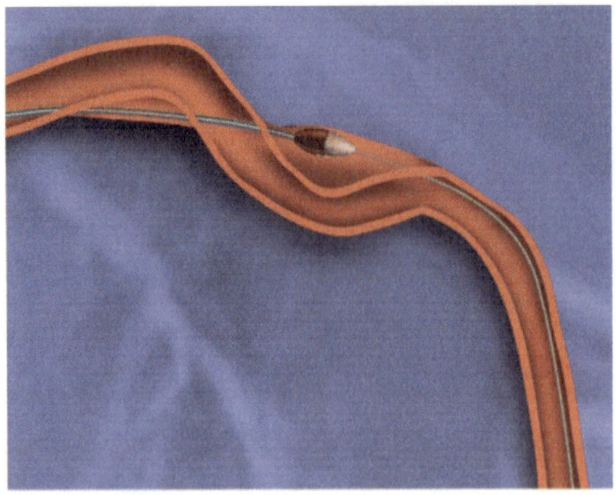

Fig. 10. Wire bias

Wire bias can occur in tortuous vessels, increasing the risk of perforation.

5. RotA contradictions

Coronary dissection, severe thrombosis and severe tortuosity are general contradictions of the method. Also RotA is relatively contraindicated in vein grafts due to the increased risk of dissection and distal embolization.

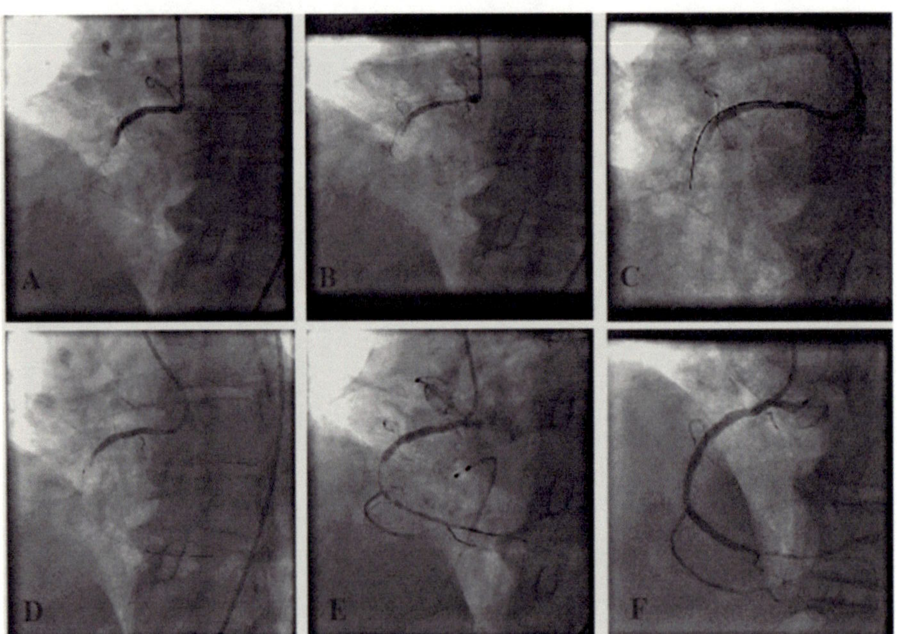

Fig. 11. Calcified chronic total occlusion of a RCA
A. Guide Wire insertion. B. Three different catheters: JR4, AL1, H-STICK. C. Inability to cross CTO with eight different balloons (diameters from 1,5 – 0,85 mm). D. Rotawire crosses the lesion. E. Rotational atherectomy with 1.25 mm burr. F. DES deployment

6. RotA in DES era

RotA followed by balloon angioplasty does not improve the rates of restenosis compared to direct balloon angioplasty, leading to high rates of restenosis and need for TLR—in up to 40% of cases (Reifart et al, 1997). RotA + balloon angioplasty strategy is better for the prevention of restenosis in small coronary vessels compared to balloon angioplasty alone (Mauri et al, 2003). BMS implantation after RotA has a high success rate, with an acceptable incidence of complications and a clearly lower incidence of angiographic restenosis compared to plain angioplasty, but the restenosis rate and need for TLR remain high, at 22.5% according to one previous study (Moussa et al, 1997).

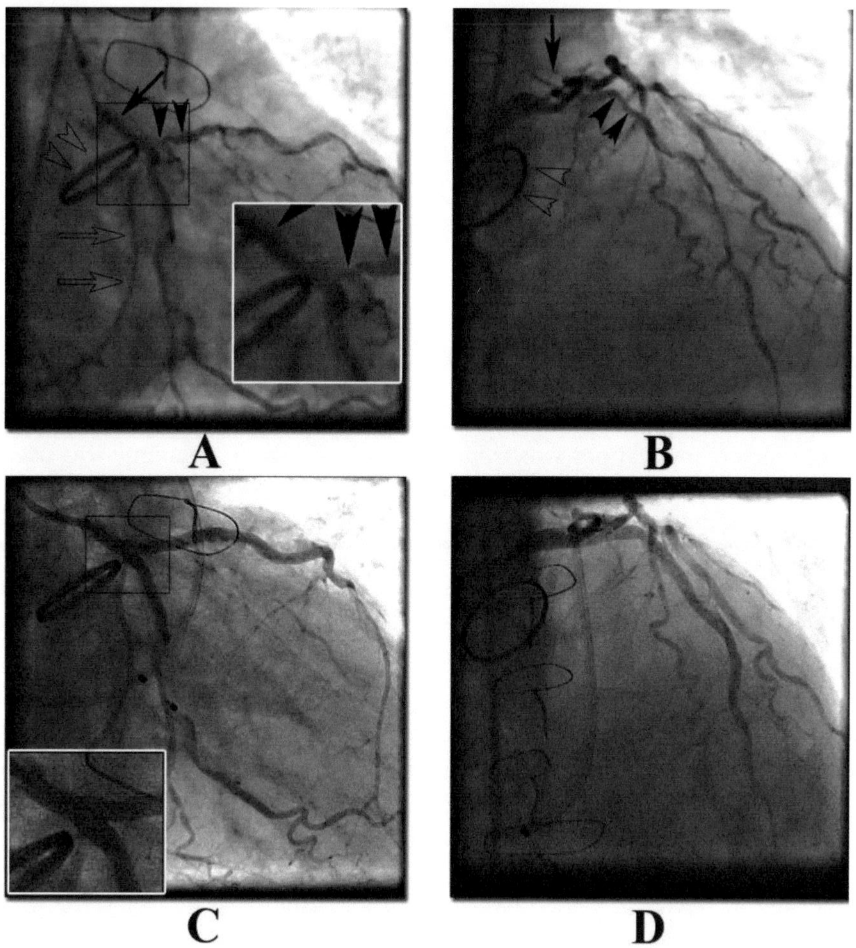

Fig. 12. Complex LMS-LAD Rotablation with ECMO support
(A- B) heavily calcified ostial LMS stenosis (black arrow), elongated 95% LAD stenosis (black head arrows)- (in magnification on the right-down corner), metallic aortic valve (white head arrows) and a collateral artery from the LAD to the occluded RCA (white arrows), in a patient with poor LV and EF 20%. (C-D) Final angiographic result after rotablation and stent implantation (in magnification on the left- down corner) with the hemodynamic support of ECMO machine.

DES reduce neointimal hyperplasia and are safer and more effective than BMS in the treatment of stable coronary lesions (Stone et al, 2007; Mauri et al, 2007). However, DES in HCCL presents a technical difficulty of stent implantation and deployment. Calcification of the lesion is already known to have a negative impact on stent deployment (MacIsaac et al, 1995). Disruption of the stent's polymer coating during forceful deployment and unsatisfactory drug elution because of extreme calcification of the lesion are the main reasons for the unsuccessful deployment and implantation of stents in HCCL. Indeed, the rates of MACE and the need for TLR were significantly higher in patients with calcified as opposed to non-calcified lesions that were treated with DES implantation (Kawaguchi et al, 2008). RotA + DES approach had better clinical and angiographic results over a 9-month follow up compared to RotA + BMS in the treatment of patients with HCCL (Khattab et al, 2007). The results from patients treated with RotA + BMS with those from a group treated with RotA + DES and another group treated with DES without RotA shows that the use of DES reduced the incidence of MACE in patients who underwent RotA, mainly because of a significant reduction in the need for TLR (Rao et al, 2006). A study compared two groups of patients with HCCL who were treated with DES, where RotA was necessary in the first group but not in the second. There was no significant difference between the groups as regards in-hospital complications or clinical outcomes (Clavijo et al, 2006). A previous study of ours showed that the therapeutic strategy of RotA + DES was effective in treating HCCL as regards both the clinical outcome and the angiographic result (Mezilis et al, 2010). The mortality and MACE rates were very low (3.3% and 11.3%, respectively) over a mean follow up of >36 months. No immediate complications related to the angioplasty were recorded, while in previous studies the incidence of such complications was from 4% to 7%. A 2-burr technique was used with a view to limiting the occurrence of the no-reflow phenomenon. Initially, a small burr was used (1.25 mm), followed by a larger burr depending on the size of the vessel. Whether this gradual approach contributed to limiting the immediate complications and to the low rate of stent thrombosis will need further investigation. Another study (Schwartz et al, 2011) reported a slightly higher rate of MACE (15.8%) and mortality (4.2%). However, in this study the authors did not describe the technique they used (i.e. burrs at one or more stages).

A recent study (Benezet et al, 2011) compared the angiographic and procedural success rates of three therapeutic strategies in patients with HCCL: RotA + only balloon angioplasty, RotA + BMS and RotA + DES. In unadjusted analysis, procedural success appears high with subsequent stent placement (DES or BMS) versus RA alone (96.4% for DES versus 95% for BMS versus 63% for no stent). However, 1 in 4 cases were not candidates for stent placement, due to reference vessel diameter < 2.25, inability to deliver DES, or desire to avert clopidogrel therapy, and the lower procedural success rate in this population should be considered prior to embarking on Rota. This rate of unsuccessful stent placement is much higher than in previous studies. Another recent study (Pagnotta et al, 2010) confirms the safety and effectiveness of Rota + DES strategy to tackle HCCL with good long-term clinical outcomes. Although the radial approach was used in 37.3% of cases, the procedure was successful in 97% of cases; this rate of success is similar to previous studies. Rotablation, when used in very high risk subsets combined with the use of short term LVADs was also proved to be efficient (Figure 12) (Dardas et al, 2011).

7. Conclusion

The combination of RotA + DES is an integrated, effective and safe method of treating HCCL. The wide use of DES may cause a renaissance of RotA and its return to daily use in the catheterization laboratory, after its decline a decade ago when it failed to show better long-term results after angioplasty. In the future, randomised studies will be needed to confirm the above results.

8. References

Benezet, J.; Díaz de la Llera, LS; Cubero, J.M.; Villa, M.; Fernández-Quero, M.; Sánchez-González, A. (2011) A Drug-eluting stents following rotational atherectomy for heavily calcified coronary lesions: long-term clinical outcomes. *J Invasive Cardiol*, Vol. 23, No. 1, pp. 28-32.

Brown, D.L.; George, C.J.; Steenkiste, A.R.; Cowley MJ, Leon, M.B.; Cleman, M.W.; Moses, J.W.; King, S.B. 3rd; Carrozza, J.P.; Holmes, D.R.; Burkhard-Meier, C.; Popma, J.J.; Brinker, J.A.; Buchbinder, M. (1997) High-speed rotational atherectomy of human coronary stenoses: acute and one-year outcomes from the New Approaches to Coronary Intervention (NACI) registry. *Am J Cardiol*, Vol. 80, No. 10A, pp. 60K-67K.

Buchbinder, M. (2001) For the SPORT Clinical Trial Investigators. Abstract presentations at TCT 2001.

Cavusoglu, E.; Kini, A.S.; Marmur, J.D.; Sharma, S.K. (2004) Current status of rotational atherectomy. *Catheter Cardiovasc Interv*, Vol. 62, No. 4, pp. 485–498.

Clavijo, L.C.; Steinberg, D.H.; Torguson, R.; Kuchulakanti, P.K.; Chu, W.W.; Fournadjiev, J.; Satler, L.F.; Kent, K.M.; Suddath, W.O.; Waksman, R.; Pichard, A.D. (2006) Sirolimus-eluting stents and calcified coronary lesions: clinical outcomes of patients treated with and without rotational atherectomy. *Catheterization Cardiovascular Interventions*, Vol. 68, No. 6, pp. 873-878.

Cutlip, D.E.; Chauhan, M.S.; Baim, D.S.; Ho, K.K.; Popma, J.J.; Carrozza, J.P.; Cohen, D.J.; Kuntz, R.E. (2002) Clinical restenosis after coronary stenting: perspectives from multicenter clinical trials. *J Am Coll Cardiol*, Vol. 18, No. 40(12), pp. 2082-208.

Dardas, P.; Mezilis, N.; Ninios, V.; Theofilogiannakos, E.K.; Tsikaderis, D.; Tsotsolis, N. Kolettas, A.; Nikoloudakis, N.; Pitsis, A.A. (2011) ECMO as a bridge to high-risk rotablation of heavily calcified coronary arteries. *Herz* 2011, July 7.

Dill, T.; Dietz, U.; Hamm, C.W.; Küchler, R.; Rupprecht, H.J.; Haude, M.; Cyran, J.; Ozbek, C.; Kuck, K.H.; Berger, J.; Erbel, R. (2000) A randomized comparison of balloon angioplasty versus rotational atherectomy in complex coronary lesions (COBRA study). *Eur Heart J*, Vol. 21, No. 21, pp. 1759-1766.

Ellis, S.G.; Popma, J.J.; Buchbinder, M.; Franco, I.; Leon, M.B.; Kent, K.M.; Pichard, A.D.; Satler, L.F.; Topol, E.J.; Whitlow, P.L. (1994) Relation of clinical presentation, stenosis morphology, and operator technique to the procedural results of rotational atherectomy and rotational atherectomy-facilitated angioplasty. *Circulation*, Vol. 89, No. 2, pp. 882-892

Fischman, D.L.; Leon, M.B.; Baim, D.S.; Schatz, R.A.; Savage, M.P.; Penn, I.; Detre, K.; Veltri, L.; Ricci, D.; Nobuyoshi M.. (1994) A randomized comparison of coronary-stent placement and balloon angioplasty in the treatment of coronary artery disease. Stent Restenosis Study Investigators. *N Engl J Med*, Vol. 25, No 331(8), pp. 496-501.

Goldberg, S.L.; Berger, P.; Cohen, D.J.; Shawl, F.; Buchbinder, M.; Fortuna, R.; O'Neill, W.; Leon, M.; Braden, G.A.; Teirstein, P.S.; Reisman, M.; Bailey, S.R.; Dauerman, H.L.; Bowers, T.; Mehran, R.; Colombo, A. (2000) Rotational atherectomy or balloon angioplasty in the treatment of intra-stent restenosis: BARASTER multicenter registry. *Catheter Cardiovasc Interv*, Vol. 51, No. 4, pp. 407-413.

Hoffmann, R.; Mintz, G.S.; Popma, J.J.; Satler, L.F.; Kent, K.M.; Pichard, A.D.; Leon, M.B. (1998) Treatment of calcified coronary lesions with Palmaz-Schatz stents. An intravascular ultrasound study. *Eur Heart, Vol.* 19, No. 8, pp. 1224-1231.

Kawaguchi, R.; Tsurugaya, H.; Hoshizaki, H.; Toyama, T.; Oshima, S.; Taniguchi, K. (2008) Impact of lesion calcification on clinical and angiographic outcome after sirolimus-eluting stent implantation in real-world patients. *Cardiovasc Revasc Med*, Vol 9, No 1, pp. 2-8.

Khattab, A.A.; Otto, A.; Hochadel, M.; Toelg, R.; Geist, V.; Richardt, G. (2007) Drug-eluting stents versus bare metal stents following rotational atherectomy for heavily calcified coronary lesions: late angiographic and clinical follow-up results. *J Interv Cardiol*, Vol. 20, No. 2, pp. 100-106.

Kovach, J.A.; Mintz, G.S.; Pichard, A.D.; Kent, K.M.; Popma, J.J.; Satler, L.F.; Leon, M.B. (1993) Sequential intravascular ultrasound characterization of the mechanisms of rotational atherectomy and adjunct balloon angioplasty. *J Am Coll Cardiol*, Vol. 22, No. 4, pp. 1024-1032.

MacIsaac, A.I.; Bass, T.A.; Buchbinder, M.; Cowley, M.J.; Leon, M.B.; Warth, D.C.; Whitlow, P.L. (1995) High speed rotational atherectomy: outcome in calcified and noncalcified coronary artery lesions. *J Am Coll Cardiol*, Vol. 26, No. 3, pp. 731-736.

Mauri, L.; Reisman, M.; Buchbinder, M.; Popma, J.J.; Sharma, S.K.; Cutlip, D.E.; Ho, K.K.; Prpic, R.; Zimetbaum, P.J.; Kuntz, R.E. (2003) Comparison of rotational atherectomy with conventional balloon angioplasty in the prevention of restenosis of small coronary arteries: results of the Dilatation vs Ablation Revascularization Trial Targeting Restenosis (DART). *Am Heart J*, Vol. 145, No. 5, pp 847-854.

Mauri, L.; Hsieh, W.H.; Massaro, J.M.; Ho, K.K.; D'Agostino, R.; Cutlip, D.E. (2007) Stent thrombosis in randomized clinical trials of drug-eluting stents. *N Engl J Med*, Vol. 356, No. 10, pp. 1020-1029.

Mezilis, N.; Dardas, P.; Ninios, V.; Tskaderis, D. (2010) Rotablation in the drug eluting era: immediate and long-term results from a single center experience. *J Interv Cardiol* Vol. 23, No.2, pp. 249-253.

Mintz, G.S.; Potkin, B.N.; Keren, G.; Satler, L.F.; Pichard, A.D.; Kent, K.M.; Popma, J.J.; Leon, M.B. (1992) Intravascular ultrasound evaluation of the effect of rotational atherectomy in obstructive atherosclerotic coronary artery disease. *Circulation*, Vol. 86, No. 5, pp. 1383-1393.

Mintz, G.S.; Popma, J.J.; Pichard, A.D.; Kent, K.M.; Satler, L.F.; Chuang, Y.C.; Ditrano, C.; Leon, M.B. (1995) Patterns of Calcification in Coronary Artery Disease. *Circulation* Vol. 91, No. 7, pp. 1959-1965.

Moses, J.W.; Leon, M.B.; Popma, J.J.; Fitzgerald, P.J.; Holmes, D.R.; O'Shaughnessy, C.; Caputo, R.P.; Kereiakes, D.J.; Williams, D.O.; Teirstein, P.S.; Jaeger, J.L.; Kuntz, R.E.; SIRIUS Investigators. (2003) Sirolimus-eluting stents versus standard stents in patients with stenosis in a native coronary artery. *N Engl J Med*, Vol. 349, No. 14, pp. 1315-1323

Moses, J.W.; Carlier, S.; Moussa, I. (2004) Lesion preparation prior to stenting. *Rev Cardiovasc Med, Vol.* 5, pp. S16-S21.

Moussa, I.; Di Mario, C.; Moses, J.; Reimers, B.; Di Francesco, L.; Martini, G.; Tobis, J.; Colombo, A. (1997) Coronary stenting after rotational atherectomy in calcified and complex lesions. Angiographic and clinical follow-up results. *Circulation*, Vol. 96, No. 1, pp. 128-136.

Pagnotta, P.; Briguori, C.; Mango, R.; Visconti, G.; Focaccio, A.; Belli, G.; Presbitero, P. (2010) Rotational atherectomy in resistant chronic total occlusions. *Catheter Cardiovasc Interv*, Vol. 76, No. 3, pp. 366-371.

Rankin, J.M.; Spinelli, J.J.; Carere, R.G.; Ricci, D.R.; Penn, I.M.; Hilton, J.D.; Henderson, M.A.; Hayden, R.I.; Buller, C.E.. (1999) Improved clinical outcome after widespread use of coronary-artery stenting in Canada. *N Engl J Med*, Vol. 341, No. 26, pp. 1957-1965.

Rao, S.V.; Honeycutt, E.; Kandzari, D. (2006) Clinical outcomes with drug-eluting stents following atheroablation therapies. *J Invasive Crdiol*, Vol. 18, No. 9, pp. 393-396.

Reisman, M. (1996) Technique and strategy of rotational atherectomy. *Cathet Cardiovasc Diagn*, Suppl. 3, pp. 2-14.

Reifart, N.; Vandormael, M.; Krajcar, M.; Göhring, S.; Preuslerm W,; Schwarz, F.; Störger, H.; Hofmann, M.; Klöpper, J.; Müller, S.;, Haase, J. (1997) Randomized comparison of angioplasty of complex coronary lesions at a single center. Excimer Laser, Rotational Atherectomy, and Balloon Angioplasty Comparison (ERBAC) Study. *Circulation*, Vol. 96, No. 1, pp. 91-98.

Schwartz, B.G.; Mayeda, G.S.; Economides, C.; Kloner, R.A.; Shavelle, D.M.; Burstein, S. (2011) Rotational atherectomy in the drug-eluting stent era: a single-center experience. *J Invasive Cardiol*, Vol. 23, No. 4, pp. 133-139.

Serruys, P.W.; de Jaegere, P.; Kiemeneij, F.; Macaya, C.; Rutsch, W.; Heyndrickx, G.; Emanuelsson, H.; Marco, J.; Legrand, V.; Materne, P.; et al. (1994) A comparison of balloon-expandable-stent implantation with balloon angioplasty in patients with coronary artery disease. Benestent Study Group. *N Engl J Med*, Vol. 331, No. 8, pp. 489-495.

Stone, G.W.; Ellis, S.G.; Cox, D.A.; Hermiller, J.; O'Shaughnessy, C.; Mann, J.T.; Turco, M.; Caputo, R.; Bergin, P.; Greenberg, J.; Popma, J.J.; Russell, M.E. TAXUS-IV Investigators. (2004) A polymer-based, paclitaxel-eluting stent in patients with coronary artery disease. *N Engl J Med*, Vol. 350, No. 3, pp. 221-231.

Stone, G.W.; Moses, J.W.; Ellis, S.G.; Schofer, J.; Dawkins, K.D.; Morice, M.C.; Colombo, A.; Schampaert, E.; Grube, E.; Kirtane, A.J.; Cutlip, D.E.; Fahy, M.; Pocock, S.J.; Mehran, R.; Leon, M.B. (2007) Safety and efficacy of sirolimus- and paclitaxel-eluting coronary stents. *N Engl J* Med , Vol. 356, No. 10, pp. 998-1008.

vom Dahl, J.; Dietz, U.; Haager, P.K.; Silber, S.; Niccoli, L.; Buettner, H.J.; Schiele, F.; Thomas, M.; Commeau, P.; Ramsdale, D.R.; Garcia, E.; Hamm, C.W.; Hoffmann, R.; Reineke, T.; Klues, H.G. (2002) Rotational atherectomy does not reduce recurrent in-stent restenosis: results of the angioplasty versus rotational atherectomy for treatment of diffuse in-stent restenosis trial (ARTIST). *Circulation* Vol. 105, No. 5, pp. 583-588.

Warth, D.C.; Leon, M.B.; O'Neill, W.; Zacca, N.; Polissar, N.L.; Buchbinder, M. (1994) Rotational atherectomy multicenter registry: acute results, complications and 6-month angiographic follow-up in 709 patients. *J Am Coll Cardiol*, Vol. 24, No. 3, pp. 641-648.

Wilensky, R.L.; Selzer, F.; Johnston, J.; Laskey, W.K.; Klugherz, B.D.; Block, P.; Cohen, H.; Detre, K.; Williams, D.O. (2002) Relation of percutaneous coronary intervention of complex lesions to clinical outcomes (from the NHLBI Dynamic Registry). *Am J Cardiol* 2002, 90: 216-221

Whitlow, P.L.; Bass, T.A.; Kipperman, R.M.; Sharaf, B.L.; Ho, K.K.; Cutlip, D.E.; Zhang, Y.; Kuntz, R.E.; Williams, D.O.; Lasorda, D.M.; Moses, J.W.; Cowley, M.J.; Eccleston, D.S.; Horrigan, M.C.; Bersin, R.M.; Ramee, S.R.; Feldman, T. (2001) Results of the study to determine rotablator and transluminal angioplasty strategy (STRATAS). *Am J Cardiol* Vol. 87, No. 6, pp. 699-705.

10

Contrast Medium-Induced Nephropathy (CIN) Gram-Iodine/GFR Ratio to Predict CIN and Strategies to Reduce Contrast Medium Doses

Ulf Nyman
Lund University
Sweden

1. Introduction

Radiographic iodine contrast media (I-CM) has been recognized as the third leading cause of hospital-acquired renal insufficiency or the most common cause among pharmaceutical agents (Nash et al., 2002) with an overall incidence of contrast medium-induced nephropathy (CIN) of 1-2% following percutaneous coronary angiography (PCA) and interventions (PCI) (Mehran & Nikolsky, 2006). The presence of multiple CIN risk factors or high-risk clinical scenarios may create a substantial risk of CIN (≈50%), acute renal failure (≈15%) requiring dialysis and an increased morbidity and mortality (Marenzi et al., 2004; McCullough et al., 2006a, 2006b). At the same time it has been argued that the risk of CIN is lower following IV administration of CM in connection with computed tomography (CT) than after IA injections during cardiac procedures (Davidson et al., 2006; Katzberg & Barrett, 2007; Katzberg & Newhouse, 2010), though there exist no comparative studies based on matched risk factors and CM doses.

Reliable prediction of pre-procedural renal function, identification of CIN risk factors, institution of adequate prophylactic regimens and to modify examination technique to reduce CM-dose are crucial to reduce patient suffering and cost since curative treatment is not available. A wide spectrum of CIN risk factors including high age, diabetes mellitus, poor cardiac function, and hemodynamic instability has been thoroughly outlined in recent reviews (McCullough et al., 2006b; Mehran & Nikolsky, 2006).

A number of prophylactic regimen studies has been performed and meta-analyzed (Kelly et al., 2008). So far no adjunctive medical pharmacological treatment has convincingly been proved to be efficacious in reducing the risk of CIN (Stacul et al., 2006) including acetylcysteine (Biondi-Zoccai et al., 2006) and hydration with sodium bicarbonate instead of saline (Zoungas et al., 2009). Haemodialysis is ineffective and hemofiltration is impractical in routine clinical practice (Stacul et al., 2006).

Thus, treating modifiable risk factors (Mehran & Nikolsky, 2006), instituting adequate intravenous volume expansion with isotonic crystalloid (Stacul et al., 2006) and withdrawal of nephrotoxic drugs, mannitol and loop diuretics are three of the four corner stones to reduce the risk of CIN (Thomsen et al., 2008a). The fourth one is to minimize the dose of the offending agent itself, i.e. the contrast medium (Davidson et al., 2006; Kane et al., 2008; Sterner et al., 2001). Though low- and iso-osmolal CM should be substituted for high-osmolal CM (Barrett & Carlisle, 1993; Rudnick et al., 1995), the benefit of iso- over low-osmolal CM is only suggestive but not statistically significant according to a recent meta-analysis (From et al., 2010).

The present chapter will focus on:

- The risk of CIN in IV versus IA CM administration.
- Using estimated glomerular filtration rate (eGFR) in absolute terms to evaluate renal function.
- Using gram iodine (g-I) to express CM-dose instead of simply volumes and promoting g-I/eGFR ratio to maximize CM doses as a predictor of CIN instead of the Cigarroa formula (Cigarroa et al., 1989).
- Potential means to reduce CM dose for CT coronary angiography (CTCA) in patients at risk of CIN.
- The potential of using iodine concentrations and doses iso-attenuating with gadolinium (Gd) CM and other means to decrease CM-doses in patients at risk of CIN.

2. IV versus IA CM administration and CIN

The alleged lower risk of CIN following CM-enhanced CT compared with PCA/PCI has lead to conclusions such as

- "In clinical settings such as CM-enhanced multidetector CT makes it defensible to consider using CM even in patients with greater levels of background risk factors (e.g. greater degree of preexisting chronic renal insufficiency) than one would be comfortable with in the IA setting" (Katzberg & Barrett, 2007) and
- "International radiologic professional organizations should revisit the basis of their practice guidelines to reduce their implications about the danger of CIN with CM-enhanced CT"s (Katzberg & Newhouse, 2010).

Such statements and conclusions may jeopardize patient safety, since they were not based on any studies comparing the risk of CIN following CM-enhanced CT and coronary interventions in patients with matched risk factors and CM-doses. In addition, a recent study showed no difference in the incidence of CIN between CT-angiography and digital subtraction angiography (DSA) of the aortofemoral arteries in the same patients. The lack of difference occurred despite that the DSA-results may have been affected by the CM load from the CT performed 3-14 days prior to the DSA (Karlsberg et al., 2011).

It seems inexplicable that the same type of CM molecules passing through the coronary arteries via the coronary sinus to the right atrium should be more nephrotoxic than if the same molecules pass via the arm veins to the right atrium and then through the pulmonary circulation to finally reach the kidneys via the aorta. As a matter of fact in the vast majority of IA injections, the CM has to pass through the venous system before reaching the kidneys (IV relative to the kidneys), i.e. carotid, subclavian, celiac, mesenteric, distal aortic and iliaco-femoral. Left ventriculography or aortography in connection with PCA/PCI is an exception. However, in this case only a minor part will reach the kidneys directly through the aortic route, i.e. about 20% of cardiac output or e.g. 2-3 grams of iodine following a left ventriculography (6-8 mL of an injected volume of 30-40 mL of 320 to 370 mg I/mL) of a total mean dose commonly ranging between 50 to 100 grams of iodine during a coronary procedures. Spill-over into the aorta also occurs during selective coronary artery injections and through side-holes of guiding catheters during PCI. However, the amount during each injection is so small that it will hardly affect plasma osmolality to cause any hypertonic renal effects and will therefore only affect the kidneys with the same pathophysiological mechanisms as an IV injection will do.

In the relatively few published reports of CIN following CM-enhanced CT the incidence may vary between 0 and 42% depending on definitions, degree of renal impairment and number and degree of risk factors (Katzberg & Newhouse, 2010; Nguyen et al., 2008; Polena et al., 2005; Tepel et al., 2000; Thomsen et al., 2008b). In a recent prospective study of unselected emergency patients 11% (n=70/633) increased their serum creatinine ≥44 μmol/L or ≥25% of whom 9% (n=6) developed CM-induced severe renal failure, which contributed to death in 4 of the 6 patients (Mitchell et al., 2010). Another CIN study showed that IV CM injections were actually associated with a higher mortality risk than IA administration (From et al., 2008). One explanation may be that the entire CM dose in CT is injected within one minute and thus may strike the kidneys at a considerable higher dose rate compared with a coronary arterial procedure that may last for 15-30-60 minutes or even longer.

It should also be noted that in randomized studies comparing renal effects of various CM, high-risk patients (e.g. unstable renal function, heart failure, uncontrolled diabetes, recent CM examinations, etc.) are often excluded (Barrett et al., 2006; Kuhn et al., 2008; Nguyen et al., 2008; Thomsen et al., 2008b). This bias in patient selection compared with coronary studies, where high-risk patients can not be excluded from life-saving procedures, may in part explain the illusive opinion that an IV CM injection implies a lesser risk of CIN than an IA. Thus, it may seem premature to consider the risk of CIN less following IV injections than after IA administration.

3. Evaluation of renal function

It is well recognized that serum creatinine is a poor predictor of renal function (Perrone et al., 1992), especially in elderly patients with decreasing muscle mass, the major source of creatinine. In one study 50% of patients ≥70 years with a normal serum creatinine had a GFR ≤50 mL/min (Duncan et al., 2001).

Measurement of GFR based on exogenous markers such as inulin and I-CM is regarded the best indices of the level of renal function in health and disease (Stevens et al., 2006), but is work-intensive, relatively expensive, time-consuming and therefore unsuitable in clinical practice prior to CM administration. Instead, GFR should be estimated (eGFR) taking into account not only serum creatinine but also anthropometric (weight and height) and/or demographic (gender and age) data as a measure of muscle mass by using dedicated GFR prediction equations (Stevens et al., 2006) such as the MDRD (Modification of Diet in Renal Disease) (Levey et al., 2007), CKD-EPI (Levey et al., 2009) and Lund-Malmö equations (Nyman et al., 2006). Consequently, newly developed CIN risk scores include eGFR using prediction equations (Bartholomew et al., 2004; Mehran et al., 2004). Before adapting a GFR prediction equation the following should be considered:

- The creatinine assay in the local laboratory must be calibrated according to the specific method used when the equation was developed, in practice isotope dilution mass spectrometry (IDMS) with modern equations (Myers et al., 2006).
- Dosing of drugs excreted by glomerular filtration should be based on GFR not adjusted for body surface area, i.e. absolute GFR in mL/min (Stevens et al., 2009). GFR adjusted to body surface area, i.e. relative GFR in mL/min/1.73 m^2, will overestimate actual GFR in small subjects, especially children, and underestimate it in large individuals. The MDRD and CKD-EPI equations primarily gives relative GFR, which can be converted to absolute GFR using a body surface area equation such as the commonly used Dubois formula (Dubois & Dubois, 1916 (DuBois & DuBois, 1916):

$$\text{Body surface area } (m^2) = \text{weight}^{0.425} \times (\text{height}^{0.725}) \times 0.007184$$

  with weight expressed in kg and height in cm.
- Estimated GFR is only within 30% of measured GFR in 80-85% of the patients (Levey et al., 2009; Nyman et al., 2006). Thus, a patient with eGFR of 50 mL/min may actually only have a real GFR of 35 mL/min.

4. Systemic drug exposure, gram-iodine/eGFR ratio and CIN

4.1 Area under the plasma concentration-time curve (AUC)

Following injection of CM, blood samples may be used to calculate AUC. It is directly proportional to CM dose and inversely correlated with GFR (Frennby & Sterner, 2002). AUC is a fundamental pharmacokinetic parameter used to estimate *systemic exposure* of drugs that are distributed and eliminated according to linear kinetics, like contrast media (Chen et al., 2001; Sherwin et al., 2005). The systemic exposure of such a drug is often well correlated with its *toxicity* and hence is generally held as an index for dose optimization (Chen et al., 2001). The clinical value of AUC as a predictor of nephrotoxicity has been shown for a variety of drugs and CM dose/GFR ratio was first proposed as a potential indicator for the risk of CIN in 1997 (Altmann et al., 1997) and later in 2005 (Nyman et al., 2005; Sherwin et al., 2005).

4.2 Gram-iodine/eGFR ratio

CM doses in CIN risk scores and recommendations to minimize the risk of CIN have for obscure reasons often been based only on volumes (Bartholomew et al., 2004; Davidson et al., 2006; Mehran et al., 2004). It should rather be expressed in terms of gram iodine (g-I) since concentrations of commercially available CM varies from 140-400 mg I/mL and it will also reflect the attenuating capacity. This also makes it easier to compare CM doses and expand the experience of CIN made from one examination or department to another if different concentrations are used. Furthermore, common g-I doses for radiography-based procedures, i.e. 10-120 g-I, are in the same numerical range as patients' GFR, i.e. 10-120 mL/min. Thus, forming a g-I/eGFR ratio combines CM volume and concentration, serum creatinine, age and body size into a single continuous risk variable, and provides the examiner with a simple numerical relationship and an expedient way to predict the risk of CIN. This implies also a more sophisticated relationship between CM dose and renal function than the Cigarroa formula (Cigarroa et al., 1989) that lacks CM concentration and uses serum creatinine instead of GFR; i.e. maximum CM volume = 5 mL × body weight/serum creatinine (mg/dL). From a female perspective, with a possible increased CIN-risk compared with males (Brown et al., 2008), the g-I/eGFR ratio is preferable since creatinine-based GFR prediction equation also contains coefficients for female gender, which is lacking in the Cigarroa formula.

Mounting evidence from coronary interventions indicate that a g-I/eGFR ratio roughly >1.0 represent a significant and independent predictor of CIN (Table 1). At a g-I/GFR ratio <1.0 the reported CIN frequency was <3% (Gurm et al, 2011; Laskey et al, 2007; Nyman et al, 2008).

First author, year	Number	Indication	Volume/ eGFR ratio	Iodine Concentration (mg I/mL)	g-I/eGFR ratio
Laskey, 2007	3179	Unselected population	3.7	350[2]	1.30[5]
Nyman, 2008	391	STEMI	2.91[1]	350	1.00
Nozue, 2009	60	Stable angina	5.1	370	1.89[5]
Worasuwannarak, 2010	248	Elective diabetics	2.60	370[3]	0.98
Mager, 2010	871	STEMI	3.7	370	1.37[5]
Liu et al, 2011	277	STEMI	2.39	370[4]	0.88[5]
Total	5026				
Weighted mean value			3.50		1.24

Table 1. Gram-iodine/eGFR ratio and CIN in coronary interventions. Studies defining CM-volume/eGFR ratio or gram-iodine/eGFR ratio as a significant and independent predictor of CIN (serum creatinine rise ≥25% or ≥44 μmol/L above baseline). Weighted mean value with individual study sizes as weights were finally calculated based on log-transformation of volume/eGFR and g-I/eGFR ratio. Absolute GFR was estimated in 3 reports (Laskey et al., 2007; Nyman et al., 2008; Worasuwannarak & Pornratanarangsi, 2010) and relative GFR in the remaining.

1. Calculated from the g-I/eGFR ratio and iodine concentration.
2. Anticipated mean concentration.
3. 96% 370 mg I/mL and 4% 320 mg I/mL (e-mail communication with the authors).
4. 271 patients 370 mg I/mL and 6 patients 320 mg I/mL (e-mail communication with the authors).
5. Calculated from the volume/eGFR ratio and iodine concentration.

A most recently published registry study involving about 50,000 patients recommended a planned gram-iodine dose restricted to 0.7 x eGFR value and not to exceed 1.0 x eGFR if a CM concentration of 350 mg I/mL for PCI is anticipated (Gurm et al., 2011).

Using a g-I/eGFR <1.0 implies a safer maximum dose compared with the Cigarroa formula. A 60-year old female with a height of 160 cm, weight 70 kg and serum creatinine of 150 μmol/mL (1.7 mg/dL) results in an eGFR of 31 mL/min if the IDMS-traceable MDRD equation is used (Levey et al., 2007). At a CM concentration of 350 mg I/mL, 31 grams of iodine will give a maximum CM volume of 88 mL (31,000/350). The corresponding figures in a male will be 41 grams of iodine and 118 mL. According to the Cigarroa formula the maximum volume will be 206 mL (5 × 70/1.7) for both females and males.

Individual patient data from CT studies are lacking, but weighted mean data from CT-studies shows an 8% incidence of CIN at a g-I/eGFR ratio of 0.9 (Table 2), indicating that the ratio should also be kept <1.0 also at CT.

First author, year	Type of CM	N	CM dose (gram iodine)	eGFR (^{A}mL/min or ^{R}mL/min/1.73 m^2)	g-I/eGFR ratio	CIN (%)
Tepel, 2000[1]	LOCM	42	23	^{A}34	0.7	21
Lufft, 2002	LOCM	33	49	^{A}63	0.8	9.1
Kolehemainen, 2003	LOCM/IOCM	50	35	$^{?}$29	1.2	16
Garcia-Ruiz, 2004	LOCM	50	48	^{A}30	1.6	4.0
Becker, 2005	LOCM	100	27	^{R}41	0.7	9.0
Barrett, 2006	LOCM/IOCM	150	40	^{A}45	1.0[2]	3.9
Thomsen, 2008b[3]	LOCM/IOCM	148	40	^{A}42	1.0	6.1
Nguyen, 2008	LOCM	56	37	^{A}53	0.7	28
Kuhn, 2008	LOCM/IOCM	248	36	^{R}49	0.7	5.2
Weisbord, 2008	LOCM	421	48	^{R}53	0.9	6.5
Total		1301				
Weighted mean data			40	47	0.9	7.8

Table 2. Gram-iodine/eGFR ratio and CIN in CT studies. Literature review of non-randomized and randomized CT-studies reporting mean gram-iodine dose (or volume and concentration), mean eGFR (A = absolute GFR, R = relative GFR), g-I/eGFR ratio (calculated by the author) and incidence of CIN (serum creatinine rise ≥25% or ≥44 μmol/L above baseline). Only results for low-osmolal contrast media (LOCM) included unless there was no significant difference between LOCM and IOCM (iso-osmolal contrast media). Weighted mean value with individual study sizes as weights were finally calculated. The weighted mean of the g-I/eGFR ratio was based on log-transformation.
1. Only control group not receiving acetylcysteine included
2. Based on individual data in the report
3. Based on the CIN definition ≥25% serum creatinine increase

Note that if GFR adjusted to body surface area is used to form the g-I/GFR ratio, a higher maximum dose may be permitted in small individuals while large individuals may tolerate a larger dose certain ratio would indicate. In addition analyzing g-I/GFR ratio as a significant independent predictor of CIN may give erroneous results. Half of the reports in Table 1 used relative eGFR (Liu et al., 2011; Mager et al., 2010; Nozue et al., 2009) and three of the ten studies in Table 2.

If a CM-based examination is deemed necessary in high risk patients, the author's strategy is to keep the g-I/GFR ratio as low as reasonably achievable, preferably below 0.5. Features classifying a patient at high risk of CIN (Kakkar et al., 2008; Mehran et al., 2004) may include:

- GFR <40 mL/min OR
- CIN risk score ≥16 (Table 3) or ≥three risk factors OR
- Congestive heart failure (NYHA III/IV) OR
- Multiple CM exposures within 72 hours

Risk factors	Integer score
Hypotension (<80 mm Hg for at least 1 h requiring inotropic support or intra-aortic balloon pump within 24 h periprocedurally)	5
Intra-aortic balloon pump	5
Congestive heart failure (New York Heart Association III/IV)	5
Age >75 years	4
Anemia (hematocrit value <39% for men and <36% for women)	3
Diabetes mellitus	3
Contrast medium volume	1 for each 100 mL
Serum creatinine >133 µmol/L (1.5 mg/dL)	4
GFR <60 mL/min/1.73 m^2 40-60 20-40 <20	2 4 6

Table 3. Mehran CIN risk score (Mehran et al., 2004).

5. Reducing CM doses in CT-angiography of azotemic patients

During the past decade, CTCA has become a clinical reality as a consequence of major advances in CT technology. Vascular enhancement in CT-angiography is dependent on a number of factors such as CM dose, injection rate, plasma volume, cardiac output (CO) and x-ray tube potential (Bae & Heiken, 2005; Fleischmann, 2003; Kormano et al., 1983; Kristiansson et al., 2010).

5.1 CM distribution volume and injected dose rate

The distribution volume of CM includes the plasma volume and the extravascular extracellular space, both related to body weight. By dosing CM in relation to body weight and using a fixed injection duration adapted to scan time, a fixed injected dose rate (mg I/kg/s) is obtained and vascular enhancement becomes essentially unrelated to body size (Awai et al., 2004a). When these principles are used, the choice of CM concentration is of no concern regarding CM enhancement (Awai et al., 2004b; Suzuki et al., 2004).

It may be anticipated that fixed CM doses irrespective of body weight have been adjusted to provide a proper enhancement in larger patients. Thus, dosing per kg implies that the risk of CIN may at least be reduced for low weight patients for the same enhancement as in a larger patient. In fact CM doses regarded sufficient for 80-100 kg patients could be halved for 40-50 kg patients to obtain the same degree of enhancement. A maximum dosing weight of 80-90 kg may be chosen, assuming that higher weights in most patients correspond to adipose tissue with minimal contribution to the distribution volume of CM.

Calculation of individual CM volumes and injection rates based on CM dose in milligram iodine/kg, concentration and injection duration can be easily done with a Microsoft Excel spreadsheet or using a dedicated computer program developed to calculate both eGFR and CM injection parameters from predefined CT protocols (OmniVis, GE Healthcare, Stockholm, Sweden).

5.2 Cardiac output and vascular CM enhancement

Arterial enhancement increases with decreasing CO (Bae et al., 1998) due to less dispersion and dilution of the CM bolus and at the same time poor cardiac function is an independent risk factor of CIN. Renal impairment may induce cardiac dysfunction and vice versa, the so called cardiorenal syndrome (Ronco et al., 2008). Since increasing age also predispose to decreasing renal function and cardiac diseases, many azotemic patients will have a reduced CO. Thus, it would be possible to decrease CM dose in most azotemic patients for the same vascular CM-enhancement as that obtained in patients with normal cardiac function. On the other hand a patient with no CIN risk factors and hyperkinetic circulation may need and tolerate a higher CM dose than normal to achieve diagnostic quality without jeopardizing renal function.

Since cardiac function may play a major role for CM-enhancement in CTCA and echocardiography results may be readily available in coronary patients, information of cardiac function should be used when tailoring the CM protocol. Another option is to use electrical velocimetry to measure CO, readily performed in the CT suite (Flinck et al., 2010). This has the advantage that measured CO will reflect cardiac function at the time of the CM injection. CO measured by echocardiography hours to days prior to CTCA may result in inadequate CM injection parameters, since CO is highly dependent on pulse rate and may vary considerably for number a of reasons.

5.3 X-ray tube potential and iodine attenuation

Attenuation of photons by iodine is highly dependent on the x-ray spectra used. As an example decreasing the x-ray tube peak kilovoltage (kVp) from commonly used 120 kVp for CT to 80 kVp brings the x-ray spectra closer to the k-edge of iodine (33.2 keV) and increases iodine attenuation by a factor 1.6 (Prokop, 2003). Thus, the CM dose may be reduced by a factor 1.6 while maintaining the attenuation at the same level as that obtained at 120 kVp.

However, the effective x-ray tube loading in terms of milliampere seconds (mAs) has to be increased by a factor four to keep image noise constant and results in 50% increase in radiation dose for the same reference object (Holmquist et al., 2009; Kristiansson et al., 2010). Thus, the diagnostic quality in terms of contrast-to-noise ratio (CNR) may be preserved. The increased radiation dose and risk of cancer induction may be of less concern in elderly azotemic patients with coronary artery disease and a limited survival time than the risk of CIN.

5.4 Halved CM doses at CT-angiography in azotemic patients

By combining CM dose tailored to body weight, a fixed injection time adapted to scan time, automatic bolus tracking, saline chaser, x-ray tube potential of 80 kVp and anticipating a decreased cardiac output in azotemic patients, it has been possible to halve the CM dose from 300 mg I/kg at 120 kVp and to 150 mg I/kg at 80 kVp when performing 16-row detector pulmonary CT-angiography in patients with eGFR <50 mL/min (Kristiansson et al., 2010). The median g-I/eGFR ratio was 0.3 and no CIN episodes were recorded. A total median dose of 10 grams of iodine was used, which is only 20-40% of non-body size related CM doses reported by those using 16-row detector for pulmonary CT-angiography at 120-140 kVp (Bae et al., 2005; Holmquist et al., 2009; Holmquist & Nyman, 2006; Johnson et al., 2007).

These principles should also be possible to adopt when performing CTCA in patients at high risk of CIN, especially with today's CT-equipments with many more detector rows, more potent x-ray tubes and dual energy options.

6. Percutaneous coronary angiography and interventions

The risk of CIN is related to the CM dose (Davidson et al., 2006; Freeman et al., 2002; Marenzi et al., 2009). Though there are numerous prophylactic studies on pharmacological agents, with hardly any unequivocally positive prophylactic effects so far (Stacul et al., 2006), studies on technical aspects of how to minimize the CM dose in coronary procedures are conspicuous by their almost total absence.

The average CM dose at PCA and/or PCI may range from 40 to 110 grams of iodine (Aspelin et al., 2003; Davidson et al., 2000; Laskey et al., 2007; Marenzi et al., 2009; Nyman et al., 2008; Rudnick et al., 1995; Worasuwannarak & Pornratanarangsi, 2010), while individual doses may range from 10 to inconceivable 500 grams of iodine (Marenzi et al., 2009).

In a Letter to the Editor Kane et al. (2008) reported on utilizing biplane angiography for PCA resulting in a mean CM dose of only 8 grams of iodine (25 mL 320 mg I/mL), half the dose used for monoplane. Despite a higher CIN risk profile among patients examined with biplane, the incidence of CIN was significantly lower compared with those studied with monoplane. Freeman et al. (2002) proposed guidelines for high-risk patients including determination of the "maximum allowed radiocontrast dose", limit necessary images (i.e. left ventriculogram or other images) and excessive "puffs", and whenever possible consider staged diagnostic and therapeutic procedures with several days in between. Another option to reduce CM dose is to use a lower concentration than the perfunctory 320 to 370 mg I/mL as discussed below.

6.1 Iodine concentration iso-attenuating with gadolinium CM

Attenuation increases with the atomic number (Z) of the atom (iodine, Z = 53; gadolinium, Z = 64). At photon energies between the k-edge of iodine (33.2 keV) and that of gadolinium (50.2 keV), iodine attenuates roughly twice as many photons as does gadolinium (Nyman et al., 2002). At all other photon energies the opposite prevail. Thus, a gadolinium (Gd) CM may be used as an x-ray CM. Before the advent of nephrogenic systemic fibrosis (NSF) (Thomsen, 2009), some investigators reported on the use of Gd-CM in a variety of diagnostic angiographic and interventional procedures (Spinosa et al., 2002; Strunk & Schild, 2004) including PCA (Barcin et al., 2006; Briguori et al., 2006; Gupta & Uretsky, 2005; Sarkis et al., 2003; Voss et al., 2004) in patients at risk of CIN due to its perceived non-nephrotoxicity (Prince et al., 1996). However, the non-nephrotoxicity of Gd-CM has been proved wrong (Buhaescu & Izzedine, 2008; Ergun et al., 2006; Sam et al., 2003). In fact, Gd-CM may have a higher, both general and renal, toxicity than I-CM in concentrations and volumes causing the same attenuation as Gd-CM (Elmståhl et al., 2004; Elmståhl et al., 2008; Nyman et al., 2002).

Moreover, the maximum dose of Gd-CM according to the manufacturers' recommendations is only 0.2-0.3 mmol/kg, though average doses used for x-ray angiographic procedures have ranged from 0.2-0.8 mmol/kg. However, average clinical I-CM doses of 40-100 grams of iodine, results in about 4-10 mmol/kg in a 75 kg individual. Thus, the use of Gd-CM is limited in terms of volume and radiodensity (Nyman et al., 2011). Despite this, diagnostic satisfactory PCA has been achieved with 1.0M Gd-CM (Briguori et al., 2006; Voss et al., 2004) or 2:1 (Barcin et al., 2006; Sarkis et al., 2003) and 1:1 mixtures (Gupta & Uretsky, 2005) of 0.5M Gd-CM and I-CM.

Angiographic experiments with a 30 cm thick water-equivalent phantom at 70 and 95 kVp indicate that iodine concentrations at 60 and 80 mg/mL, respectively, are iso-attenuating with 0.5M Gd-CM (Nyman et al., 2011). The attenuation of the 1.0M Gd-CM and the mixtures between 0.5M Gd-CM and I-CM at 320 or 350 mg I/mL would correspond to about 140-200 mg I/mL of a pure I-CM at 70-95 kVp, concentrations that are commercially available. Thus, it seems possible to perform coronary procedures with half or even one third of the standard concentrations, not at least in thinner patients patients in whom automatic or manual down-regulation of the x-ray tube potential will increase attenuation by iodine.

Precautions and techniques to save contrast media during PCA/PCI in azotemic patients are summarized as follows:

- If possible, delay examination, treat risk factors and institute hydration.
- Substitute echocardiography for left ventriculography.
- Use biplane technique if available.
- Consider to use commercially available concentrations in the range of 140-200 mg I/mL, especially in thinner patients.
- Avoid excessive "puffs" and scrutinize each series before the next one to avoid unnecessary standard projections.
- Substitute measurements with pressure wires of indeterminate stenotic lesions for multiple projections.

- Whenever possible consider staged diagnostic and therapeutic procedures with several days in between.

7. Conclusion

- Scientific evidence is lacking regarding the opinion that IV administration of CM should be less nephrotoxic than IA administration.
- Renal function should be estimated taking into account not only serum creatinine but also anthropometric (weight and height) and/or demographic (gender and age) by using dedicated GFR prediction equations.
- CM dose should be expressed in grams of iodine instead of simply volumes since it also takes into account concentration and serves as an index of diagnostic capacity.
- A g-I/eGFR ratio ≥1.0 appears to a significant and independent predictor of CIN in coronary interventions but it may also be valid for CT-angiography.
- If a CM examination is deemed necessary in patients at high risk of CIN, the author's goal is to keep the dose as low as reasonably achievable, preferably below a g-I/eGFR ratio of 0.5, which may be possible by applying a meticulous examination technique and the following CM doses and concentrations:
  - CT-angiography: 100-150 mg I/kg by using 80 kVp, mAs-compensation for constant CNR, fixed injection duration adapted to scan time, automatic bolus tracking and a saline chaser.
  - Coronary arteriography and interventions: 140-200 mg I/mL, especially in thinner patients in whom automatic or manual down-regulation of the x-ray tube potential will increase iodine attenuation.

8. References

Altmann DB, Zwas D, Spatz A, Bergman G, Spokojny A, Riva S, Sanborn TA (1997). Use of the contrast volume estimated creatinine clearance ratio to predict renal failure after angiography. *J Interv Cardiol,* Vol.10, pp. 113-119

Aspelin P, Aubry P, Fransson SG, Strasser R, Willenbrock R, Berg KJ (2003). Nephrotoxic effects in high-risk patients undergoing angiography. *N Engl J Med,* Vol.348, No.6, (2003 Feb 6), pp. 491-499, ISSN 1533-4406 (Electronic)

Awai K, Hiraishi K, Hori S (2004a). Effect of contrast material injection duration and rate on aortic peak time and peak enhancement at dynamic CT involving injection protocol with dose tailored to patient weight. *Radiology,* Vol.230, No.1, (2004 Jan), pp. 142-150, ISSN 0033-8419 (Print)

Awai K, Inoue M, Yagyu Y, Watanabe M, Sano T, Nin S, Koike R, Nishimura Y, Yamashita Y (2004b). Moderate versus high concentration of contrast material for aortic and hepatic enhancement and tumor-to-liver contrast at multi-detector row CT. *Radiology,* Vol.233, No.3, (2004 Dec), pp. 682-688, ISSN 0033-8419 (Print)

Bae KT, Heiken JP (2005). Scan and contrast administration principles of MDCT. *Eur Radiol,* Vol.15(Suppl 5), pp. E46-E59

Bae KT, Heiken JP, Brink JA (1998). Aortic and hepatic contrast medium enhancement at CT. Part II. Effect of reduced cardiac output in a porcine model. *Radiology,* Vol.207, No.3, (1998 Jun), pp. 657-662, ISSN 0033-8419 (Print)

Bae KT, Mody GN, Balfe DM, Bhalla S, Gierada DS, Gutierrez FR, Menias CO, Woodard PK, Goo JM, Hildebolt CF (2005). CT depiction of pulmonary emboli: display window settings. *Radiology,* Vol.236, No.2, (2005 Aug), pp. 677-684, ISSN 0033-8419 (Print)

Barcin C, Kursaklioglu H, Iyisoy A, Kose S, Tore HF, Isik E (2006). Safety of gadodiamide mixed with a small quantity of iohexol in patients with impaired renal function undergoing coronary angiography. *Heart Vessels,* Vol.21, No.3, (2006 May), pp. 141-145, ISSN 0910-8327 (Print)

Barrett BJ, Carlisle EJ (1993). Metaanalysis of the relative nephrotoxicity of high- and low-osmolality iodinated contrast media. *Radiology,* Vol.188, No.1, (1993 Jul), pp. 171-178, ISSN 0033-8419 (Print)

Barrett BJ, Katzberg RW, Thomsen HS, Chen N, Sahani D, Soulez G, Heiken JP, Lepanto L, Ni ZH, Nelson R (2006). Contrast-induced nephropathy in patients with chronic kidney disease undergoing computed tomography: a double-blind comparison of iodixanol and iopamidol. *Invest Radiol,* Vol.41, No.11, (2006 Nov), pp. 815-821, ISSN 0020-9996 (Print)

Bartholomew BA, Harjai KJ, Dukkipati S, Boura JA, Yerkey MW, Glazier S, Grines CL, O'Neill WW (2004). Impact of nephropathy after percutaneous coronary intervention and a method for risk stratification. *Am J Cardiol,* Vol.93, No.12, (2004 Jun 15), pp. 1515-1519, ISSN 0002-9149 (Print)

Becker CR, Reiser MF (2005). Use of iso-osmolar nonionic dimeric contrast media in multidetector row computed tomography angiography for patients with renal impairment. *Invest Radiol,* Vol.40, No.10, (2005 Oct), pp. 672-675, ISSN 0020-9996 (Print)

Biondi-Zoccai GG, Lotrionte M, Abbate A, Testa L, Remigi E, Burzotta F, Valgimigli M, Romagnoli E, Crea F, Agostoni P (2006). Compliance with QUOROM and quality of reporting of overlapping meta-analyses on the role of acetylcysteine in the prevention of contrast associated nephropathy: case study. *BMJ,* Vol.332, No.7535, (Jan 28), pp. 202-209, ISSN 1468-5833 (Electronic), 0959-535X (Linking)

Briguori C, Colombo A, Airoldi F, Melzi G, Michev I, Carlino M, Montorfano M, Chieffo A, Bellanca R, Ricciardelli B (2006). Gadolinium-based contrast agents and nephrotoxicity in patients undergoing coronary artery procedures. *Catheter Cardiovasc Interv,* Vol.67, No.2, (2006 Feb), pp. 175-180, ISSN 1522-1946 (Print)

Brown JR, DeVries JT, Piper WD, Robb JF, Hearne MJ, Ver Lee PM, Kellet MA, Watkins MW, Ryan TJ, Silver MT, Ross CS, MacKenzie TA, O'Connor GT, Malenka DJ (2008). Serious renal dysfunction after percutaneous coronary interventions can be predicted. *Am Heart J,* Vol.155, No.2 pp. 260-266, ISSN 1097-6744 (Electronic), 0002-8703 (Linking)

Buhaescu I, Izzedine H (2008). Gadolinium-induced nephrotoxicity. *Int J Clin Pract,* Vol.62, No.7, (2008 Jul), pp. 1113-1118, ISSN 1742-1241 (Electronic), 1368-5031 (Linking)

Chen M-L, Lekso L, Williams R (2001). Measures of exposure versus measures of rate and extent of absorption. *Clin Pharmacokinet,* Vol.40, pp. 565-572

Cigarroa RG, Lange RA, Williams RH, Hillis LD (1989). Dosing of contrast material to prevent contrast nephropathy in patients with renal disease. *Am J Med,* Vol.86, No.6 Pt 1, (1989 Jun), pp. 649-652, ISSN 0002-9343 (Print)

Davidson CJ, Laskey WK, Hermiller JB, Harrison JK, Matthai W, Jr., Vlietstra RE, Brinker JA, Kereiakes DJ, Muhlestein JB, Lansky A, Popma JJ, Buchbinder M, Hirshfeld JW, Jr.

(2000). Randomized trial of contrast media utilization in high-risk PTCA: the COURT trial. *Circulation,* Vol.101, No.18 pp. 2172-2177, ISSN 1524-4539 (Electronic), 0009-7322 (Linking)

Davidson CJ, Stacul F, McCullough PA, Tumlin J, Adam A, Lameire N, Becker CR (2006). Contrast medium use. *Am J Cardiol,* Vol.98, No.6A, (2006 Sep 18), pp. 42K-58K, ISSN 0002-9149 (Print)

DuBois D, DuBois E (1916). A formula to estimate the approximate surface area if height and weight be known. *Arch Intern Med,* Vol.17, pp. 863-871

Duncan L, Heathcote J, Djurdjev O, Levin A (2001). Screening for renal disease using serum creatinine: who are we missing? *Nephrol Dial Transplant,* Vol.16, No.5, (2001 May), pp. 1042-1046, ISSN 0931-0509 (Print)

Elmståhl B, Nyman U, Leander P, Chai CM, Frennby B, Almén T (2004). Gadolinium contrast media are more nephrotoxic than a low osmolar iodine medium employing doses with equal X-ray attenuation in renal arteriography: an experimental study in pigs. *Acad Radiol,* Vol.11, No.11, (2004 Nov), pp. 1219-1228, ISSN 1076-6332 (Print)

Elmståhl B, Nyman U, Leander P, Golman K, Chai CM, Grant D, Doughty R, Pehrson R, Bjork J, Almen T (2008). Iodixanol 320 results in better renal tolerance and radiodensity than do gadolinium-based contrast media: arteriography in ischemic porcine kidneys. *Radiology,* Vol.247, No.1, (2008 Apr), pp. 88-97, ISSN 1527-1315 (Electronic)

Ergun I, Keven K, Uruc I, Ekmekci Y, Canbakan B, Erden I, Karatan O (2006). The safety of gadolinium in patients with stage 3 and 4 renal failure. *Nephrol Dial Transplant,* Vol.21, No.3, (2006 Mar), pp. 697-700, ISSN 0931-0509 (Print)

Fleischmann D (2003). Use of high-concentration contrast media in multiple-detector-row CT: principles and rationale. *Eur Radiol,* Vol.13 Suppl 5, (2003 Dec), pp. M14-20, ISSN 0938-7994 (Print)

Flinck M, Graden A, Milde H, Flinck A, Hellstrom M, Bjork J, Nyman U (2010). Cardiac output measured by electrical velocimetry in the CT suite correlates with coronary artery enhancement: a feasibility study. *Acta Radiol,* Vol.51, No.8, (Oct), pp. 895-902, ISSN 1600-0455 (Electronic), 0284-1851 (Linking)

Freeman RV, O'Donnell M, Share D, Meengs WL, Kline-Rogers E, Clark VL, DeFranco AC, Eagle KA, McGinnity JG, Patel K, Maxwell-Eward A, Bondie D, Moscucci M (2002). Nephropathy requiring dialysis after percutaneous coronary intervention and the critical role of an adjusted contrast dose. *Am J Cardiol,* Vol.90, No.10 pp. 1068-1073, ISSN 0002-9149 (Print), 0002-9149 (Linking)

Frennby B, Sterner G (2002). Contrast media as markers of GFR. *Eur Radiol,* Vol.12, No.2, (2002 Feb), pp. 475-484, ISSN 0938-7994 (Print)

From AM, Al Badarin FJ, McDonald FS, Bartholmai BJ, Cha SS, Rihal CS (2010). Iodixanol versus low-osmolar contrast media for prevention of contrast induced nephropathy: meta-analysis of randomized, controlled trials. *Circ Cardiovasc Interv,* Vol.3, No.4 pp. 351-358, ISSN 1941-7632 (Electronic), 1941-7640 (Linking)

From AM, Bartholmai BJ, Williams AW, Cha SS, McDonald FS (2008). Mortality associated with nephropathy after radiographic contrast exposure. *Mayo Clin Proc,* Vol.83, No.10, (2008 Oct), pp. 1095-1100, ISSN 1942-5546 (Electronic)

Garcia-Ruiz C, Martinez-Vea A, Sempere T, Sauri A, Olona M, Peralta C, Oliver A (2004). Low risk of contrast nephropathy in high-risk patients undergoing spiral computed tomography angiography with the contrast medium iopromide and prophylactic oral hydratation. *Clin Nephrol,* Vol.61, No.3, (Mar), pp. 170-176, ISSN 0301-0430 (Print), 0301-0430 (Linking)

Gupta R, Uretsky BF (2005). Gadodiamide-based coronary angiography in a patient with severe renal insufficiency. *J Interv Cardiol,* Vol.18, No.5, (2005 Oct), pp. 379-383, ISSN 0896-4327 (Print)

Gurm HS, Dixon SR, Smith DE, Share D, LaLonde T, Greenbaum A, Moscucci M (2011). Renal function-based contrast dosing to define safe limits of radiographic contrast media in patients undergoing percutaneous coronary interventions. *J Am Coll Cardiol,* Vol.58, pp. 907-914.

Holmquist F, Hansson K, Pasquariello F, Bjork J, Nyman U (2009). Minimizing Contrast Medium Doses to Diagnose Pulmonary Embolism with 80-kVp Multidetector Computed Tomography in Azotemic Patients. *Acta Radiol,* Vol.50, (2009 Jan 23), pp. 181-193, ISSN 1600-0455 (Electronic)

Holmquist F, Nyman U (2006). Eighty-peak kilovoltage 16-channel multidetector computed tomography and reduced contrast-medium doses tailored to body weight to diagnose pulmonary embolism in azotaemic patients. *Eur Radiol,* Vol.16, No.5, (2006 May), pp. 1165-1176, ISSN 0938-7994 (Print)

Johnson PT, Naidich D, Fishman EK (2007). MDCT for suspected pulmonary embolism: multi-institutional survey of 16-MDCT data acquisition protocols. *Emerg Radiol,* Vol.13, No.5, (2007 Feb), pp. 243-249, ISSN 1070-3004 (Print)

Kakkar R, Sobieszczyk P, Binkert CA, Faxon DP, Mortele KJ, Singh AK (2008). Prevention of intravenous contrast-induced nephropathy in hospital inpatients. *Crit Pathw Cardiol,* Vol.7, No.1, (Mar), pp. 1-4, ISSN 1535-2811 (Electronic), 1535-2811 (Linking)

Kane GC, Doyle BJ, Lerman A, Barsness GW, Best PJ, Rihal CS (2008). Ultra-low contrast volumes reduce rates of contrast-induced nephropathy in patients with chronic kidney disease undergoing coronary angiography. *J Am Coll Cardiol,* Vol.51, No.1, (2008 Jan 1), pp. 89-90, ISSN 1558-3597 (Electronic), 0735-1097 (Linking)

Karlsberg RP, Dohad SY, Sheng R (2011). Contrast Medium-induced Acute Kidney Injury: Comparison of Intravenous and Intraarterial Administration of Iodinated Contrast Medium. *J Vasc Interv Radiol,* pp. 1-7, Epub ahead of print, doi: 10.1016/j.jvir.2011.03.020, ISSN 1535-7732 (Electronic), 1051-0443 (Linking)

Katzberg RW, Barrett BJ (2007). Risk of iodinated contrast material--induced nephropathy with intravenous administration. *Radiology,* Vol.243, No.3, (2007 Jun), pp. 622-628, 0033-8419 (Print)

Katzberg RW, Newhouse JH (2010). Intravenous contrast medium-induced nephrotoxicity: is the medical risk really as great as we have come to believe? *Radiology,* Vol.256, No.1, (Jul), pp. 21-28, ISSN 1527-1315 (Electronic), 0033-8419 (Linking)

Kelly AM, Dwamena B, Cronin P, Bernstein SJ, Carlos RC (2008). Meta-analysis: effectiveness of drugs for preventing contrast-induced nephropathy. *Ann Intern Med,* Vol.148, No.4, (2008 Feb 19), pp. 284-294, ISSN 1539-3704 (Electronic)

Kolehemainen H, Sovia M (2003). Comparison of Xenetix 300 and Visipaque 320 in patients with renal failure (P27). 10th European Symposium on Urogenital Radiology. *Euro Radiol,* Vol.13, pp. B32-B33

Kormano M, Partanen K, Soimakallio S, Kivimaki T (1983). Dynamic contrast enhancement of the upper abdomen: effect of contrast medium and body weight. *Invest Radiol,* Vol.18, No.4, (1983 Jul-Aug), pp. 364-367, ISSN 0020-9996 (Print)

Kristiansson M, Holmquist F, Nyman U (2010). Ultralow contrast medium doses at CT to diagnose pulmonary embolism in patients with moderate to severe renal impairment. A feasibility study. *Eur Radiol,* Vol.20, No.6, pp. 1321-1330

Kuhn MJ, Chen N, Sahani DV, Reimer D, van Beek EJ, Heiken JP, So GJ (2008). The PREDICT study: a randomized double-blind comparison of contrast-induced nephropathy after low- or isoosmolar contrast agent exposure. *AJR Am J Roentgenol,* Vol.191, No.1, (2008 Jul), pp. 151-157, ISSN 1546-3141 (Electronic)

Laskey WK, Jenkins C, Selzer F, Marroquin OC, Wilensky RL, Glaser R, Cohen HA, Holmes DR, Jr. (2007). Volume-to-creatinine clearance ratio: a pharmacokinetically based risk factor for prediction of early creatinine increase after percutaneous coronary intervention. *J Am Coll Cardiol,* Vol.50, No.7, (2007 Aug 14), pp. 584-590, ISSN 1558-3597 (Electronic)

Levey AS, Coresh J, Greene T, Marsh J, Stevens LA, Kusek JW, Van Lente F (2007). Expressing the Modification of Diet in Renal Disease Study equation for estimating glomerular filtration rate with standardized serum creatinine values. *Clin Chem,* Vol.53, No.4, (2007 Apr), pp. 766-772, ISSN 0009-9147 (Print)

Levey AS, Stevens LA, Schmid CH, Zhang YL, Castro AF, 3rd, Feldman HI, Kusek JW, Eggers P, Van Lente F, Greene T, Coresh J (2009). A new equation to estimate glomerular filtration rate. *Ann Intern Med,* Vol.150, No.9, (2009 May 5), pp. 604-612, ISSN 1539-3704 (Electronic), 1539-3704 (Linking)

Liu Y, Tan N, Zhou YL, He PC, Luo JF, Chen JY (2011). The contrast medium volume to estimated glomerular filtration rate ratio as a predictor of contrast-induced nephropathy after primary percutaneous coronary intervention. *Int Urol Nephrol,* (Feb 20), Epub ahead of print, doi:10.1007/s11255-11011-19910-11254, ISSN 1573-2584 (Electronic), 0301-1623 (Linking)

Lufft V, Hoogestraat-Lufft L, Fels LM, Egbeyong-Baiyee D, Tusch G, Galanski M, Olbricht CJ (2002). Contrast media nephropathy: intravenous CT angiography versus intraarterial digital subtraction angiography in renal artery stenosis: a prospective randomized trial. *Am J Kidney Dis,* Vol.40, No.2, (Aug), pp. 236-242, ISSN 1523-6838 (Electronic), 0272-6386 (Linking)

Mager A, Assa HV, Lev EI, Bental T, Assali A, Kornowski R (2010). The ratio of contrast volume to glomerular filtration rate predicts outcomes after percutaneous coronary intervention for ST-segment elevation acute myocardial infarction. *Catheter Cardiovasc Interv,* (Oct 14), Epub ahead of print, doi: 10.1002/ccd.22828, ISSN 1522-726X (Electronic), 1522-1946 (Linking)

Marenzi G, Assanelli E, Campodonico J, Lauri G, Marana I, De Metrio M, Moltrasio M, Grazi M, Rubino M, Veglia F, Fabbiocchi F, Bartorelli AL (2009). Contrast volume during primary percutaneous coronary intervention and subsequent contrast-induced nephropathy and mortality. *Ann Intern Med,* Vol.150, No.3 pp. 170-177, ISSN 1539-3704 (Electronic), 0003-4819 (Linking)

Marenzi G, Lauri G, Assanelli E, Campodonico J, De Metrio M, Marana I, Grazi M, Veglia F, Bartorelli AL (2004). Contrast-induced nephropathy in patients undergoing primary angioplasty for acute myocardial infarction. *J Am Coll Cardiol,* Vol.44, No.9, (2004 Nov 2), pp. 1780-1785, ISSN 0735-1097 (Print)

McCullough PA, Adam A, Becker CR, Davidson C, Lameire N, Stacul F, Tumlin J (2006a). Epidemiology and prognostic implications of contrast-induced nephropathy. *Am J Cardiol,* Vol.98, No.6A, (2006 Sep 18), pp. 5K-13K, ISSN 0002-9149 (Print)

McCullough PA, Adam A, Becker CR, Davidson C, Lameire N, Stacul F, Tumlin J (2006b). Risk prediction of contrast-induced nephropathy. *Am J Cardiol,* Vol.98, No.6A, (2006 Sep 18), pp. 27K-36K, ISSN 0002-9149 (Print)

Mehran R, Aymong ED, Nikolsky E, Lasic Z, Iakovou I, Fahy M, Mintz GS, Lansky AJ, Moses JW, Stone GW, Leon MB, Dangas G (2004). A simple risk score for prediction of contrast-induced nephropathy after percutaneous coronary intervention: development and initial validation. *J Am Coll Cardiol,* Vol.44, No.7, (2004 Oct 6), pp. 1393- ISSN 1399, 0735-1097 (Print)

Mehran R, Nikolsky E (2006). Contrast-induced nephropathy: definition, epidemiology, and patients at risk. *Kidney Int Suppl,* Vol.69, No.100, (2006 Apr), pp. S11-15, ISSN 0098-6577 (Print)

Mitchell AM, Jones AE, Tumlin JA, Kline JA (2010). Incidence of contrast-induced nephropathy after contrast-enhanced computed tomography in the outpatient setting. *Clin J Am Soc Nephrol,* Vol.5, No.1 pp. 4-9, ISSN 1555-905X (Electronic), 1555-9041 (Linking)

Myers GL, Miller WG, Coresh J, Fleming J, Greenberg N, Greene T, Hostetter T, Levey AS, Panteghini M, Welch M, Eckfeldt JH (2006). Recommendations for improving serum creatinine measurement: a report from the Laboratory Working Group of the National Kidney Disease Education Program. *Clin Chem,* Vol.52, No.1, (2006 Jan), pp. 5-18, ISSN 0009-9147 (Print)

Nash K, Hafeez A, Hou S (2002). Hospital-acquired renal insufficiency. *Am J Kidney Dis,* Vol.39, No.5, (2002 May), pp. 930-936, ISSN 1523-6838 (Electronic)

Nguyen SA, Suranyi P, Ravenel JG, Randall PK, Romano PB, Strom KA, Costello P, Schoepf UJ (2008). Iso-osmolality versus low-osmolality iodinated contrast medium at intravenous contrast-enhanced CT: effect on kidney function. *Radiology,* Vol.248, No.1, (2008 Jul), pp. 97-105, ISSN 1527-1315 (Electronic)

Nozue T, Michishita I, Iwaki T, Mizuguchi I, Miura M (2009). Contrast medium volume to estimated glomerular filtration rate ratio as a predictor of contrast-induced nephropathy developing after elective percutaneous coronary intervention. *J Cardiol,* Vol.54, No.2, (Oct), pp. 214-220, ISSN 1876-4738 (Electronic), 0914-5087 (Linking)

Nyman U, Almen T, Aspelin P, Hellström M, Kristiansson M, Sterner G (2005). Contrast-medium-Induced nephropathy correlated to the ratio between dose in gram iodine and estimated GFR in ml/min. *Acta Radiol,* Vol.46, No.8, (2005 Dec), pp. 830-842, ISSN 0284-1851 (Print)

Nyman U, Björk J, Aspelin P, Marenzi G (2008). Contrast medium dose-to-GFR ratio: A measure of systemic exposure to predict contrast-induced nephropathy after percutaneous coronary intervention. *Acta Radiol* Vol.49, pp. 658-667,

Nyman U, Björk J, Sterner G, Bäck SE, Carlson J, Lindström V, Bakoush O, Grubb A (2006). Standardization of p-creatinine assays and use of lean body mass allow improved prediction of calculated glomerular filtration rate in adults: a new equation. *Scand J Clin Lab Invest,* Vol.66, No.6, (2006), pp. 451-468, ISSN 0036-5513 (Print)

Nyman U, Elmstahl B, Geijer H, Leander P, Almen T, Nilsson M (2011). Iodine contrast iso-attenuating with diagnostic gadolinium doses in CTA and angiography results in ultra-low iodine doses. A way to avoid both CIN and NSF in azotemic patients? *Eur Radiol,* Vol.21, (Aug 29), pp. 326-336, ISSN 1432-1084 (Electronic), 0938-7994 (Linking)

Nyman U, Elmståhl B, Leander P, Nilsson M, Golman K, Almén T (2002). Are gadolinium-based contrast media really safer than iodinated media for digital subtraction angiography in patients with azotemia? *Radiology*, Vol.223, No.2, (2002 May), pp. 311-318; discussion 328-319, ISSN 0033-8419 (Print)

Perrone RD, Madias NE, Levey AS (1992). Serum creatinine as an index of renal function: new insights into old concepts. *Clin Chem*, Vol.38, No.10, (1992 Oct), pp. 1933-1953, ISSN 0009-9147 (Print)

Polena S, Yang S, Alam R, Gricius J, Gupta JR, Badalova N, Chuang P, Gintautas J, Conetta R (2005). Nephropathy in critically Ill patients without preexisting renal disease. *Proc West Pharmacol Soc*, Vol.48, (2005), pp. 134-135, ISSN 0083-8969 (Print)

Prince MR, Arnoldus C, Frisoli JK (1996). Nephrotoxicity of high-dose gadolinium compared with iodinated contrast. *J Magn Reson Imaging*, Vol.6, No.1, (1996 Jan-Feb), pp. 162-166, ISSN 1053-1807 (Print), 1053-1807 (Linking)

Prokop M (2003). Image analysis In: *Spiral and multislice computed tomography of the body*. Prokop M, Galanski M, Van der Molen AJ, Schaefer-Prokop C, Thieme, ISBN 3-13-116481-6, Stuttgart

Ronco C, Haapio M, House AA, Anavekar N, Bellomo R (2008). Cardiorenal syndrome. *J Am Coll Cardiol*, Vol.52, No.19, (Nov 4), pp. 1527-1539, ISSN 1558-3597 (Electronic), 0735-1097 (Linking)

Rudnick MR, Goldfarb S, Wexler L, Ludbrook PA, Murphy MJ, Halpern EF, Hill JA, Winniford M, Cohen MB, VanFossen DB (1995). Nephrotoxicity of ionic and nonionic contrast media in 1196 patients: a randomized trial. The Iohexol Cooperative Study. *Kidney Int*, Vol.47, No.1, (1995 Jan), pp. 254-261, ISSN 0085-2538 (Print)

Sam AD, 2nd, Morasch MD, Collins J, Song G, Chen R, Pereles FS (2003). Safety of gadolinium contrast angiography in patients with chronic renal insufficiency. *J Vasc Surg*, Vol.38, No.2, (2003 Aug), pp. 313-318, ISSN 0741-5214 (Print)

Sarkis A, Badaoui G, Azar R, Sleilaty G, Bassil R, Jebara VA (2003). Gadolinium-enhanced coronary angiography in patients with impaired renal function. *Am J Cardiol*, Vol.91, No.8, (2003 Apr 15), pp. 974-975, A974, ISSN 0002-9149 (Print)

Sherwin PF, Cambron R, Johnson JA, Pierro JA (2005). Contrast dose-to-creatinine clearance ratio as a potential indicator of risk for radiocontrast-induced nephropathy: correlation of D/CrCL with area under the contrast concentration-time curve using iodixanol. *Invest Radiol*, Vol.40, No.9, (2005 Sep), pp. 598-603, ISSN 0020-9996 (Print)

Spinosa DJ, Angle JF, Hartwell GD, Hagspiel KD, Leung DA, Matsumoto AH (2002). Gadolinium-based contrast agents in angiography and interventional radiology. *Radiol Clin North Am*, Vol.40, No.4, (2002 Jul), pp. 693-710, ISSN 0033-8389 (Print), 0033-8389 (Linking)

Stacul F, Adam A, Becker CR, Davidson C, Lameire N, McCullough PA, Tumlin J (2006). Strategies to reduce the risk of contrast-induced nephropathy. *Am J Cardiol*, Vol.98, No.6A, (2006 Sep 18), pp. 59K-77K, ISSN 0002-9149 (Print)

Sterner G, Nyman U, Valdes T (2001). Low risk of contrast-medium-induced nephropathy with modern angiographic technique. *J Intern Med*, Vol.250, No.5, (2001 Nov), pp. 429-434, ISSN 0954-6820 (Print), 0954-6820 (Linking)

Stevens LA, Coresh J, Greene T, Levey AS (2006). Assessing kidney function--measured and estimated glomerular filtration rate. *N Engl J Med*, Vol.354, No.23, (2006 Jun 8), pp. 2473-2483, ISSN 1533-4406 (Electronic)

Stevens LA, Nolin TD, Richardson MM, Feldman HI, Lewis JB, Rodby R, Townsend R, Okparavero A, Zhang YL, Schmid CH, Levey AS (2009). Comparison of drug dosing recommendations based on measured GFR and kidney function estimating equations. *Am J Kidney Dis,* Vol.54, No.1 pp. 33-42, ISSN 1523-6838 (Electronic), 0272-6386 (Linking)

Strunk HM, Schild H (2004). Actual clinical use of gadolinium-chelates for non-MRI applications. *Eur Radiol,* Vol.14, No.6, (2004 Jun), pp. 1055-1062, ISSN 0938-7994 (Print), 0938-7994 (Linking)

Suzuki H, Oshima H, Shiraki N, Ikeya C, Shibamoto Y (2004). Comparison of two contrast materials with different iodine concentrations in enhancing the density of the the aorta, portal vein and liver at multi-detector row CT: a randomized study. *Eur Radiol,* Vol.14, No.11, (2004 Nov), pp. 2099-2104, ISSN 0938-7994 (Print)

Tepel M, van der Giet M, Schwarzfeld C, Laufer U, Liermann D, Zidek W (2000). Prevention of radiographic-contrast-agent-induced reductions in renal function by acetylcysteine. *N Engl J Med,* Vol.343, No.3, (Jul 20), pp. 180-184, ISSN 0028-4793 (Print), 0028-4793 (Linking)

Thomsen HS (2009). Nephrogenic systemic fibrosis: history and epidemiology. *Radiol Clin North Am,* Vol.47, No.5, (2009 Sep), pp. 827-831, ISSN 1557-8275 (Electronic), 1557-8275 (Linking)

Thomsen HS, Morcos SK, Almén T, Aspelin P, Liss P, Bellin M-F, Oyen R, den Braber ET, Flaten H, Idée J-M, Löwe A, Jakobsen JÅ, Spinazzi A, Stacul F, Webb JA, van der Molen A (2008a). European Society of Urogenital Radiology Contrast Media Safety Committee. ESUR guidelines on contrast media version 7.0. 23.06.2011, Available from http://www.esur.org

Thomsen HS, Morcos SK, Erley CM, Grazioli L, Bonomo L, Ni Z, Romano L (2008b). The ACTIVE Trial: Comparison on the effects on renal function of iomeprol-400 and iodixanol-320 in patients with chronic kidney disease undergoing abdominal computed tomography. *Invest Radiol,* Vol.43, pp. 170-178

Voss R, Grebe M, Heidt M, Erdogan A (2004). Use of gadobutrol in coronary angiography. *Catheter Cardiovasc Interv,* Vol.63, No.3, (2004 Nov), pp. 319-322, ISSN 1522-1946 (Print)

Weisbord SD, Mor MK, Resnick AL, Hartwig KC, Palevsky PM, Fine MJ (2008). Incidence and outcomes of contrast-induced AKI following computed tomography. *Clin J Am Soc Nephrol,* Vol.3, No.5, (2008 Sep), pp. 1274-1281, ISSN 1555-905X (Electronic)

Worasuwannarak S, Pornratanarangsi S (2010). Prediction of contrast-induced nephropathy in diabetic patients undergoing elective cardiac catheterization or PCI: role of volume-to-creatinine clearance ratio and iodine dose-to-creatinine clearance ratio. *J Med Assoc Thai,* Vol.93 Suppl 1, (Jan), pp. S29-34, ISSN 0125-2208 (Print), 0125-2208 (Linking)

Zoungas S, Ninomiya T, Huxley R, Cass A, Jardine M, Gallagher M, Patel A, Vasheghani-Farahani A, Sadigh G, Perkovic V (2009). Systematic review: sodium bicarbonate treatment regimens for the prevention of contrast-induced nephropathy. *Ann Intern Med,* Vol.151, No.9, (Nov 3), pp. 631-638, ISSN 1539-3704 (Electronic), 0003-4819 (Linking)

11

Pharmacotherapy During Percutaneous Coronary Interventions

David C. Yang and Dmitriy N. Feldman
Greenberg Division of Cardiology, New York Presbyterian Hospital, Weill Cornell Medical College, New York, NY USA

1. Introduction

Percutaneous arterial catheterization and transluminal dilatation of stenotic vessels were first described by Charles T. Dotter and Melvin P. Judkins in their seminal paper published in 1964 (1). With the advent of contemporary coronary angioplasty and stenting techniques for patients with coronary artery disease (CAD) and acute coronary syndromes (ACS), the procedure has now been termed percutaneous coronary intervention (PCI). While PCI has done much in the modern era to improve patient outcomes in the face of acute myocardial infarction as well as in disabling cardiac angina, its benefits can still be limited by peri-procedural complications such as acute vessel closure and stent thrombosis as well as conditions occurring after 30 days post-PCI, such as in-stent restenosis or late stent thrombosis. Additionally, catheter and wire associated thrombus formation can occur during PCI in the absence of adequate anticoagulation. Excess anticoagulation on the other hand carries a risk of major gastrointestinal or intracranial bleeding as well as vascular access bleeding complications. Stent thrombosis is a rare, but serious complication of PCI and usually presents as death or ST-elevation myocardial infarction. Coronary stents are generally made of stainless steel or cobalt chromium alloys rendering them thrombogenic until they are completely covered by endothelial tissue. The timing of complete endothelialization is variable and depends on whether the implanted stent is bare metal or drug-eluting, as well as which type of anti-proliferative drug the stent is coated with. Stent thrombosis can be described based on its timing relative to stent placement and is associated with a number of different risk factors (Table 1). Acute stent thrombosis occurs within 24 hours of PCI and in one pooled analysis, approximately 80 percent of all bare metal stent (BMS) thromboses occurred within this acute period (2). Subacute stent thrombosis occurs up to 30 days after PCI and this time period encompasses the majority of all thrombotic events observed in both BMS and drug-eluting stents (DES) (3). Stent thrombosis after 30 days and up to one year post-PCI is referred to as late stent thrombosis and seems to occur with equal frequency in BMS and DES, particularly in the absence or cessation of dual anti-platelet therapy with aspirin or clopidogrel (4-5). Occurring even less commonly at greater than one year post-PCI, very late stent thrombosis appears to be associated with DES more than BMS and is thought to be related to delayed neo-intimal coverage as well as ongoing vessel inflammation (6). Current ACC/AHA guidelines make a number of recommendations regarding the concurrent use of antiplatelet, antithrombotic, and thrombolytic pharmacotherapy during PCI to prevent such complications. The goal of this chapter will be to describe different therapeutic agents available to clinicians during PCI and to summarize the most current guidelines regarding their use.

2. Anti-platelet agents

2.1 Aspirin

Aspirin causes an irreversible inactivation of the cyclooxygenase-1 enzyme required for prostaglandin and thromboxane synthesis, which in turn diminishes platelet aggregation. The use of aspirin for secondary prevention has been shown to decrease overall mortality in patients with established CAD or a CAD equivalent such as diabetes (7-10). Meanwhile, the net benefit for its use in primary prevention is less certain and needs to be weighed against individual risk for major gastrointestinal or extra-cranial bleeding (11). Extensive studies have also shown significant reductions in mortality and morbidity with the use of aspirin in unstable angina (UA) as well as in both non-ST-elevation myocardial infarction (NSTEMI) and ST-elevation myocardial infarction (STEMI). In one of the earliest trials from the Results of a Veterans Administration Cooperative Study, Lewis et al. reported a 51% reduction in incidence of death or acute MI as well as a 50% reduction in rates of nonfatal MI in patients with UA who received aspirin (12). These findings were reproduced in subsequent studies and helped to solidify the role for the use of aspirin in UA (13-14). The RISC trial evaluated the role of aspirin in both NSTEMI and UA patients and again demonstrated that aspirin was associated with a significant reduction in the combined endpoint of death and MI with differences persisting beyond one-year providing evidence for the long-term benefit of aspirin in NSTE-ACS (15). The landmark trial ISIS-2 then expanded the role of aspirin use to standard therapy in STEMI (16). ISIS-2 randomized 17,187 patients presenting with acute STEMI to streptokinase, aspirin, both therapies, or neither, and demonstrated an additive effect of aspirin to thrombolytic therapy. Currently, the ACC/AHA guidelines for the management of UA, NSTEMI and STEMI recommend immediate treatment with aspirin for all patients for indefinite duration (17). The recommendations for the use of aspirin in PCI with stenting are derived from several early clinical trials in which treatment with high dose aspirin (650 mg to 990 mg/day) along with dipyridamole or ticlopidine in percutaneous transluminal coronary angioplasty (PTCA) was compared to placebo. Patients who were treated with aspirin-based regimens uniformly had better outcomes with significant reductions in peri-procedural complications including abrupt vessel closure, dissection or MI (18-19). Pre-treatment with aspirin monotherapy was tested against aspirin plus dipyridamole and shown to have an independent beneficial effect (20). Subsequent studies comparing high-dose versus low-dose aspirin (1500 mg vs. 80 mg/day) prior to PTCA showed no difference in the incidence of MI or in the rate of major complications and restenosis (21). The most current ACC/AHA recommendations for the use of aspirin in PCI are that higher dose aspirin (300 mg to 325 mg) be given at least 2 hours before PCI as well as for at least 1 month after BMS implantation, 3 months after sirolimus-eluting stent implantation, and 6 months after paclitaxel-eluting stent implantation (17).

2.2 Ticlopidine

Thienopyridines block the adenosine diphosphate (ADP) receptor P2Y12 on platelet surfaces thereby decreasing platelet activation and aggregation (see section on platelet function testing below). Ticlopidine was the first widely used thienopyridine that began to have an antiplatelet effect within 24 to 48 hours after its administration. The STAIG trial was one of the first multicenter trials to evaluate the role of thienopyridines, particularly ticlopidine, in ACS (22). 652 patients with UA were randomized within 48 hours of presentation to conventional medical therapy alone versus ticlopidine in addition to conventional treatment. Ticlopidine use was associated with a reduction in vascular mortality by 46.8% (4.8% vs. 8.9%) and MI by 53.2% (5.1% vs. 10.9%). Further randomized trials such as STARS, MATTIS, ISAR, and FANTASTIC compared antiplatelet therapy with ticlopidine and aspirin to conventional anticoagulant therapy with heparin or warfarin in PCI with bare metal stenting and demonstrated a clear reduction in stent thrombosis, death, MI, or emergent CABG (23-26). Ticlopidine use, however, has been associated with significant side effects including thrombocytopenia, neutropenia and thrombotic thrombocytopenic purpura-hemolytic uremic syndrome (TTP-HUS); thus it is crucial that biweekly monitoring of blood counts be performed for four months after initiation of ticlopidine (27-28).

2.3 Clopidogrel

Due to the unfavorable side effect profile of ticlopidine, interest began to develop in clopidogrel as a potential thienopyridine alternative. The efficacy of clopidogrel in the treatment of CAD had already been demonstrated in the CAPRIE trial in which clopidogrel use significantly reduced the combined endpoint of ischemic stroke, MI and vascular death in patients with atherosclerotic disease (29). Clopidogrel's overall safety benefit as compared to ticlopidine was then convincingly demonstrated in the CLASSICS trial and a meta-analysis later found that clopidogrel use was at least as efficacious as ticlopidine with fewer major adverse cardiac events (MACE) as well as a lower incidence of mortality (30-31). Based on these findings, clopidogrel replaced ticlopidine as the thienopyridine of choice in combination with aspirin as standard therapy after PCI. Several landmark trials then fully expanded the application of clopidogrel therapy to ACS and PCI. Investigators in the CURE trial found a 20% reduction in the primary combined endpoint of cardiovascular death, MI, or stroke (9.3% vs. 11.4%) in 12,562 patients with NSTE-ACS when treated with combined aspirin and clopidogrel as compared to aspirin alone (32). When the subset of patients undergoing PCI was analyzed separately in the PCI-CURE substudy, pre-treatment with clopidogrel plus aspirin prior to PCI led to both immediate and long-term benefits in reducing ischemic vascular events and death (33-34). The CREDO trial later confirmed the benefit of upstream clopidogrel therapy in more than 2,100 patients who were randomized to receive either clopidogrel at a 300 mg loading dose or placebo 3 to 24 hours before elective PCI, followed by 75 mg/day for 28 days in both groups and then either clopidogrel or placebo out to one year according to the original randomization (35). The results from CREDO also proved the benefits of long-term clopidogrel therapy by finding a 26.9% relative risk reduction in the combined end point of death, MI, or stroke at one year (8.5% vs. 11.5%, 95% CI 3.9-44.4). Two additional randomized trials, CLARITY-TIMI 28 and COMMIT/CCS-2, then demonstrated that clopidogrel therapy when added to aspirin also improved outcomes in patients with STEMI being treated with fibrinolytics and heparin (36-37).

With the role of clopidogrel now clearly defined in all forms of ACS as well as PCI, the timing and dose of clopidogrel pre-treatment for PCI came under question. In a pre-specified sub-group analysis, the PCI-CLARITY trial found that early treatment with clopidogrel (300 mg) led to significantly better outcomes in all time groups ranging from within 6 hours before PCI to as far as 96 hours ahead of PCI (38). A substudy from CREDO, however, found that the benefit was only seen if clopidogrel (300 mg) was given 10 to 12 hours before PCI and did not become significant unless given >15 hours prior to PCI, with a maximum effect seen at 24 hours (39).

Since pre-treatment with clopidogrel for >15 hours prior to PCI is not always practical in situations of ACS or ad hoc decisions to stent at the time of diagnostic angiography, the issue was raised as to whether higher loading doses of clopidogrel could be beneficial by increasing the level of platelet inhibition or by decreasing the time required until its maximum antiplatelet effects were achieved. In an unselected cohort of over 1,000 patients, who were given a 600 mg dose of clopidogrel, in vitro studies found that maximum platelet inhibition was seen by two hours and additional testing showed that clopidogrel 600 mg dosing seemed to achieve more intense levels of peak platelet inhibition when compared with the conventional 300 mg dose (40-41). Several large studies then sought to evaluate whether these pharmacodynamic differences could translate into improved patient outcomes. The ARMYDA-2 trial randomized 255 patients with stable angina or NSTE-ACS to either 600 mg or 300 mg of clopidogrel given four to eight hours prior to PCI (42). By 30 days, the composite endpoint of death, MI, or target vessel revascularization (TVR) occurred in only 4% of the 600 mg group as compared to 12% in the 300-mg group, a difference that was entirely driven by rates of peri-procedural MI ($p < 0.05$). No differences were reported in the rates of major bleeding between the two groups. The benefit of a clopidogrel 600 mg loading dose was seen again in a subgroup analysis from the HORIZONS-AMI trial in which 3,602 patients with STEMI undergoing primary PCI were randomized to either bivalirudin or unfractionated heparin (UFH) plus a glycoprotein (GP) IIb/IIIa inhibitor (43). Clopidogrel loading doses of either 300 mg (1,153 patients) or 600 mg (2,158 patients) were chosen at the clinician's discretion and after multivariable analysis, the 600 mg dose was found to be an independent predictor of lower rates of 30-day MACE without higher bleeding. The CURRENT-OASIS 7 trial then randomized over 25,000 patients with ACS (29.2% STEMI) who were referred for an invasive strategy and compared the regimen of double dose clopidogrel (600 mg loading dose followed by 150 mg daily for six days and then 75 mg daily thereafter) versus standard dose clopidogrel (300 mg loading dose followed by 75 mg daily) (44). The investigators found that while there was no significant difference in the primary outcome of cardiovascular death, MI or stroke at 30 days (4.2% in the double dose group vs. 4.4% in the standard dose group; HR 0.94; 95% CI 0.83-1.06; $p = 0.30$), double dose clopidogrel was associated with a significant reduction in the secondary outcome of stent thrombosis in the greater than 17,000 patients who underwent PCI (1.6% vs. 2.3%; HR 0.68; 95% CI 0.55-0.85; $p=0.001$). Notably, major bleeding occurred significantly more in the double dose group (2.5% vs. 2.0%; HR 1.24; 95% CI 1.05-1.46; $p=0.01$). Several subsequent smaller studies including ISAR-CHOICE, ALBION, and PREPAIR have attempted to look at whether even higher loading doses of clopidogrel (900 mg and 1200 mg) might carry additional benefit when compared to the 600 mg and 300 mg doses (45-47). These studies found that while treatment with increasing doses of clopidogrel did in fact result in greater levels of platelet inhibition, clinical endpoints such as MACE and troponin release were not statistically different. At this point, larger prospective trials evaluating clinical outcomes are needed before clopidogrel loading doses above 600 mg can be justified.

With regards to timing of double-dose clopidogrel pre-treatment, the ISAR-REACT trial showed that among 2,159 patients undergoing PCI, a clopidogrel 600 mg loading dose could be given as early as as 2 hours prior to PCI without detrimental effects when compared to longer durations of pre-treatment (2 to 3 hours, 3 to 6 hours, 6 to 12 hours, > 12 hours) (48). Similarly, the PRAGUE-8 and ARMYDA-5 PRELOAD trials reported no differences in outcomes when clopidogrel 600 mg was given to patients with stable angina or NSTE-ACS either before (mean of 19 and 6 hours respectively) or immediately after diagnostic coronary angiography, but prior to PCI (49-50).

The RELOAD and ARMYDA-4 RELOAD trials attempted to address the question of whether an additional loading dose of clopidogrel was required prior to PCI in stable and ACS patients who were already receiving chronic clopidogrel therapy (51-52). The trials found that although clopidogrel reloading produced significantly greater levels of platelet inhibition, there was no difference in the primary endpoint of MACE. A subgroup analysis, however, showed that when reloaded with clopidogrel 600 mg, there was a significant benefit in patients with ACS who underwent PCI. While there is not enough evidence to make definitive recommendations regarding this issue, it may be reasonable to reload patients receiving chronic clopidogrel therapy with clopidogrel 600 mg prior to PCI for ACS or if their risk for stent thrombosis is high.

2.4 Prasugrel

Despite the increasing use of higher doses of clopidogrel, there are still many cases of breakthrough thrombotic events in patients receiving standard dual antiplatelet therapy (32). Limitations of clopidogrel therapy are thought to be due to its delayed onset of action, modest platelet inhibition effects, and a wide range of inter-individual variability with regards to platelet responsiveness. Prasugrel is a third-generation thienopyridine and like clopidogrel, also requires biotransformation to its active metabolite before binding to P2Y12 receptors and inhibiting platelet aggregation. In contrast to clopidogrel however, prasugrel has been shown to achieve greater levels of platelet inhibition more rapidly and more consistently among healthy individuals as well as in patients with CAD and those who are undergoing PCI (53-55). The JUMBO-TIMI 26 trial was a phase 2 randomized study of 904 patients designed to assess the safety of prasugrel when administered at the time of PCI and the results of this trial showed no difference in the rates of clinically significant bleeding events (56). In PRINCIPLE-TIMI 44, 201 subjects were randomized to either prasugrel 60 mg or clopidogrel 600 mg as a loading dose one half hour prior to elective PCI, and then to either prasugrel 10 mg or clopidogrel 150 mg as a maintenance dose (57). The prasugrel groups were found to achieve significantly greater levels of platelet inhibition in both the loading and maintenance phases. To assess prasugrel's clinical efficacy, the landmark TRITON-TIMI 38 trial enrolled 13,608 patients with moderate- to high-risk ACS (including both NSTE-ACS and STEMI) undergoing PCI and randomly assigned patients to either prasugrel (60 mg loading dose followed by 10 mg maintenance dose) or clopidogrel (300 mg loading dose followed by 75 mg maintenance dose) (58). At 15 month follow-up, prasugrel reduced the composite endpoint of death, nonfatal MI or nonfatal stroke by 20% in comparison to clopidogrel (9.9% vs. 12.1%; HR 0.81; 95% CI 0.73-0.90; $p<0.001$) with the majority of the difference driven by lower rates of nonfatal MI (7.4% vs. 9.7%). Stent thrombosis was also significantly reduced with prasugrel (1.1% vs. 2.4%; $p<0.001$), however, the risk for bleeding in all categories was significantly increased including major bleeding (2.4% vs. 1.8%; $p=0.03$), life-threatening bleeding (1.4% vs. 0.9%; $p=0.01$), and fatal hemorrhage (0.4% vs. 0.1%; $p=0.002$). Risk factors for bleeding included age ≥75 years, history of stroke or TIA, and body weight <60 kg. Overall mortality did not differ significantly between the treatment groups.

The 2009 ACC/AHA Joint STEMI/PCI updated guidelines recommend that in patients with ACS in whom PCI is planned, a loading dose of either clopidogrel of at least 300 to 600 mg (Class I, Level of Evidence C) or prasugrel 60 mg (provided there are no contraindications) (Class I, Level of Evidence B) be given as soon as possible. For STEMI patients who have received fibrinolytic therapy, clopidogrel at a loading dose of either 300 or 600 mg should be given followed by clopidogrel as the thienopyridine of choice for maintenance therapy (Class I, Level of Evidence C). The choice and duration of maintenance therapy for ACS patients receiving a BMS or DES should be either clopidogrel 75 mg daily (Class I, Level of Evidence B) or prasugrel 10 mg daily (provided there are no contraindications) (Class I, Level of Evidence B) for at least 12 months unless the risk of morbidity due to bleeding outweighs the anticipated benefit of thienopyridine therapy, at which point earlier discontinuation should be considered (Class I, Level of Evidence C). In patients in whom coronary artery bypass grafting (CABG) is planned and can be delayed, it is recommended that clopidogrel be withdrawn for at least 5 days (Class I, Level of Evidence B) and prasugrel for at least 7 days (Class I, Level of Evidence C) unless the need for revascularization and/or the net benefit of the thienopyridine outweighs the risks of bleeding (Class I, Level of Evidence C). Age ≥ 75 years, history of TIA or stroke, and active major bleeding are contraindications to prasugrel therapy. Body weight < 60 kg is a relative contraindication to prasugrel therapy and consideration of lowering the maintenance dose from 10 mg to 5 mg daily should be given, though the safety and efficacy of the 5 mg dose have not been established (17).

2.5 Ticragrelor

Ticragrelor is an oral antiplatelet agent from the cyclopentyltriazolopyrimidine class that reversibly binds the ADP-P2Y12 platelet receptor. Like prasugrel, it is known to produce a more rapid and intense reduction in platelet function when compared to clopidogrel. In the PLATO trial, 18,624 patients with ACS (38% STEMI) were randomized to either ticragrelor (180 mg loading dose followed by 90 mg twice daily) or clopidogrel (300 to 600 mg loading dose followed by 75 mg daily) in addition to chronic aspirin therapy (59). At 12 months, ticragrelor therapy was associated with a significant reduction in the primary efficacy endpoint of cardiovascular death, MI or stroke (9.8% vs. 11.7%; HR 0.84; 95% CI 0.77-0.92; $p<0.001$). Importantly, the rate of death from any cause was reduced in the ticagrelor group (4.5% vs. 5.9% with clopidogrel, $p<0.001$). Furthermore, there were no significant differences in the rates of major bleeding, although ticagrelor was associated with a higher rate of bleeding not related to CABG. The STEMI patients in PLATO, when analyzed separately, also showed a benefit of ticagrelor over clopidogrel with trends consistent with the overall PLATO trial. In addition, ticagrelor reduced rates of MI alone, total mortality, and stent thrombosis. The reductions in stent thrombosis (ST) for ticagrelor versus clopidogrel were 1.6% vs. 2.4% (definite ST, $p=0.03$), 2.6% vs. 3.4% (definite or probable ST), and 3.3% vs. 4.3% (definite, probable, or possible ST). A subgroup analysis of patients with chronic kidney disease found that ticragrelor produced a more pronounced reduction in the primary endpoint when compared to patients with normal renal function as well as an overall decrease in total mortality (60).

3. Anti-thrombotic agents

3.1 Unfractionated heparin

Unfractionated heparin (UFH) inhibits platelet aggregation and fibrin formation by accelerating the action of antithrombin, which in turn inactivates factors IIa, IXa, and Xa. The evidence for UFH therapy in UA and NSTE-ACS has been well defined in early trials such as RISC and ATACS (61-65), however, the benefits in acute STEMI are less clear. Current ACC/AHA guidelines on the management of acute STEMI recommend intravenous UFH therapy for all patients treated with a fibrin-specific fibrinolytic agent (alteplase, tenecteplase, reteplase) or a non-fibrin-specific agent (streptokinase, urokinase, anistreplase) if the risk for systemic embolization is high (large or anterior MI, atrial fibrillation, prior embolus, or known left ventricular thrombus). The goal for activated partial thromboplastin time (aPTT) should be 1.5 to 2.0 times control or between 50-70 seconds. The benefit of adjunctive UFH with fibrinolytic therapy is thought to be due to its effect on maintaining infarct vessel patency as there is limited data regarding any improvements in either mortality or reinfarction (66-69). In patients being referred for PCI, current guidelines recommend intravenous treatment with UFH (17). UFH use during PCI is believed to reduce the risk for acute vessel closure as well as catheter or wire thrombosis and has been extrapolated from data obtained from PTCA prior to the era of coronary stenting and dual anti-platelet therapy (70). The 2005 ACC/AHA/SCAI guidelines for PCI recommend that in patients not receiving a glycoprotein (GP) IIb/IIIa inhibitor, UFH should be given using a bolus of 70 to 100 IU/kg to target an activated clotting time (ACT) between 250 to 350 seconds. For patients who are receiving a GP IIb/IIIa inhibitor, heparin bolus should be lowered to 50 to 70 IU/kg to achieve an ACT of 200 to 250 seconds (71). Heparin monitoring during PCI is generally done with ACT instead of aPTT as the anticoagulation levels required during the procedure are frequently too high for aPTT to track. An alternative strategy endorsed by the 2005 European Society of Cardiology guidelines for PCI was a single bolus of 100 IU/kg without ACT monitoring (72). The routine use of UFH after uncomplicated procedures has not been shown to reduce stent thrombosis and is not recommended given its association with increased rates of bleeding and vascular access complications. UFH use can cause autoimmune heparin-induced thrombocytopenia, a rare but potentially lethal complication associated with thrombosis. Treatment includes prompt withdrawal of UFH or low molecular weight heparin (LMWH) and initiation of alternative anticoagulation therapy (argatroban, lepirudin, bivalirudin).

3.2 Low-Molecular-Weight Heparin

Low-molecular-weight heparin (LMWH), like UFH, prevents clot propagation, but possesses several advantages over UFH due to different mechanisms of action. The ratio of anti-Xa/anti-IIa activity is significantly higher in LMWH compared to UFH, thereby inhibiting thrombin generation more effectively with potentially less bleeding. Suppression of the release of von Willebrand factor also augments LMWH's anticoagulant effect.

Increased bioavailability leads to a longer duration of systemic anticoagulation and less binding to plasma proteins and produces a more consistent anticoagulant effect. Several trials including FRISC, FRIC, FRAXIS, TIMI 11-B, and ESSENCE have found that treatment with LMWH is at least as effective as UFH across a spectrum of ACS patients while maintaining a comparable safety profile (73-79). The efficacy and safety of LMWH in PCI as compared to UFH was studied in over 10,000 patients with NSTE-ACS being referred for early invasive strategy in the SYNERGY trial (80). While enoxaparin use was shown to be non-inferior to UFH, it was associated with a significantly higher rate of major bleeding (9.1% vs. 7.6%). STEEPLE, a trial designed to assess the safety of enoxaparin (a single intravenous bolus of either 0.50 or 0.75 mg/kg prior to PCI) compared to UFH in over 2,500 patients undergoing elective PCI was terminated early due to an excess mortality rate among the patients receiving lower dose enoxaparin (81). As such, the 2005 ACC/AHA/SCAI guideline update for PCI recommends UFH as first line antithrombotic therapy in patients undergoing PCI except in patients with heparin-induced thrombocytopenia (Class I, Level of Evidence C). LMWH is a reasonable alternative in patients with UA/NSTEMI (Class IIa, Level of Evidence B) and in patients with STEMI (Class IIb, Level of Evidence B) (71).

3.3 Fondaparinux

Fondaparinux, a selective inhibitor of factor Xa, was tested against UFH in 350 patients undergoing urgent or elective PCI in the ASPIRE pilot trial and was found to have similar efficacy and safety outcomes (82). This issue was further examined in the much larger OASIS-6 trial, which included over 12,000 STEMI patients split into two strata based on whether UFH was indicated or not (83). Stratum 1 in which UFH was not indicated consisted of 5,658 patients most of whom had received fibrinolytic therapy with streptokinase and in whom adequate reperfusion was achieved and PCI was not planned. Stratum 2 consisted of 6,434 patients in whom UFH was indicated (those who received a fibrin-specific fibrinolytic agent, those in whom adequate reperfusion was not achieved, or those in whom primary PCI was planned). Patients in each stratum were then randomized to receive either fondaparinux or placebo. Although there was an overall decrease in the primary endpoint of death or reinfarction with fondaparinux (9.7% vs. 11.2%), investigators found that this effect was driven mainly by a significant reduction in events in the stratum that did not receive heparin or primary PCI and that there was actually a trend towards worse outcomes with fondaparinux in the stratum of patients who received heparin and were treated with primary PCI. Fondaparinux use was also associated with a higher rate of catheter related thrombosis as well as coronary complications during PCI such as acute vessel closure, no reflow phenomenon, and dissection. Therefore, the 2007 focused update of the ACC/AHA/SCAI guidelines for PCI do not recommend fondaparinux use as the sole anticoagulant to support PCI and when used should be supplemented with another agent that has anti-IIa activity such as UFH or bivalirudin (84).

3.4 Direct thrombin inhibitors

Direct thrombin inhibitors (e.g., hirudin, bivalirudin, lepirudin) inactivate thrombin by binding directly to its catalytic site and hold several advantages over UFH in that antithrombin is not required as a cofactor allowing clot-bound thrombin to be inactivated

(85). Additionally, there is no thrombin-mediated activation of platelets. Hirudin, a naturally occurring peptide derived from the saliva of the medicinal leech has been studied in patients with ACS undergoing reperfusion therapy with fibrinolytics or PCI (TIMI-9B, GUSTO-IIB, HELVETICA) and found to have no benefit when compared to UFH with comparable rates of major bleeding (86-88). The pilot trial HERO reproduced a similar finding with bivalirudin, a synthetic peptide that directly inhibits free and clot-bound thrombin (89). When given concurrently with streptokinase, bivalirudin was more effective than UFH in producing early infarct-related artery patency (TIMI grade 3 flow) without increasing the risk of major bleeding. The follow up HERO-2 mortality trial found that bivalirudin had similar rates of mortality at 30 days (10.5% vs. 10.9% with UFH, OR 0.99) with a small reduction in reinfarction at 96 hours (1.6% vs. 2.3%) and a nonsignificant trend toward more severe bleeding (0.6% vs. 0.4%) (90). The 2004 AHA/ACC guidelines on the management of STEMI state that it is reasonable to consider bivalirudin as an alternative to UFH in patients with heparin-induced thrombocytopenia and who are treated with streptokinase.

The role of bivalirudin in primary PCI was evaluated in the HORIZONS-AMI trial in which 3,602 patients with STEMI undergoing primary PCI were randomized to receive treatment with either UFH plus a GP IIb/IIIa inhibitor or to treatment with bivalirudin alone with provisional GP IIb/IIIa inhibitor (91). The investigators found that anticoagulation with bivalirudin alone resulted in lower rates of MACE at 30 days (9.2% vs. 12.1%; RR 0.76; 95% CI 0.63-0.92; p=0.005), major bleeding (4.9% vs. 8.3%; RR 0.60; 95% CI 0.46-0.77; p<0.001), 30-day death from cardiac causes (1.8% vs. 2.9%; RR 0.62; 95% CI 0.40-0.95; p=0.03), and 30-day overall mortality (2.1% vs. 3.1%; RR 0.66; 95% CI 0.44-1.00; p=0.047). There was a concern about a significant 1% increase in acute stent thrombosis seen within 24 hours, however, the rates for stent thrombosis at 30 days were similar in both groups. Bivalirudin was further examined in the REPLACE-2, ISAR-REACT 3, and ACUITY randomized trials evaluating patients across a broad spectrum of disease (stable CAD to high-risk ACS) undergoing PCI (92-94). The results of these trials solidified bivalirudin's favorable safety and efficacy profile when compared to UFH plus a GP IIb/IIIa inhibitor by demonstrating the non-inferiority of bivalirudin in preventing ischemic complications after PCI along with a reduction in rates of major bleeding. Additionally, a meta-analysis of randomized trials revealed that bivalirudin use provided greater absolute benefits in the prevention of ischemic and bleeding complications in patients with renal insufficiency (95). In the 2009 Focused Update of the ACC/AHA guidelines for the management of patients with STEMI/PCI, bivalirudin was added as an acceptable anticoagulant for primary PCI (Class I, Level of Evidence B) as well as in STEMI patients undergoing PCI who are at high risk of bleeding (Class IIa, Level of Evidence B) (17).

3.5 Glycoprotein IIb/IIIa inhibitors

Glycoprotein (GP) IIb/IIIa is an integrin receptor expressed on the surface membrane of platelets that undergoes a conformational change following platelet activation allowing it to bind to fibrinogen and cross-link with other platelets. This forms the basis for platelet aggregation and the pathologic vascular thrombosis seen in ACS. Three GP IIb/IIIa inhibitors are currently approved for use in ACS and PCI although much of the evidence supporting their use was established in the era prior to dual oral antiplatelet therapy.

Abciximab is the Fab fragment of a human-murine monoclonal antibody directed at the GP IIb/IIIa receptor. A number of clinical trials have attempted to evaluate its use in patients undergoing PCI for stable angina or ACS. These include EPIC, EPILOG, CAPTURE, RAPPORT, ADMIRAL, ISAR-2, ISAR-REACT, ISAR-SWEET, CADILLAC, ACE, EPISTENT, and ERASER (96-107). Pooled analyses of several of these trials have found that abciximab significantly reduced the incidence of 30-day death and MI when compared to placebo (HR 0.55; 95% CI 0.43-0.69; p<0.001) (108). This benefit was found regardless of the type of coronary intervention used including balloon angioplasty, elective stenting, bail-out stenting, and directional atherectomy, without an increase in significant bleeding complications. Protection from major adverse outcomes with abciximab continued out to six months and was independent of gender and a significant mortality benefit persisted at three years (6.4% vs. 5.0%; HR 0.78; 95% CI 0.63-0.98; p=0.03) (109-110). In the BRAVE-3 study, 800 patients presenting within 24 hours of STEMI were treated with aspirin, clopidogrel 600 mg, and randomized to either abciximab or placebo given prior to primary PCI. There were no significant differences between the two groups with respect to the primary endpoint of infarct size as measured by single-photon emission computed tomography (SPECT) or in 30 day MACE (111).

Tirofiban is a non-peptide molecule that exhibits dose dependent inhibition of the GP IIb/IIIa receptor. The RESTORE trial randomized 2,139 patients with ACS undergoing PTCA with balloon angioplasty or directional atherectomy to either placebo or tirofiban (10 µg/kg/3 min intravenous bolus followed by continuous infusion of 0.15 µg/kg/min for 36 hours) (112). The composite end point (death from any cause, MI, bypass surgery for angioplasty failure or recurrent ischemia necessitating repeat PCI) was reduced by tirofiban at two days (RR 38%; p<0.005) and at seven days (RR 27%; p=0.022) post-PTCA however this reduction was no longer statistically significant at 30 days (10.3% vs. 12.2%; p=0.16) and at 6 month follow up (113). The ADVANCE trial then evaluated whether higher doses of tirofiban would confer a benefit in 202 patients with ACS undergoing primary PCI (114). Patients were randomly assigned to either placebo or tirofiban (25 µg/kg/3 min bolus plus 0.15 µg/kg/min continuous infusion for 24 to 48 hours). The results of this study showed that treatment with high dose tirofiban produced a significant reduction in the primary endpoint of death, MI, target vessel revascularization, or bailout use of a GP IIb/IIIa inhibitor (35% vs. 20%; HR 0.51; 95% CI 0.29-0.88; p=0.01). The difference was driven by a reduction in MI and bailout use of GP IIb/IIIa inhibitors with no significant effect on mortality. Bleeding rates were comparable between tirofiban and placebo. Subgroup analyses found that while patients with ACS benefited from tirofiban use, those with stable angina did not. Diabetics also appeared to gain a benefit with tirofiban while nondiabetics did not. Upstream use of tirofiban prior to PCI in patients with STEMI was evaluated in three trials: TIGER-PA, ON-TIME, and ON-TIME 2 (115-117). These trials demonstrated that tirofiban use was generally associated with improved electrocardiographic endpoints such as resolution of ST-segment elevations with no increase in the risk of major or minor bleeding. In the ON-TIME 2 trial, approximately 1,000 patients with STEMI were randomized to pre-treatment with either high dose tirofiban or placebo prior to PCI and while there was an improvement in ST-segment resolution in the tirofiban group, there was no significant difference between the two groups in angiographic variables such as Thrombolysis in Myocardial Infarction (TIMI) grade 3 flow or blush grade. Later results from ON-TIME 2 however reported a significant reduction in 30 day MACE in the tirofiban group (5.8% vs. 8.6%; p=0.043) that was maintained at 1-year follow up (3.7% vs. 5.8%; p=0.08) (118).

Eptifibatide is a synthetic, nonimmunogenic cyclic heptapeptide inhibitor of GP IIb/IIIa with an active pharmacophore which is derived from the structure of barbourin, a GP IIb/IIIa inhibitor isolated from the venom of the Southeastern pigmy rattlesnake (119). It has a rapid onset of action with a plasma half-life of 10-15 minutes making its antiplatelet effect rapidly reversible. Its use in ACS and PCI has been evaluated in several clinical trials. In the PURSUIT trial, 10,948 patients were randomized to eptifibatide or placebo in conjunction with UFH and aspirin (120). By four days, the combined endpoint of death and nonfatal MI were reduced by 1.5% in the eptifibatide group (14.2% vs. 15.7%; p=0.04). More remarkably, this benefit was apparent as early as 96 hours and persisted through 30 days with a greater benefit observed in patients undergoing early angioplasty (121). In the IMPACT-II trial of 4,010 patients undergoing elective, urgent or emergent PCI, treatment with eptifibatide during PCI reduced the rates of early abrupt vessel closure and ischemic events by 30 days (122). The benefits of eptifibatide have also been shown in patients undergoing elective PCI, as seen in the ESPRIT trial that randomized 2,064 patients to pre-treatment with placebo or ebtifibatide prior to PCI (123). The trial was terminated early for efficacy as pre-treatment with ebtifibatide led to a significant reduction in the primary end point of death, MI, urgent revascularization, or need for bail-out GP IIb/IIIa inhibitor at 48 hours (6.6% vs. 10.5%; p=0.0015) as well as at 30 days (6.8% vs. 10.5%; p=0.0034). With regards to safety endpoints, bleeding rates with eptifibatide were equivalent to placebo in IMPACT-II (4.8% vs. 5.1%), although severe bleeding without hemorrhagic stroke was increased in PURSUIT (11.6% vs. 9.2%) (104, 106). Additionally, a pooled analysis of eight randomized control trials showed that eptifibatide did not significantly increase the rate of thrombocytopenia compared to placebo (124).

The general benefits of intravenous GP IIb/IIIa inhibitors have been evaluated in a meta-analysis pooling data from 21 trials involving patients with a broad range of CAD (125). The study reported that GP IIb/IIIa inhibitor use produced significant reductions in the combined end point of 30-day death, MI, or urgent revascularization in patients undergoing PCI (7.8% vs. 11.6%), patients with NSTE-ACS (11.4% vs. 12.8%), and patients with acute STEMI who underwent angioplasty (3.9% vs. 7.8%). The benefits of adjunctive GP IIb/IIIa inhibitors in acute STEMI remain uncertain however. As discussed in the section on bivalirudin, the HORIZONS-AMI trial randomized 3,602 patients with STEMI undergoing primary PCI to UFH with a GP IIb/IIIa inhibitor (either abciximab or eptifibatide) or to bivalirudin alone with provisional GP IIb/IIIa (91). All patients were treated with aspirin and a thienopyridine prior to PCI. Of the 1,661 patients who were randomized to treatment with UFH, 757 received a double bolus of eptifibatide and 863 received abciximab. In the bivalirudin alone plus provisional GP IIb/IIIa arm, only 53 of 1,674 patients received eptifibatide and 72 received abciximab. At 30 days, the primary endpoint of MACE as well as major bleeding was higher in the group that received UFH and a GP IIb/IIIa inhibitor as compared to bivalirudin alone. A subgroup analysis of the UFH plus GP IIb/IIIa group compared those treated with eptifibatide and abciximab and found that there was no significant difference in the incidence of stent thrombosis at one year (126).

With regards to the timing of adjunctive GP IIb/IIIa use in patients undergoing PCI for acute STEMI, a meta-analysis of six randomized trials including TIGER-PA and ON-TIME found that early administration (prior to transfer to catheterization laboratory) as compared to late (at the time of PCI) improved measures of coronary patency as well as clinical outcomes (127). The FINESSE trial also addressed the issue of timing of GP IIb/IIIa inhibitor therapy. In the trial, 2,453 patients with STEMI were randomized to pre-PCI treatment with a half-dose fibrinolytic agent plust abciximab, pre-PCI abciximab alone, or abciximab at the time of PCI (128). The primary endpoint was composite death, ventricular fibrillation occurring over 48 hours after randomization, cardiogenic shock and congestive heart failure during the first 90 days after randomization. The results of this trial showed no benefit and perhaps a trend towards more bleeding with abciximab pre-treatment as compared to abciximab given at the time of PCI.

With regards to its safety profile, there does appear to be an increased risk of bleeding with the use of intravenous GP IIb/IIIa inhibitors, however a pooled analysis of 14 randomized trials including approximately 28,000 patients found no difference in the incidence of intracerebral hemorrhage when comparing heparin plus any GP IIb/IIIa inhibitor to heparin plus placebo (0.12% vs. 0.09%, OR 1.3), or when comparing a GP IIb/IIIa inhibitor alone with heparin alone (129).

When deciding between agents for use in PCI, it is unclear whether one GP IIb/IIIa inhibitor holds any significant advantage in clinical efficacy over another. It is likely that the level of platelet inhibition achieved at two hours is similar between all three agents although there is some suggestion that the current recommended dosing regimen for tirofiban produces relatively less platelet inhibition in the first 15 to 60 minutes after coronary intervention (130). One of the few clinical trials to compare the clinical efficacy of two GP IIb/IIIa inhibitors head to head was the TARGET trial in which 4,809 patients undergoing elective PCI were randomly assigned to either abciximab or tirofiban (131). The study showed that abciximab (0.25 mg/kg bolus followed by 0.125 µg/kg [maximum 10 µg/min] for 12 hours) was significantly superior to tirofiban (10 µg/kg bolus followed by 0.15 µg/kg for 18 to 24 hours) in reducing the composite end point of death, MI, or urgent revascularization at 30 days (6% vs. 7.6%; HR 0.79). The difference appeared to be driven mainly by less procedure related MIs in the abciximab group (5.4% vs. 6.9%). A subgroup analysis found that this benefit was limited to patients who had ACS or were non-diabetic. At six months however, there was no longer any difference in the primary composite endpoint between the two drugs and by one year, the benefit of abciximab in the subgroup of patients with ACS had disappeared (132-133). A higher tirofiban bolus dose regimen (25 µg/kg bolus over three minutes followed by 0.15 µg/kg/min for 18 hours) given prior to PCI is being compared with pre-treatment with abciximab in the ongoing TENACITY trial. MULTISTRATEGY was an open-label, multi-center European trial which randomized 745 patients with STEMI undergoing primary PCI in a 2-by-2 factorial design to pre-treatment with either high dose tirofiban or abciximab and sirolimus-eluting stent versus bare-metal stent (134). All patients received dual oral anti-platelet therapy with aspirin and clopidogrel as well as with UFH. There was no significant difference between the GP IIb/IIIa groups in the primary end points of ST-segment resolution at 90 minutes after PCI (RR 1.020; 97.5% CI 0.958-1.086; p=0.001 for non-inferiority) and the rate of MACE at 8 months. Rates of major and minor bleeding complications were similar, however the incidence of moderate or severe thrombocytopenia was increased with abciximab (4.0% vs. 0.8%; p=0.004). To date abciximab has not been directly compared to ebtifibatide to evaluate relative clinical efficacy, although one study showed that compared to tirofiban, ebtifibatide was as effective as abciximab in achieving a greater proportion of patients in whom there was greater than 80% inhibition of platelet activation at 15 minutes (135). A retrospective analysis of 452 patients with STEMI undergoing primary PCI who received adjunctive therapy with either abciximab or eptifibatide found no significant differences in clinical outcomes including reinfarction (2% vs. 3% for eptifibatide and abciximab respectively), repeat revascularization (3% vs. 4%), bleeding complications (8% vs. 12%), congestive heart failure (5% vs. 3%), cerebrovascular accidents (0% vs. 2%), renal failure (2% vs. 3%), and all-cause mortality at discharge (5% vs. 4%) as well as at 6 months (6.5% vs. 6.4%; HR 0.976; 95% CI 0.43-2.23; log-rank, p=0.95) (136).

Given the above evidence, the 2009 ACC/AHA Focused Updates of the STEMI and PCI guidelines concluded that in the setting of dual antiplatelet therapy with aspirin and a thienopyridine plus either UFH or bivalirudin as the anticoagulant, GP IIb/IIIa inhibitors can be useful at the time of primary PCI but cannot be recommended as routine therapy. In select cases such as for the patient with a large thrombus burden or for patients who have not received adequate thienopyridine loading, adjunctive treatment with a GP IIb/IIIa inhibitor (abciximab [Level of Evidence A], tirofiban [Level of Evidence B], or eptifibatide [Level of Evidence B]) may be of more benefit (Class IIa) (17).

3.6 Fibrinolytic therapy

Fibrinolytic therapy restores blood flow in the infarct-related artery and has been shown to improve mortality in STEMI patients who are not able to receive timely PCI, though not in patients with NSTE-ACS. The mortality benefit of fibrinolytic therapy was first demonstrated with streptokinase in the GISSI-2 and ISIS-2 landmark trials (137-141). Streptokinase is a single chain polypeptide derived from beta-hemolytic streptococcus that binds to and cleaves peptide bonds on plasminogen causing an indirect conformational change that then activates plasmin. Streptokinase is antigenic and can infrequently cause an immunologic sensitization and allergic reaction with repeated use exposure. Increased doses are required to neutralize the body's anti-streptococcal antibodies.

Alteplase (recombinant tissue-type plasminogen activator, t-PA) is a serine protease that is naturally produced by endothelial cells and possesses no antigenic features. In contrast to streptokinase (nonfibrin-specific), t-PA is one of several fibrin-specific agents whose ability to convert plasminogen to plasmin is greatly enhanced after binding preferentially to fibrin in a thrombus with resultant local fibrinolysis. The results of the clinical trial GUSTO-I comparing streptokinase and t-PA in 41,000 patients with STEMI demonstrated an absolute survival benefit of 1% with t-PA at 30 days (6.3% vs. 7.3%) that persisted at one year (9.1% vs. 10.1%) with the most benefit seen in patients less than 75 years old and in those with anterior wall infarctions (142-143). Streptokinase however remains the most widely used fibrinolytic agent worldwide. Although it is less efficacious than alteplase, it maintains a reasonable efficacy to safety ratio with a lower risk of intra-cranial hemorrhage and is significantly less expensive.

Two other genetically engineered fibrin-specific agents currently approved in the US for use in the treatment of acute STEMI include reteplase (r-PA) and tenecteplase (TNK). Like t-PA, these agents are not antigenic and have no associated risk of allergic reaction. r-PA is a recombinant nonglycosylated form of human tissue plasminogen activator. In comparison to t-PA, r-PA has a longer half-life and binds fibrin with lower affinity improving its ability to penetrate into clots, though clinical trials (RAPID I and II, GUSTO III, INJECT) have generally demonstrated similar outcomes with r-PA and t-PA (144-148). The newest of these, tenecteplase (TNK) is a recombinant plasminogen activator derived from the native t-PA. It possesses 14 times more specificity to fibrin and is 80 times more resistant to inhibition by plasminogen activator inhibitor 1 (PAI-1) (149). It has a longer plasma half-life, allowing for easier and faster treatment with a single intravenous bolus injection and has been shown in several clinical trials including TIMI 10A and 10B, ASSENT-1 and ASSENT-2 to be as effective as t-PA with a significant reduction in non-cerebral bleeding (150-153).

Lanoteplase (n-PA) is another genetically engineered mutant of wild-type t-PA, however, it is not currently approved for use due to an increase in hemorrhagic stroke (154-155). Anistreplase (APSAC) is another fibrinolytic agent that has a significantly longer half-life compared to streptokinase (90 to 100 minutes versus 18-23 minutes). Like streptokinase and staphylokinase, it is antigenic leading to restrictions in repeated use. Though its efficacy and safety profiles were similar to streptokinase, anistreplase is no longer available. Urokinase is a non-fibrin specific fibrinolytic and is a nonselective activator of plasminogen. Urokinase is currently used only in the treatment of pulmonary embolism.

Absolute contraindications to fibrinolytic therapy include any history of intracranial hemorrhage, history of ischemic stroke within the preceding three months, presence of a cerebral vascular malformation or a primary or metastatic intracranial malignancy, symptoms or signs suggestive of an aortic dissection, a bleeding diathesis or active bleeding with the exception of menses, and a significant closed-head trauma within the preceding three months (156). Furthermore, combination therapy with fibrinolytic agents and GP IIb/IIIa inhibitors is not recommended owing to a lack of mortality benefit with significantly higher rates of bleeding seen in the GUSTO V and ASSENT-3 trials (157-162).

In patients with acute STEMI, PCI has been shown to be more effective than fibrinolytic therapy in preventing death, reinfarction, and stroke (163). However, many patients are unable to receive prompt PCI, particularly those who first present to a hospital without PCI capabilities. In such cases, it is recommended that patients who are eligible receive early fibrinolytic therapy. The issue of whether and when to perform coronary angiography and PCI in patients who have received fibrinolytic therapy is complex and has been examined extensively in clinical trials. Evidence suggests that patients who are able to attain normalization of blood flow (TIMI grade 3) in the infarct-related artery after fibrinolysis tend to have the most favorable outcomes (164-165). Although fibrinolytic therapy restores patency (TIMI grade 2 or 3) in 80% of infarct-related arteries, it only restores normalization of flow (TIMI grade 3) in 50-60% of arteries. This provides the rationale for performing PCI following the administration of fibrinolytic therapy. Two trials, GRACIA-2 and FAST-MI, have demonstrated equivalency in efficacy and safety when comparing fibrinolytic therapy followed by PCI to primary PCI (166-167). Previously used terms describing specific reperfusion strategies with PCI after fibrinolytic therapy have included *facilitated PCI* and *rescue PCI*, however, the 2009 STEMI/PCI Focused Update considered these labels potentially misleading. Though these terms are no longer used in the recommendations, many of the previous supporting trials refer to these strategies so a brief review will be necessary.

Facilitated PCI involves initial treatment with full or half dose fibrinolytic agent or a combination of fibrinolytic and GP IIb/IIIa agents followed by immediate PCI. Two large, randomized clinical trials have addressed this issue. The trial ASSENT-4-PCI was intended to randomize 4,000 patients with STEMI who presented within 6 hours of symptom onset to full-dose tenecteplase or placebo prior to primary PCI (168). The trial was terminated early due to a significant increase in the primary endpoint of death, heart failure, or shock within 90 days in the tenecteplase group (19% vs. 13%, RR 1.39, 95% CI 1.11-1.74), along with increased mortality (6% vs. 3%), in-hospital stroke (1.8% vs. 0%; mostly intra-cranial hemorrhage), as well as reinfarction (6% vs. 4%) and target vessel revascularization (7% vs. 3%) at 90 days. The FINESSE trial, described in more detail in the GP IIb/IIIa section, showed that there was no benefit in the treatment of acute STEMI with half-dose reteplase and abciximab prior to PCI with trends toward an increase in intra-cranial hemorrhage as well as major and minor bleeding (128). One possible explanation for the poor outcomes seen with facilitated PCI is the immediate nature of planned PCI after fibrionlytic therapy (median time period of 104 minutes between tenecteplase and PCI in the ASSENT-4- PCI trial). Recanalization of the infarct artery occurs 30-45 minutes after tenecteplase injection, so the relatively short time gain from the point of recanalization until PCI likely exposes the patient to more bleeding risk associated with full-dose fibrinolytic and antithrombotic therapy relative to any potential smaller benefit of PCI. A subgroup analysis showing a trend toward better outcomes when tenecteplase was given in the ambulance compared to much worse outcomes when given at a PCI center is consistent with this theory. The results of these and various smaller trials, as well as a 2006 meta-analysis have led most major society guidelines to recommend against facilitated PCI with full dose fibrinolytic therapy, though the 2007 PCI Focused Update makes a weak recommendation for the consideration of facilitated PCI using regimens other than full-dose fibrinolytic therapy in patients with high-risk STEMI in whom bleeding risk is low and PCI is not immediately available within 90 minutes (Class IIb, Level of Evidence: C) (84).

Rescue PCI refers to the strategy of performing PCI only if there are clinical or electrocardiographic signs of failed reperfusion of the infarct artery after treatment with fibrinolytics. The 2007 PCI Focused Update makes a Class I recommendation for rescue PCI or emergency CABG for cardiogenic shock in patients less than 75 years of age (Level of Evidence: B), severe congestive heart failure and/or pulmonary edema (Killip class III) (Level of Evidence: B), or hemodynamically compromising ventricular arrhythmias (Level of Evidence: C). Rescue PCI is also reasonable for cardiogenic shock in patients 75 years of age or older if they are suitable candidates for revascularization (Level of Evidence: B), hemodynamic or electrical instability (Level of Evidence: C), persistent ischemic symptoms (Level of Evidence: C), or for <50% ST-segment resolution in the lead that showed the greatest degree of ST elevation at presentation at 90 minutes after initiation of fibrinolytic therapy and a moderate or large area of myocardium at risk (anterior MI, inferior MI with right ventricular involvement or precordial ST-segment depression) (Level of Evidence: B) (Class IIa). These recommendations were based largely on results from the REACT trial as well as a subsequent meta-analysis of 8 rescue PCI trials demonstrating a clear benefit of rescue PCI over repeated doses of fibrinolytic therapy or medical management for failed fibrinolysis (169-172).

As stated above, the 2009 STEMI/PCI Focused Update has abandoned the potentially confusing terms facilitated PCI (immediate planned PCI usually performed within 2 hours of fibrinolytic or fibrinolytic plus GP IIb/IIIa therapy) and rescue PCI (PCI reserved for only those who fail fibrinolysis) in favor of a *pharmacoinvasive strategy* (17). Several trials have provided valuable evidence informing the 2009 STEMI/PCI Focused Update on this matter. In the CARESS-in-AMI trial, 600 STEMI patients 75 years of age or younger with one or more high-risk features (extensive ST-segment elevation, new left bundle branch block, previous MI, Killip class >2, or left ventricular ejection fraction ≥35%) were treated with half-dose reteplase, abciximab, heparin, and aspirin, and randomly assigned to immediate transfer for PCI or to standard medical management at the local hospital with transfer only for rescue PCI (173). The primary outcome was a composite of death, reinfarction, or refractory ischemia at 30 days. PCI was performed in 85.6% of the patients assigned to immediate transfer for PCI and rescue PCI was performed in 30.3% of the standard care/rescue PCI group. The primary outcome occurred significantly less in the immediate PCI group compared to standard care/rescue PCI (4.4% vs. 10.7%; HR 0.40; 95% CI 0.21-0.76; log rank p=0.004). There was no difference in major bleeding or strokes between the two groups. In the TRANSFER-AMI trial, 1,059 high-risk STEMI patients who were treated with tenecteplase within two hours of symptom onset were then randomized to either immediate transfer for cardiac catheterization (PCI within 6 hours) or to standard medical care (174). High-risk STEMI was defined as ST segment elevation ≥2 mm in two anterior leads or ST-segment elevation ≥1 mm in two inferior leads plus one or more of the following: systolic blood pressure <100 mmHg, heart rate >100 beats/min, Killip class II or III, ST-segment depression ≥2 mm in the anterior leads, or ST-segment ≥1 mm in right sided lead (V4R). Standard care included rescue PCI if required, or delayed angiography >24 hours after STEMI. All patients received aspirin, tenecteplase, and heparin or enoxaparin with a recommendation for clopidogrel. The primary endpoint was the composite of death, reinfarction, recurrent ischemia, new or worsening congestive heart failure, or cardiogenic shock within 30 days. Cardiac catheterization PCI were performed in 98.5% and 84.9% of the patients assigned to early PCI at a median of 2.8 hours after randomization and in 88.7% and 67.4% of the patients assigned to standard treatment at a median of 32.5 hours after randomization. At 30 days, the primary endpoint was significantly reduced in the early PCI group (11.0% vs. 17.2%; RR 0.64; 95% CI 0.47-0.87; p=0.004) with no significant differences between the groups in the incidence of major bleeding. Several other trials have evaluated the timing of PCI after fibrinolysis with an early pharmacoinvasive therapy compared to standard care including GRACIA-1, NORDISTEMI, and SIAM III (175-177). Each had a different study design and thus examined slightly different patient populations but all have confirmed the observations seen in CARESS-in-AMI and TRANSFER-AMI that a pharmacoinvasive strategy with immediate or early PCI after fibrinolytic therapy (within 3 to 24 hours) produces better outcomes than standard medical care with rescue PCI or routine late PCI (over 24 hours).

Based on the above evidence, a pharmacoinvasive approach to the management of STEMI patients who present to a hospital without PCI capabilities has been developed, which includes routine use of a pharmacologic agent (either fibrinolytic therapy or a GP IIb/IIIa inhibitor) prior to transfer to a PCI-capable hospital for diagnostic angiogram and consideration of PCI (17). Patients with STEMI who present to a PCI capable hospital are not recommended to receive fibrinolytic therapy and should undergo prompt PCI no later than 90 minutes after presentation. STEMI patients who present to a hospital without PCI capability should be triaged to either immediate transfer for PCI or to receive fibrinolytic therapy if deemed an appropriate candidate. Those with high-risk STEMI features (congestive heart failure, cardiogenic shock, electrical instability, etc.), elevated bleeding risk with fibrinolytic therapy, or presenting more than 4 hours after symptom onset may be better suited for immediate transfer for PCI without delay for fibrinolytic therapy if the time required for transport to the receiving hospital is not prolonged. STEMI patients who present early after symptom onset with low bleeding risk are the most suitable candidates for fibrinolytic therapy. If after receiving the fibrinolytic agent the patient is deemed to have high-risk features, the patient should then be immediately transferred for PCI with the intention to perform diagnostic catheterization with possible PCI within 3 to 24 hours of presentation. Patients who are not judged to be high-risk may be transferred to a PCI-capable hospital after receiving antithrombotic therapy or may be observed in the initial facility.

3.7 Platelet function testing (P2Y12 testing)

Several studies have shown that patients with high platelet reactivity despite being treated with clopidogrel have a higher incidence of cardiovascular events after PCI (178). This has led to a departure from the "one size fits all" paradigm in clopidogrel use during PCI as well as investigations into the different genetic and clinical factors that affect individual response in platelet reactivity. Clopidogrel is a prodrug which requires biotransformation to its active thiol metabolite via the hepatic cytochrome P450 system (179). It exerts its antiplatelet effect by irreversibly binding the adenosine diphosphate receptor P2Y12, a G-protein coupled receptor found on the platelet surface, which mediates inhibition of adenylyl cyclase resulting in the final activation of the GPIIb/IIIa receptor (180). Blockade of this pathway with clopidogrel inhibits platelet aggregation and along with the co-administration of aspirin has contributed to a substantial reduction in thrombotic complications peri-PCI (181). Pharmacokinetic and pharmacodynamic data have revealed significant inter-individual variability in platelet response to clopidogrel, with reports of clopidogrel "non-responsiveness" in up to 30% of Caucasian patients (182-183). There are many potential causes of clopidogrel response variability with recent studies focusing on genetic variations in hepatic CYP isoenzymes, in particular single-nucleotide polymorphisms of CYP2C19. In a genetic substudy from the TRITON-TIMI 38 trial, patients with a reduced function CYP2C19 allele who were treated with clopidogrel had lower serum levels of active clopidogrel metabolite as well as diminished platelet inhibition leading to higher rates of major adverse cardiovascular events including stent thrombosis when compared to noncarriers of the CYP2C19 allele (12.1% vs. 8.0%; HR 1.53; 95% CI 1.07 to 2.19; p = 0.01) (184). Additionally, variants in ABCB1, a gene encoding for efflux pump P-glycoprotein expressed on intestinal epithelial cells, have been reported to affect clopidogrel absorption and efficacy. Carriers of the specific ABCB1 polymorphism 3435C→T, particularly those who are TT homozygotes have lower serum levels of active metabolite when treated with clopidogrel as well as higher rates of a combined endpoint of cardiovascular death, myocardial infarction, or stroke (12.9% vs. 7.8%; HR 1.72; 95% CI 1.22–2.44; p=0.002) (185). Further studies are needed to determine how much a role

ABCB1 variants play in clopidogrel response variability. Genome-wide association studies have shown that the heritability of platelet response to clopidogrel may be as high as 70%, with the reduced function CYP2C19*2 polymorphism accounting for only 12% of the clopidogrel response variability (186). As such, much of the inter-individual variability cannot be explained by genotype differences alone. Given the complexity of testing for multiple genetic polymorphisms along with its as yet uncertain yield, there has been increasing interest recently in the direct assessment of platelet reactivity peri-procedurally.

A number of different methods exist for the laboratory quantification of platelet inhibition. Light transmittance aggregometry (LTA) analyzes percent inhibition by measuring the amount of transmitted light through a vial of platelet plasma before and after the addition of ADP, which induces platelet aggregation. LTA is considered the "gold standard" for measurement of platelet aggregation but the test is very labor intensive and thus limits its routine use for guiding clinical care. Other tests for platelet inhibition include flow cytometry, platelet function analyzer (PFA-100), vasodilator-stimulated phosphoprotein (VASP) phosphorylation assay, and the bedside VerifyNow P2Y12 assay, which measures the aggregation of platelets to fibrinogen-coated beads. A study by Price et al. reported that the optimal cut-off value for post-PCI platelet reactivity as measured by the VerifyNow P2Y12 assay is 235 PRU (P2Y12 reactivity units) (187). Patients with increased residual platelet reactivity (measured at ≥235 PRU) after PCI had significantly higher rates of cardiovascular death (2.8% vs 0%, p=0.04), stent thrombosis (4.6% vs 0%, p=0.004), and the combined ischemic endpoints (6.5% vs 1.0%, p=0.008) at 6 months. Due to its high predictive value for post-PCI outcomes and its ease of use as a point-of-care platelet function assay, the use of VerifyNow P2Y12 assay as a clinical guide for intensified platelet inhibition therapy was recently evaluated in the large multi-center trial, GRAVITAS (188). Investigators in the GRAVITAS trial randomized patients with stable CAD or NSTE-ACS and high on-treatment platelet reactivity as defined by a PRU value of ≥230 after PCI to treatment with either high-dose clopidogrel (first-day loading dose of 600mg, followed by 150mg daily for 6 months) or standard-dose clopidogrel (required to have received either 300mg loading dose at the time of PCI or at least 75mg daily for seven days preceding PCI and standard maintanence 75mg dose for 6 months). The results of the trial failed to demonstrate a reduction in the incidence of cardiovascular death, non-fatal MI, or stent thrombosis with the use of high-dose clopidogrel (2.3% vs 2.3%; HR 1.01; 95% CI 0.58-1.76; p=0.97) (11). A second trial, TRIGGER—PCI, intended to compare the use of clopidogrel versus prasugrel in patients undergoing stenting for stable CAD with high post-PCI residual platelet reactivity (defined as a PRU>208 utilizing the VerifyNow P2Y12 assay). Unfortunately, the trial was terminated early due to an unexpected low rate of primary endpoint events in both groups, reported to be even less than the low event rates seen in the GRAVITAS trial. It has been hypothesized that these two trials were negative mainly because the patient population studied was at low risk for cardiovascular complications - patients with stable CAD undergoing successful uncomplicated PCI with contemporary drug-eluting stents. Based on the results of these two trials, it may be argued that platelet function testing in these low-risk situations has limited value as there is little to be gained from more potent platelet inhibition. Whether a personalized approach to intensified platelet inhibition therapy can be beneficial in higher risk groups such as patients with acute coronary syndromes, patients with diabetes, patients with complex coronary anatomy and complex interventions as well as clopidogrel "hypo-responsiveness" remains to be determined and requires further prospective investigation.

Absence or termination of dual anti-platelet therapy
Stent under-expansion
Inflow or outflow obstruction (CAD >50%)
Greater stent length
Small vessel diameter
Emergent PCI or ACS
Residual thrombus or stent edge dissection
Subtherapeutic peri-procedural anticoagulation
Severe left ventricular dysfunction
History of brachytherapy
Cocaine use
Post-procedure TIMI flow grade <3
Bifurcation lesions
Malignancy
Genetic polymorphisms in hepatic enzymes involved in clopidogrel metabolism
High on-treatment platelet reactivity (with clopidogrel)

Table 1. Factors associated with increased risk of stent thrombosis

4. References

[1] Dotter CT, Judkins MP. Transluminal treatment of arteriosclerotic obstruction. Circulation 1964; 30(5):654–70.

[2] Cutlip DE, Baim DS, Ho KK, et al. Stent thrombosis in the modern era: a pooled analysis of multicenter coronary stent clinical trials. Circulation 2001; 103(15):1967.

[3] van Werkum JW, Heestermans AA, Zomer AC, et al. Predictors of coronary stent thrombosis: the Dutch Stent Thrombosis Registry. J Am Coll Cardiol 2009; 53(16):1399.

[4] Iakovou I, Schmidt T, Bonizzoni E, et al. Incidence, predictors, and outcome of thrombosis after successful implantation of drug-eluting stents. JAMA 2005; 293(17):2126.

[5] Finn AV, Joner M, Nakazawa G, et al. Pathological correlates of late drug-eluting stent thrombosis: strut coverage as a marker of endothelialization. Circulation 2007; 115(18):2435.

[6] Joner M, Finn AV, Farb A, et al. Pathology of drug-eluting stents in humans: delayed healing and late thrombotic risk. J Am Coll Cardiol 2006; 48(1):193.

[7] Antithrombotic Trialists' Collaboration. Collaborative meta-analysis of randomised trials of antiplatelet therapy for prevention of death, myocardial infarction, and stroke in high risk patients. BMJ 2002; 324(7329):71

[8] Berger JS, Brown DL, Becker RC. Low-dose aspirin in patients with stable cardiovascular disease: a meta-analysis. Am J Med 2008; 121(1):43.

[9] Standards of medical care in diabetes. American Diabetes Association. Diabetes Care 2004; 27 Suppl 1:S15
[10] Hennekens CH, Knatterud GL, Pfeffer MA, et al. Use of aspirin to reduce risks of cardiovascular disease in patients with diabetes: clinical and research challenges. Diabetes Care 2004; 27(11):2752.
[11] Baigent C, Blackwell L, Collins R, et al. Aspirin in the primary and secondary prevention of vascular disease: collaborative meta-analysis of individual participant data from randomised trials. Lancet 2009; 373(9678):1849.
[12] Lewis HD, Davis JW, Archibald DG, et al. Protective effects of aspirin against acute myocardial infarction and death in men with unstable angina. Results of a Veterans Administration Cooperative Study. N Engl J Med 1983; 309(7):396–403.
[13] Cairns JA, Gent M, Singer J, et al. Aspirin, sulfinpyrazone, or both in unstable angina. Results of a Canadian multicenter trial. N Engl J Med 1985; 313(22):1369–75.
[14] Theroux P, Ouimet H, McCans J, et al. Aspirin, heparin, or both to treat acute unstable angina. N Engl J Med 1988; 319(17):1105–11.
[15] Risk of myocardial infarction and death during treatment with low dose aspirin and intravenous heparin in men with unstable coronary artery disease. The RISC Group. Lancet 1990; 336(8719):827–30.
[16] Randomised trial of intravenous streptokinase, oral aspirin, both, or neither among 17,187 cases of suspected acute myocardial infarction: ISIS–2. ISIS–2 (Second International Study of Infarct Survival) Collaborative Group. Lancet 1988; 2(8607):349–60.
[17] Kushner FG, Hand M, Smith SC Jr, et al. 2009 Focused Updates: ACC/AHA Guidelines for the Management of Patients With ST-Elevation Myocardial Infarction (updating the 2004 Guideline and 2007 Focused Update) and ACC/AHA/SCAI Guidelines on Percutaneous Coronary Intervention (updating the 2005 Guideline and 2007 Focused Update): a report of the American College of Cardiology Foundation/American Heart Association Task Force on Practice Guidelines. Circulation 2009; 120:2271.
[18] Schwartz L, Bourassa MG, Lespérance J, et al. Aspirin and dipyridamole in the prevention of restenosis after percutaneous transluminal coronary angioplasty. N Engl J Med. 1988;318:1714.
[19] Wilson RF, White CW. Does coronary artery bypass surgery restore normal maximal coronary flow reserve? The effect of diffuse atherosclerosis and focal obstructive lesions. Circulation 1987; 76:563.
[20] Lembo NJ, Black AJ, Roubin GS, et al. Effect of pretreatment with aspirin versus aspirin plus dipyridamole on frequency and type of acute complications of percutaneous transluminal coronary angioplasty. Am J Cardiol 1990; 65:422.
[21] Mufson, L, Black, A, Roubin, G, et al. A randomized trial of aspirin in PTCA: effect of high dose versus low dose aspirin on major complications and restenosis (abstract). J Am Coll Cardiol 1988; 11:236A.
[22] Balsano F, Rizzon P, Violi F, et al. Antiplatelet treatment with ticlopidine in unstable angina. A controlled multicenter clinical trial. The Studio della Ticlopidina nell'Angina Instabile Group. Circulation 1990; 82(1):17–26.
[23] Leon MB, Baim DS, Popma JJ, et al. A clinical trial comparing three antithrombotic-drug regimens after coronary-artery stenting. Stent Anticoagulation Restenosis Study Investigators. N Engl J Med 1998; 339:1665.

[24] Schömig A, Neumann FJ, Kastrati A, et al. A randomized comparison of antiplatelet and anticoagulant therapy after the placement of coronary-artery stents. N Engl J Med 1996; 334:1084.

[25] Bertrand ME, Legrand V, Boland J, et al. Randomized multicenter comparison of conventional anticoagulation versus antiplatelet therapy in unplanned and elective coronary stenting. The full anticoagulation versus aspirin and ticlopidine (fantastic) study. Circulation 1998; 98:1597.

[26] Urban P, Macaya C, Rupprecht HJ, et al. Randomized evaluation of anticoagulation versus antiplatelet therapy after coronary stent implantation in high-risk patients: the multicenter aspirin and ticlopidine trial after intracoronary stenting (MATTIS). Circulation 1998; 98:2126.

[27] Bennett CL, Davidson CJ, Raisch DW, et al. Thrombotic thrombocytopenic purpura associated with ticlopidine in the setting of coronary artery stents and stroke prevention. Arch Intern Med 1999; 159:2524.

[28] Steinhubl SR, Tan WA, Foody JM, Topol EJ. Incidence and clinical course of thrombotic thrombocytopenic purpura due to ticlopidine following coronary stenting. EPISTENT Investigators. Evaluation of Platelet IIb/IIIa Inhibitor for Stenting. JAMA 1999; 281:806.

[29] CAPRIE Steering Committee. A randomised, blinded, trial of clopidogrel versus aspirin in patients at risk of ischaemic events (CAPRIE). Lancet 1996; 348(9038):1329–39.

[30] Bertrand ME, Rupprecht HJ, Urban P, et al. Double-blind study of the safety of clopidogrel with and without a loading dose in combination with aspirin compared with ticlopidine in combination with aspirin after coronary stenting: the clopidogrel aspirin stent international cooperative study (CLASSICS). Circulation 2000; 102:624.

[31] Bhatt DL, Bertrand ME, Berger PB, et al. Meta-analysis of randomized and registry comparisons of ticlopidine with clopidogrel after stenting. J Am Coll Cardiol 2002; 39:9.

[32] Yusuf S, Zhao F, Mehta SR, et al. Clopidogrel in Unstable Angina to Prevent Recurrent Events Trial Investigators. Effects of clopidogrel in addition to aspirin in patients with acute coronary syndromes without ST-segment elevation. N Engl J Med 2001; 345(7):494–502.

[33] Mehta SR, Yusuf S, Peters R, et al. Effects of pretreatment with clopidogrel and aspirin followed by long-term therapy in patients undergoing percutaneous coronary intervention: the PCI-CURE study. Lancet 2001; 358(9281):527–33.

[34] Yusuf S, Mehta SR, Zhao F, et al. Early and late effects of clopidogrel in patients with acute coronary syndromes. Circulation 2003; 107(7):966–72.

[35] Steinhubl SR, Berger PB, Mann JT 3rd, et al. Early and sustained dual oral antiplatelet therapy following percutaneous coronary intervention: a randomized controlled trial. JAMA 2002; 288(19):2411–20.

[36] Sabatine MS, Cannon CP, Gibson CM, et al, for the CLARITY-TIMI 28 investigators. Addition of clopidogrel to aspirin and fibrinolytic therapy for myocardial infarction with ST-segment elevation. N Engl J Med 2005; 352(12):1179–89.

[37] www.commit-ccs2.org (Accessed 7/3/11).

[38] Sabatine MS, Cannon CP, Gibson CM, et al. Effect of clopidogrel pretreatment before percutaneous coronary intervention in patients with ST-elevation myocardial infarction treated with fibrinolytics: the PCI-CLARITY study. JAMA 2005; 294:1224.

[39] Steinhubl SR, Berger PB, Brennan DM, et al. Optimal timing for the initiation of pre-treatment with 300 mg clopidogrel before percutaneous coronary intervention. J Am Coll Cardiol 2006; 47:939.

[40] Hochholzer W, Trenk D, Frundi D, et al. Time dependence of platelet inhibition after a 600-mg loading dose of clopidogrel in a large, unselected cohort of candidates for percutaneous coronary intervention. Circulation 2005; 111:2560.

[41] Angiolillo DJ, Fernández-Ortiz A, Bernardo E, et al. High clopidogrel loading dose during coronary stenting: effects on drug response and interindividual variability. Eur Heart J 2004; 25:1903.

[42] Patti G, Colonna G, Pasceri V, et al. Randomized trial of high loading dose of clopidogrel for reduction of periprocedural myocardial infarction in patients undergoing coronary intervention: results from the ARMYDA-2 (Antiplatelet therapy for Reduction of MYocardial Damage during Angioplasty) study. Circulation 2005; 111:2099.

[43] Dangas G, Mehran R, Guagliumi G, et al. Role of clopidogrel loading dose in patients with ST-segment elevation myocardial infarction undergoing primary angioplasty: results from the HORIZONS-AMI (harmonizing outcomes with revascularization and stents in acute myocardial infarction) trial. J Am Coll Cardiol 2009; 54:1438.

[44] CURRENT-OASIS 7 Investigators, Mehta SR, Bassand JP, et al. Dose comparisons of clopidogrel and aspirin in acute coronary syndromes. N Engl J Med 2010; 363:930.

[45] von Beckerath N, Taubert D, Pogatsa-Murray G, et al. Absorption, metabolization, and antiplatelet effects of 300-, 600-, and 900-mg loading doses of clopidogrel: results of the ISAR-CHOICE (Intracoronary Stenting and Antithrombotic Regimen: Choose Between 3 High Oral Doses for Immediate Clopidogrel Effect) Trial. Circulation 2005; 112:2946.

[46] Montalescot G, Sideris G, Meuleman C, et al. A randomized comparison of high clopidogrel loading doses in patients with non-ST-segment elevation acute coronary syndromes: the ALBION (Assessment of the Best Loading Dose of Clopidogrel to Blunt Platelet Activation, Inflammation and Ongoing Necrosis) trial. J Am Coll Cardiol 2006; 48:931.

[47] L'Allier PL, Ducrocq G, Pranno N, et al. Clopidogrel 600-mg double loading dose achieves stronger platelet inhibition than conventional regimens: results from the PREPAIR randomized study. J Am Coll Cardiol 2008; 51:1066.

[48] Kandzari DE, Berger PB, Kastrati A, et al. Influence of treatment duration with a 600-mg dose of clopidogrel before percutaneous coronary revascularization. J Am Coll Cardiol 2004; 44:2133.

[49] Widimsky P, Motovská Z, Simek S, et al. Clopidogrel pre-treatment in stable angina: for all patients > 6 h before elective coronary angiography or only for angiographically selected patients a few minutes before PCI? A randomized multicentre trial PRAGUE-8. Eur Heart J 2008; 29:1495.

[50] Di Sciascio G, Patti G, Pasceri V, et al. Effectiveness of in-laboratory high-dose clopidogrel loading versus routine pre-load in patients undergoing percutaneous coronary intervention: results of the ARMYDA-5 PRELOAD (Antiplatelet therapy for Reduction of MYocardial Damage during Angioplasty) randomized trial. J Am Coll Cardiol 2010; 56:550.

[51] Collet JP, Silvain J, Landivier A, et al. Dose effect of clopidogrel reloading in patients already on 75-mg maintenance dose: the Reload with Clopidogrel Before Coronary

Angioplasty in Subjects Treated Long Term with Dual Antiplatelet Therapy (RELOAD) study. Circulation 2008; 118:1225.

[52] Di Sciascio G, Patti G, Pasceri V, et al. Clopidogrel reloading in patients undergoing percutaneous coronary intervention on chronic clopidogrel therapy: results of the ARMYDA-4 RELOAD (Antiplatelet therapy for Reduction of MYocardial Damage during Angioplasty) randomized trial. Eur Heart J 2010; 31:1337.

[53] Brandt JT, Payne CD, Wiviott SD, et al. A comparison of prasugrel and clopidogrel loading doses on platelet function: magnitude of platelet inhibition is related to active metabolite formation. Am Heart J 2007; 153:66.e9-66.e16.

[54] Jernberg T, Payne CD, Winters KJ, et al. Prasugrel achieves greater inhibition of platelet aggregation and a lower rate of non-responders compared with clopidogrel in aspirin-treated patients with stable coronary artery disease. Eur Heart J 2006; 27:1166-73.

[55] Varenhorst C, Braun O, James S, et al. Greater inhibition of platelet aggregation with prasugrel 60 mg loading dose compared with a clopidogrel 600 mg loading dose in aspirin-treated patients. Eur Heart J 2007; 28:Suppl:189. abstract.

[56] Wiviott SD, Antman EM, Winters KJ, et al. Randomized comparison of prasugrel (CS-747, LY640315), a novel thienopyridine P2Y12 antagonist, with clopidogrel in percutaneous coronary intervention: results of the Joint Utilization of Medications to Block Platelets Optimally (JUMBO)-TIMI 26 trial. Circulation 2005; 111:3366.

[57] Wiviott SD, Trenk D, Frelinger AL, et al. Prasugrel compared with high loading- and maintenance-dose clopidogrel in patients with planned percutaneous coronary intervention: the Prasugrel in Comparison to Clopidogrel for Inhibition of Platelet Activation and Aggregation-Thrombolysis in Myocardial Infarction 44 trial. Circulation 2007; 116:2923.

[58] Wiviott SD, Braunwald E, McCabe CH, et al. Prasugrel versus clopidogrel in patients with acute coronary syndromes. N Engl J Med 2007; 357:2001.

[59] Wallentin L, Becker RC, Budaj A, et al. Ticagrelor versus clopidogrel in patients with acute coronary syndromes. N Engl J Med 2009; 361:1045.

[60] James S, Budaj A, Aylward P, et al. Ticagrelor versus clopidogrel in acute coronary syndromes in relation to renal function: results from the Platelet Inhibition and Patient Outcomes (PLATO) trial. Circulation 2010; 122:1056.

[61] Theroux P, Ouimet H, McCans J, et al. Aspirin, heparin, or both to treat acute unstable angina. N Engl J Med 1988; 319(17):1105–11.

[62] Risk of myocardial infarction and death during treatment with low dose aspirin and intravenous heparin in men with unstable coronary artery disease. The RISC Group. Lancet 1990; 336(8719):827–30.

[63] Oler A, Whooley MA, Oler J, et al. Adding heparin to aspirin reduces the incidence of myocardial infarction and death in patients with unstable angina. A meta-analysis. JAMA 1996; 276(10):811–15.

[64] Cohen M, Adams PC, Parry G, et al. Combination antithrombotic therapy in unstable rest angina and non-Q-wave infarction in nonprior aspirin users. Primary end points analysis from the ATACS trial. Antithrombotic Therapy in Acute Coronary Syndromes Research Group. Circulation 1994; 89(1):81–8.

[65] Eikelboom JW, Anand SS, Malmberg K, et al. Unfractionated heparin and low-molecular-weight heparin in acute coronary syndrome without ST elevation: a meta-analysis. Lancet 2000; 355(9219):1936–42.

[66] de Bono DP, Simoons ML, Tijssen J, et al. Effect of early intravenous heparin on coronary patency, infarct size, and bleeding complications after alteplase thrombolysis: results of a randomised double blind European Cooperative Study Group trial. Br Heart J 1992; 67:122.

[67] Arnout J, Simoons M, de Bono D, et al. Correlation between level of heparinization and patency of the infarct-related coronary artery after treatment of acute myocardial infarction with alteplase (rt-PA). J Am Coll Cardiol 1992; 20:513.

[68] Eikelboom JW, Quinlan DJ, Mehta SR, et al. Unfractionated and low-molecular-weight heparin as adjuncts to thrombolysis in aspirin-treated patients with ST-elevation acute myocardial infarction: a meta-analysis of the randomized trials. Circulation 2005; 112:3855.

[69] An international randomized trial comparing four thrombolytic strategies for acute myocardial infarction. The GUSTO investigators. N Engl J Med 1993; 329:673.

[70] Popma JJ, Weitz J, Bittl JA, et al. Antithrombotic therapy in patients undergoing coronary angioplasty. Chest 1998; 114:728S.

[71] Smith SC Jr, Feldman TE, Hirshfeld JW Jr, et al. ACC/AHA/SCAI 2005 guideline update for percutaneous coronary intervention: a report of the American College of Cardiology/American Heart Association Task Force on Practice Guidelines (ACC/AHA/SCAI Writing Committee to Update the 2001 Guidelines for Percutaneous Coronary Intervention). J Am Coll Cardiol 2006; 47:e1.

[72] Silber S, Albertsson P, Avilés FF, et al. Guidelines for percutaneous coronary interventions. The Task Force for Percutaneous Coronary Interventions of the European Society of Cardiology. Eur Heart J 2005; 26:804.

[73] Low-molecular-weight heparin during instability in coronary artery disease, Fragmin during Instability in Coronary Artery Disease (FRISC) study group. Lancet 1996; 347(9001):561–8.

[74] Klein W, Buchwald A, Hillis SE, et al. Comparison of low-molecular-weight heparin with unfractionated heparin acutely and with placebo for 6 weeks in the management of unstable coronary artery disease. Fragmin in unstable coronary artery disease study (FRIC). Circulation 1997; 96(1):61–8.

[75] Comparison of two treatment durations (6 days and 14 days) of a low molecular weight heparin with a 6-day treatment of unfractionated heparin in the initial management of unstable angina or non-Q wave myocardial infarction: FRAX.I.S. (FRAxiparine in Ischaemic Syndrome). Eur Heart J 1999; 20(21):1553–62.

[76] Antman EM, Cohen M, Radley D, et al. Assessment of the treatment effect of enoxaparin for unstable angina/non-Q-wave myocardial infarction. TIMI 11B-ESSENCE meta-analysis. Circulation 1999; 100(15):1602–8.

[77] Murphy SA, Gibson CM, Morrow DA, et al. Efficacy and safety of the low-molecular weight heparin enoxaparin compared with unfractionated heparin across the acute coronary syndrome spectrum: a meta-analysis. Eur Heart J 2007; 28(17):2077–86.

[78] Antman EM, McCabe CH, Enrique P, et al. Enoxaparin Prevents Death and Cardiac Ischemic Events in Unstable Angina/Non–Q-Wave Myocardial Infarction: Results of the Thrombolysis In Myocardial Infarction (TIMI) 11B Trial. Circulation 1999; 100(15):1593–601.

[79] Cohen M, Demers C, Gurfinkel EP, et al. A comparison of low-molecular-weight heparin with unfractionated heparin for unstable coronary artery disease. Efficacy

and Safety of Subcutaneous Enoxaparin in Non-Q-Wave Coronary Events Study Group. N Engl J Med 1997; 337(7):447–52.

[80] Ferguson JJ, Califf RM, Antman EM, et al. Enoxaparin vs unfractionated heparin in high-risk patients with non-ST-segment elevation acute coronary syndromes managed with an intended early invasive strategy: primary results of the SYNERGY randomized trial. JAMA 2004; 292(1):45–54.

[81] Montalescot G, White HD, Gallo R, et al. Enoxaparin versus unfractionated heparin in elective percutaneous coronary intervention. N Engl J Med 2006; 355:1006.

[82] Mehta SR, Steg PG, Granger CB, et al. Randomized, blinded trial comparing fondaparinux with unfractionated heparin in patients undergoing contemporary percutaneous coronary intervention: Arixtra Study in Percutaneous Coronary Intervention: a Randomized Evaluation (ASPIRE) Pilot Trial. Circulation 2005; 111:1390.

[83] Yusuf S, Mehta SR, Chrolavicius S, et al. Effects of fondaparinux on mortality and reinfarction in patients with acute ST-segment elevation myocardial infarction: the OASIS-6 randomized trial. JAMA 2006; 295:1519.

[84] King, SB, 3rd, Smith, SC Jr, Hirshfeld, JW Jr, et al. 2007 focused update of the ACC/AHA/SCAI 2005 guideline update for percutaneous coronary intervention: a report of the American College of Cardiology/American Heart Association task force on practice guidelines: 2007 writing group to review new evidence and update the ACC/AHA/SCAI 2005 guideline update for percutaneous coronary intervention, writing on behalf of the 2005 writing committee. Circulation 2008; 117:261.

[85] Weitz JI, Hudoba M, Massel D, et al. Clot-bound Thrombin is Protected from Inhibition by Heparin –Antithrombin III but is Susceptible to Inactivation by Antithrombin III-independent Inhibitors. J Clin Invest 1990; 86:385-391.

[86] Antman EM. Hirudin in acute myocardial infarction. Thrombolysis and Thrombin Inhibition in Myocardial Infarction (TIMI) 9B trial. Circulation 1996; 94:911.

[87] A comparison of recombinant hirudin with heparin for the treatment of acute coronary syndromes. The Global Use of Strategies to Open Occluded Coronary Arteries (GUSTO) IIb investigators. N Engl J Med 1996; 335:775.

[88] Serruys PW, Herrman JP, Simon R, et al. A comparison of hirudin with heparin in the prevention of restenosis after coronary angioplasty. Helvetica Investigators. N Engl J Med 1995; 333(12):757–63.

[89] White HD, Aylward PE, Frey MJ, et al. Randomized, Double-blind Comparison of Hirulog Versus Heparin in Patients Receiving Streptokinase and Aspirin for Acute Myocardial Infarction (HERO). Circulation 1997; 96(7):2155–61.

[90] White H, Hirulog and Early Reperfusion or Occlusion (HERO)-2 Trial Investigators. Thrombin-specific anticoagulation with bivalirudin versus heparin in patients receiving fibrinolytic therapy for acute myocardial infarction: the HERO-2 randomised trial. Lancet 2001; 358:1855.

[91] Stone GW, Witzenbichler B, Guagliumi G, et al. Bivalirudin during primary PCI in acute myocardial infarction. N Engl J Med 2008; 358:2218.

[92] Lincoff AM, Bittl JA, Harrington RA, et al. Bivalirudin and provisional glycoprotein IIb/IIIa blockade compared with heparin and planned glycoprotein IIb/IIIa blockade during percutaneous coronary intervention: REPLACE-2 randomized trial. JAMA 2003; 289:853.

[93] Kastrati A, Neumann FJ, Mehilli J, et al. Bivalirudin versus unfractionated heparin during percutaneous coronary intervention. N Engl J Med 2008; 359:688.

[94] Stone GW, McLaurin BT, Cox DA, et al. Bivalirudin for patients with acute coronary syndromes. N Engl J Med 2006; 355:2203.
[95] Chew DP, Bhatt DL, Kimball W, et al. Bivalirudin provides increasing benefit with decreasing renal function: a meta-analysis of randomized trials. Am J Cardiol 2003; 92:919.
[96] Use of a monoclonal antibody directed against the platelet glycoprotein IIb/IIIa receptor in high-risk coronary angioplasty. The EPIC Investigation. N Engl J Med 1994; 330:956.
[97] Lincoff AM, Tcheng JE, Califf RM, et al. Sustained suppression of ischemic complications of coronary intervention by platelet GP IIb/IIIa blockade with abciximab: one-year outcome in the EPILOG trial. Evaluation in PTCA to Improve Long-term Outcome with abciximab GP IIb/IIIa blockade. Circulation 1999; 99:1951.
[98] Randomised placebo-controlled trial of abciximab before and during coronary intervention in refractory unstable angina: the CAPTURE Study. Lancet 1997; 349:1429.
[99] Brener SJ, Barr LA, Burchenal JE, et al. Randomized, placebo-controlled trial of platelet glycoprotein IIb/IIIa blockade with primary angioplasty for acute myocardial infarction. ReoPro and Primary PTCA Organization and Randomized Trial (RAPPORT) Investigators. Circulation 1998; 98:734.
[100] Montalescot G, Barragan P, Wittenberg O, et al. Platelet glycoprotein IIb/IIIa inhibition with coronary stenting for acute myocardial infarction. N Engl J Med 2001; 344:1895.
[101] Neumann FJ, Kastrati A, Schmitt C, et al. Effect of glycoprotein IIb/IIIa receptor blockade with abciximab on clinical and angiographic restenosis rate after the placement of coronary stents following acute myocardial infarction. J Am Coll Cardiol 2000; 35:915.
[102] Stone GW, Grines CL, Cox DA, et al. Comparison of angioplasty with stenting, with or without abciximab, in acute myocardial infarction. N Engl J Med 2002; 346:957.
[103] Antoniucci D, Rodriguez A, Hempel A, et al. A randomized trial comparing primary infarct artery stenting with or without abciximab in acute myocardial infarction. J Am Coll Cardiol 2003; 42:1879.
[104] EPISTENT Investigators. Randomised placebo-controlled and balloon-angioplasty-controlled trial to assess safety of coronary stenting with use of platelet glycoprotein-IIb/IIIa blockade. Lancet 1998; 352:87.
[105] Kastrati A, Mehilli J, Schühlen H, et al. A clinical trial of abciximab in elective percutaneous coronary intervention after pretreatment with clopidogrel. N Engl J Med 2004; 350:232.
[106] Mehilli J, Kastrati A, Schühlen H, et al. Randomized clinical trial of abciximab in diabetic patients undergoing elective percutaneous coronary interventions after treatment with a high loading dose of clopidogrel. Circulation 2004; 110:3627.
[107] Acute platelet inhibition with abciximab does not reduce in-stent restenosis (ERASER study). The ERASER Investigators. Circulation 1999; 100:799.
[108] Bhatt DL, Lincoff AM, Califf RM, et al. The benefit of abciximab in percutaneous coronary revascularization is not device-specific. Am J Cardiol 2000; 85:1060.
[109] Cho L, Topol EJ, Balog C, et al. Clinical benefit of glycoprotein IIb/IIIa blockade with Abciximab is independent of gender: pooled analysis from EPIC, EPILOG and EPISTENT trials. Evaluation of 7E3 for the Prevention of Ischemic Complications.

Evaluation in Percutaneous Transluminal Coronary Angioplasty to Improve Long-Term Outcome with Abciximab GP IIb/IIIa blockade. Evaluation of Platelet IIb/IIIa Inhibitor for Stent. J Am Coll Cardiol 2000; 36:381.

[110] Topol EJ, Lincoff AM, Kereiakes DJ, et al. Multi-year follow-up of abciximab therapy in three randomized, placebo-controlled trials of percutaneous coronary revascularization. Am J Med 2002; 113:1.

[111] Mehilli J, Kastrati A, Schulz S, et al. Abciximab in patients with acute ST-segment-elevation myocardial infarction undergoing primary percutaneous coronary intervention after clopidogrel loading: a randomized double-blind trial. Circulation 2009; 119:1933.

[112] Effects of platelet glycoprotein IIb/IIIa blockade with tirofiban on adverse cardiac events in patients with unstable angina or acute myocardial infarction undergoing coronary angioplasty. The RESTORE Investigators. Randomized Efficacy Study of Tirofiban for Outcomes and REstenosis. Circulation 1997; 96:1445.

[113] Gibson CM, Goel M, Cohen DJ, et al. Six-month angiographic and clinical follow-up of patients prospectively randomized to receive either tirofiban or placebo during angioplasty in the RESTORE trial. Randomized Efficacy Study of Tirofiban for Outcomes and Restenosis. J Am Coll Cardiol 1998; 32:28.

[114] Valgimigli M, Percoco G, Barbieri D, et al. The additive value of tirofiban administered with the high-dose bolus in the prevention of ischemic complications during high-risk coronary angioplasty: the ADVANCE Trial. J Am Coll Cardiol 2004; 44:14.

[115] Lee DP, Herity NA, Hiatt BL, et al. Adjunctive platelet glycoprotein IIb/IIIa receptor inhibition with tirofiban before primary angioplasty improves angiographic outcomes: results of the TIrofiban Given in the Emergency Room before Primary Angioplasty (TIGER-PA) pilot trial. Circulation 2003; 107:1497.

[116] van 't Hof AW, Ernst N, de Boer MJ, et al. Facilitation of primary coronary angioplasty by early start of a glycoprotein 2b/3a inhibitor: results of the ongoing tirofiban in myocardial infarction evaluation (On-TIME) trial. Eur Heart J 2004; 25:837.

[117] Van't Hof AW, Ten Berg J, Heestermans T, et al. Prehospital initiation of tirofiban in patients with ST-elevation myocardial infarction undergoing primary angioplasty (On-TIME 2): a multicentre, double-blind, randomised controlled trial. Lancet 2008; 372:537.

[118] ten Berg JM, van 't Hof AW, Dill T, et al. Effect of early, pre-hospital initiation of high bolus dose tirofiban in patients with ST-segment elevation myocardial infarction on short- and long-term clinical outcome. J Am Coll Cardiol 2010; 55:2446.

[119] Phillips DR, Scarborough RM. Clinical pharmacology of eptifibatide. Am J Cardiol 1997; 80:11B.

[120] Inhibition of platelet glycoprotein IIb/IIIa with eptifibatide in patients with acute coronary syndromes. The PURSUIT Trial Investigators. Platelet Glycoprotein IIb/IIIa in Unstable Angina: Receptor Suppression Using Integrilin Therapy. N Engl J Med 1998; 339:436.

[121] Kleiman NS, Lincoff AM, Flaker GC, et al. Early percutaneous coronary intervention, platelet inhibition with eptifibatide, and clinical outcomes in patients with acute coronary syndromes. PURSUIT Investigators. Circulation 2000; 101:751.

[122] Randomised placebo-controlled trial of effect of eptifibatide on complications of percutaneous coronary intervention: IMPACT-II. Integrilin to Minimise Platelet Aggregation and Coronary Thrombosis-II. Lancet 1997; 349:1422.

[123] ESPRIT Investigators. Enhanced Suppression of the Platelet IIb/IIIa Receptor with Integrilin Therapy. Novel dosing regimen of eptifibatide in planned coronary stent implantation (ESPRIT): a randomised, placebo-controlled trial. Lancet 2000; 356:2037.

[124] Dasgupta H, Blankenship JC, Wood GC, et al. Thrombocytopenia complicating treatment with intravenous glycoprotein IIb/IIIa receptor inhibitors: a pooled analysis. Am Heart J 2000; 140:206.

[125] Sabatine MS, Jang IK. The use of glycoprotein IIb/IIIa inhibitors in patients with coronary artery disease. Am J Med 2000; 109:224.

[126] Dangas GD, Lansky AJ, Brodie BR. Predictors of Stent Thrombosis After Primary Angioplasty in Acute Myocardial Infarction: The HORIZONS-AMI Trial. Available at: http://www.cardiosource.com/rapidnewssummaries/summary.asp?SumID=406. Accessed July 14, 2011.

[127] Montalescot G, Borentain M, Payot L, et al. Early vs late administration of glycoprotein IIb/IIIa inhibitors in primary percutaneous coronary intervention of acute ST-segment elevation myocardial infarction: a meta-analysis. JAMA 2004; 292:362.

[128] Ellis SG, Tendera M, de Belder MA, et al. Facilitated PCI in patients with ST-elevation myocardial infarction. N Engl J Med. 2008; 358:2205–17.

[129] Memon MA, Blankenship JC, Wood GC, et al. Incidence of intracranial hemorrhage complicating treatment with glycoprotein IIb/IIIa receptor inhibitors: a pooled analysis of major clinical trials. Am J Med 2000; 109:213.

[130] Batchelor WB, Tolleson TR, Huang Y, et al. Randomized COMparison of platelet inhibition with abciximab, tiRofiban and eptifibatide during percutaneous coronary intervention in acute coronary syndromes: the COMPARE trial. Comparison Of Measurements of Platelet aggregation with Aggrastat, Reopro, and Eptifibatide. Circulation 2002; 106:1470.

[131] Topol EJ, Moliterno DJ, Herrmann HC, et al. Comparison of two platelet glycoprotein IIb/IIIa inhibitors, tirofiban and abciximab, for the prevention of ischemic events with percutaneous coronary revascularization. N Engl J Med 2001; 344:1888.

[132] Moliterno DJ, Yakubov SJ, DiBattiste PM, et al. Outcomes at 6 months for the direct comparison of tirofiban and abciximab during percutaneous coronary revascularisation with stent placement: the TARGET follow-up study. Lancet 2002; 360:355.

[133] Mukherjee D, Topol EJ, Bertrand ME, et al. Mortality at 1 year for the direct comparison of tirofiban and abciximab during percutaneous coronary revascularization: do tirofiban and ReoPro give similar efficacy outcomes at trial 1-year follow-up. Eur Heart J 2005; 26:2524.

[134] Valgimigli M, Campo G, Percoco G, et al. Comparison of angioplasty with infusion of tirofiban or abciximab and with implantation of sirolimus-eluting or uncoated stents for acute myocardial infarction: the MULTISTRATEGY randomized trial. JAMA 2008; 299:1788 –99.

[135] Batchelor WB, Tolleson TR, Huang Y, et al. Randomized COMparison of platelet inhibition with abciximab, tiRofiban and eptifibatide during percutaneous coronary intervention in acute coronary syndromes: the COMPARE trial. Comparison Of

Measurements of Platelet aggregation with Aggrastat, Reopro, and Eptifibatide. Circulation 2002; 106:1470.
[136] Midei MG, Coombs VJ, Lowry DR, et al. Clinical outcomes comparing eptifibatide and abciximab in ST elevation acute myocardial infarction patients undergoing percutaneous coronary interventions. Cardiology 2007; 107:172.
[137] Effectiveness of intravenous thrombolytic treatment in acute myocardial infarction. Gruppo Italiano per lo Studio della Streptochinasi nell'Infarto Miocardico (GISSI). Lancet 1986; 1:397.
[138] Boersma E, Maas AC, Deckers JW, Simoons ML. Early thrombolytic treatment in acute myocardial infarction: reappraisal of the golden hour. Lancet 1996; 348:771.
[139] Franzosi MG, Santoro E, De Vita C, et al. Ten-year follow-up of the first megatrial testing thrombolytic therapy in patients with acute myocardial infarction: results of the Gruppo Italiano per lo Studio della Sopravvivenza nell'Infarto-1 study. The GISSI Investigators. Circulation 1998; 98:2659.
[140] Randomised trial of intravenous streptokinase, oral aspirin, both, or neither among 17,187 cases of suspected acute myocardial infarction: ISIS-2. ISIS-2 (Second International Study of Infarct Survival) Collaborative Group. Lancet 1988; 2:349.
[141] Baigent C, Collins R, Appleby P, et al. ISIS-2: 10 year survival among patients with suspected acute myocardial infarction in randomised comparison of intravenous streptokinase, oral aspirin, both, or neither. The ISIS-2 (Second International Study of Infarct Survival) Collaborative Group. BMJ 1998; 316:1337.
[142] An international randomized trial comparing four thrombolytic strategies for acute myocardial infarction. The GUSTO investigators. N Engl J Med 1993; 329:673.
[143] Califf RM, White HD, Van de Werf F, et al. One-year results from the Global Utilization of Streptokinase and TPA for Occluded Coronary Arteries (GUSTO-I) trial. GUSTO-I Investigators. Circulation 1996; 94:1233.
[144] Smalling RW, Bode C, Kalbfleisch J, et al. More rapid, complete, and stable coronary thrombolysis with bolus administration of reteplase compared with alteplase infusion in acute myocardial infarction. RAPID Investigators. Circulation 1995; 91:2725.
[145] Bode C, Smalling RW, Berg G, et al. Randomized comparison of coronary thrombolysis achieved with double-bolus reteplase (recombinant plasminogen activator) and front-loaded, accelerated alteplase (recombinant tissue plasminogen activator) in patients with acute myocardial infarction. The RAPID II Investigators. Circulation 1996; 94:891.
[146] A comparison of reteplase with alteplase for acute myocardial infarction. The Global Use of Strategies to Open Occluded Coronary Arteries (GUSTO III) Investigators. N Engl J Med 1997; 337:1118.
[147] Topol EJ, Ohman EM, Armstrong PW, et al. Survival outcomes 1 year after reperfusion therapy with either alteplase or reteplase for acute myocardial infarction: results from the Global Utilization of Streptokinase and t-PA for Occluded Coronary Arteries (GUSTO) III Trial. Circulation 2000; 102:1761.
[148] Randomised, double-blind comparison of reteplase double-bolus administration with streptokinase in acute myocardial infarction (INJECT): trial to investigate equivalence. International Joint Efficacy Comparison of Thrombolytics. Lancet 1995; 346:329.

[149] Keyt BA, Paoni NF, Refino CJ, et al. A faster-acting and more potent form of tissue plasminogen activator. Proc Natl Acad Sci U S A 1994; 91:3670.

[150] Cannon CP, McCabe CH, Gibson CM, et al. TNK-tissue plasminogen activator in acute myocardial infarction. Results of the Thrombolysis in Myocardial Infarction (TIMI) 10A dose-ranging trial. Circulation 1997; 95:351.

[151] Cannon CP, Gibson CM, McCabe CH, et al. TNK-tissue plasminogen activator compared with front-loaded alteplase in acute myocardial infarction: results of the TIMI 10B trial. Thrombolysis in Myocardial Infarction (TIMI) 10B Investigators. Circulation 1998; 98:2805.

[152] Van de Werf F, Cannon CP, Luyten A, et al. Safety assessment of single-bolus administration of TNK tissue-plasminogen activator in acute myocardial infarction: the ASSENT-1 trial. The ASSENT-1 Investigators. Am Heart J 1999; 137:786.

[153] Assessment of the Safety and Efficacy of a New Thrombolytic (ASSENT-2) Investigators, Van De Werf F, Adgey J, et al. Single-bolus tenecteplase compared with front-loaded alteplase in acute myocardial infarction: the ASSENT-2 double-blind randomised trial. Lancet 1999; 354:716.

[154] den Heijer P, Vermeer F, Ambrosioni E, et al. Evaluation of a weight-adjusted single-bolus plasminogen activator in patients with myocardial infarction: a double-blind, randomized angiographic trial of lanoteplase versus alteplase. Circulation 1998; 98:2117.

[155] InTIME-II Investigators. Intravenous NPA for the treatment of infarcting myocardium early; InTIME-II, a double-blind comparison of single-bolus lanoteplase vs accelerated alteplase for the treatment of patients with acute myocardial infarction. Eur Heart J 2000; 21:2005.

[156] Antman EM, Hand M, Armstrong PW, et al. 2007 Focused Update of the ACC/AHA 2004 guidelines for the Management of Patients with ST-Elevation Myocardial Infacrtion. Circulation 2008; 117(2):296–329.

[157] Topol EJ, GUSTO V Investigators. Reperfusion therapy for acute myocardial infarction with fibrinolytic therapy or combination reduced fibrinolytic therapy and platelet glycoprotein IIb/IIIa inhibition: the GUSTO V randomised trial. Lancet 2001; 357:1905.

[158] Savonitto S, Armstrong PW, Lincoff AM, et al. Risk of intracranial haemorrhage with combined fibrinolytic and glycoprotein IIb/IIIa inhibitor therapy in acute myocardial infarction. Dichotomous response as a function of age in the GUSTO V trial. Eur Heart J 2003; 24:1807.

[159] Assessment of the Safety and Efficacy of a New Thrombolytic Regimen (ASSENT)-3 Investigators. Efficacy and safety of tenecteplase in combination with enoxaparin, .abciximab, or unfractionated heparin: the ASSENT-3 randomised trial in acute myocardial infarction. Lancet 2001; 358:605.

[160] Lincoff AM, Califf RM, Van de Werf F, et al. Mortality at 1 year with combination platelet glycoprotein IIb/IIIa inhibition and reduced-dose fibrinolytic therapy vs conventional fibrinolytic therapy for acute myocardial infarction: GUSTO V randomized trial. JAMA 2002; 288:2130.

[161] Gurm HS, Lincoff AM, Lee D, et al. Outcome of acute ST-segment elevation myocardial infarction in diabetics treated with fibrinolytic or combination reduced fibrinolytic therapy and platelet glycoprotein IIb/IIIa inhibition: lessons from the GUSTO V trial. J Am Coll Cardiol 2004; 43:542.

[162] Sinnaeve PR, Alexander JH, Bogaerts K, et al. Efficacy of tenecteplase in combination with enoxaparin, abciximab, or unfractionated heparin: one-year follow-up results of the Assessment of the Safety of a New Thrombolytic-3 (ASSENT-3) randomized trial in acute myocardial infarction. Am Heart J 2004; 147:993.

[163] Keeley EC, Boura JA, Grines CL. Primary angioplasty versus intravenous thrombolytic therapy for acute myocardial infarction: a quantitative review of 23 randomised trials. Lancet 2003; 361:13.

[164] An international randomized trial comparing four thrombolytic strategies for acute myocardial infarction. The GUSTO investigators. N Engl J Med 1993; 329:673.

[165] Ross AM, Coyne KS, Moreyra E, et al. Extended mortality benefit of early postinfarction reperfusion. GUSTO-I Angiographic Investigators. Global Utilization of Streptokinase and Tissue Plasminogen Activator for Occluded Coronary Arteries Trial. Circulation 1998; 97:1549.

[166] Fernández-Avilés F, Alonso JJ, Peña G, et al. Primary angioplasty vs. early routine post-fibrinolysis angioplasty for acute myocardial infarction with ST-segment elevation: the GRACIA-2 non-inferiority, randomized, controlled trial. Eur Heart J 2007; 28:949.

[167] Danchin N, Coste P, Ferrières J, et al. Comparison of thrombolysis followed by broad use of percutaneous coronary intervention with primary percutaneous coronary intervention for ST-segment-elevation acute myocardial infarction: data from the french registry on acute ST-elevation myocardial infarction (FAST-MI). Circulation 2008; 118:268.

[168] Assessment of the Safety and Efficacy of a New Treatment Strategy with Percutaneous Coronary Intervention (ASSENT-4 PCI) investigators. Primary versus tenecteplase-facilitated percutaneous coronary intervention in patients with ST-segment elevation acute myocardial infarction (ASSENT-4 PCI): randomised trial. Lancet 2006; 367:569.

[169] Alp NJ, Gershlick AH, Carver A, et al. Rescue angioplasty for failed thrombolysis in older patients: insights from the REACT trial. Int J Cardiol 2008; 125:254–7.74.

[170] Gershlick AH, Stephens-Lloyd A, Hughes S, et al. Rescue angioplasty after failed thrombolytic therapy for acute myocardial infarction. N Engl J Med 2005; 353:2758–68.75.

[171] Collet JP, Montalescot G, Le May M, et al. Percutaneous coronary intervention after fibrinolysis: a multiple meta-analyses approach according to the type of strategy. J Am Coll Cardiol 2006; 48:1326–35.76.

[172] Wijeysundera HC, Vijayaraghavan R, Nallamothu BK, et al. Rescue angioplasty or repeat fibrinolysis after failed fibrinolytic therapy for ST-segment myocardial infarction: a meta-analysis of randomized trials. J Am Coll Cardiol 2007; 49:422–30.

[173] Di Mario C, Dudek D, Piscione F, et al. Immediate angioplasty versus standard therapy with rescue angioplasty after thrombolysis in the Combined Abciximab REteplase Stent Study in Acute Myocardial Infarction (CARESS-in-AMI): an open, prospective, randomised, multicentre trial. Lancet 2008; 371:559.

[174] Cantor WJ, Fitchett D, Borgundvaag B, et al. Routine early angioplasty after fibrinolysis for acute myocardial infarction. N Engl J Med 2009; 360:2705.

[175] Fernandez-Avilés F, Alonso JJ, Castro-Beiras A, et al. Routine invasive strategy within 24 hours of thrombolysis versus ischaemia-guided conservative approach for acute

myocardial infarction with ST-segment elevation (GRACIA-1): a randomised controlled trial. Lancet 2004; 364:1045.

[176] Bøhmer E, Hoffmann P, Abdelnoor M, et al. Efficacy and safety of immediate angioplasty versus ischemia-guided management after thrombolysis in acute myocardial infarction in areas with very long transfer distances results of the NORDISTEMI (NORwegian study on DIstrict treatment of ST-elevation myocardial infarction). J Am Coll Cardiol 2010; 55:102.

[177] Scheller B, Hennen B, Hammer B, et al. Beneficial effects of immediate stenting after thrombolysis in acute myocardial infarction. J Am Coll Cardiol 2003; 42:634.

[178] Bonello L, Tantry US, Marcucci R et al. Consensus and Future Directions on the Definition of High On-Treatment Platelet Reactivity to Adenosine Diphosphate. J Am Coll Cardiol 2010; 56:919-933.

[179] Kazui M, Nishiya Y, Ishizuka T, et al. Identification of the human cytochrome P450 enzymes involved in the two oxidative steps in the bioactivation of clopidogrel to its pharmacologically active metabolite. Drug Metab Dispos 2010; 38:92–99.

[180] Hollopeter G, Jantzen HM, Vincent D, et al. Identification of platelet ADP receptor targeted by antithrombotic drugs. Nature 2001; 409:202–7.

[181] Investigators CURE. Clopidogrel in unstable angina to prevent recurrent events trial effects of pretreatment with clopidogrel and aspirin followed by long-term therapy in patients undergoing percutaneous coronary intervention: the PCI-CURE study. Lancet 2001; 358:527–33.

[182] Järemo P, Lindahl TL, Fransson SG, Richter A. Individual variations of platelet inhibition after loading doses of clopidogrel. J Intern Med. 2002; 252:233–8.

[183] Gurbel PA, Becker RC, Mann KG, Steinhubl SR, Michelson AD. Platelet function monitoring in patients with coronary artery disease. J Am Coll Cardiol 2007; 50:1822–1834.

[184] Mega JL, Close SL, Wiviott SD, et al. Cytochrome p-450 polymorphisms and response to clopidogrel. N Engl J Med 2009; 360:354–362.

[185] Mega JL, Close SL, Wiviott SD, et al. Genetic variants in ABCB1 and CYP2C19 and cardiovascular outcomes after treatment with clopidogrel and prasugrel in the TRITON-TIMI 38 trial: a pharmacogenetic analysis. Lancet 2010; 376:1312-19.

[186] Shuldiner AR, O'Connell JR, Bliden KP, et al. Association of cytochrome P450 2C19 genotype with the antiplatelet effect and clinical efficacy of clopidogrel therapy. JAMA 2009; 302:849

[187] Price MJ, Endemann S, Gollapudi RR, et al. Prognostic significance of postclopidogrel platelet reactivity assessed by a point-of-care assay on thrombotic events after drug-eluting stent implantation. Eur Heart J 2008; 29:992–1000.

[188] Price MJ, Berger PB, Teirstein PS, et al. (GRAVITAS Investigators). Standard- vs high-dose clopidogrel based on platelet function testing after percutaneous coronary intervention: the GRAVITAS randomized trial. JAMA 2011; 305:1097-1105. http://clinicaltrials.gov/ct2/show/NCT00910299